Urogynecology

Urogynecology

Edited by GRETCHEN M LENTZ, MD

Assistant Professor, Department of Obstetrics and Gynecology, and Associate Director of the Women's Health Care Center, University of Washington School of Medicine, Seattle, Washington, USA

A member of the Hodder Headline Group
LONDON
Co-published in the USA by
Oxford University Press Inc., New York

First published in Great Britain in 2000 by
Arnold, a member of the Hodder Headline Group,
338 Euston Road, London NW1 3BH

http://www.arnoldpublishers.com

Co-published in the USA by
Oxford University Press Inc.,
198 Madison Avenue, New York, NY10016
Oxford is a registered trademark of Oxford University Press

Whilst the advice and information in this book are believed to be true and
accurate at the date of going to press, neither the author[s] nor the publisher
can accept any legal responsibility or liability for any errors or omissions
that may be made. In particular (but without limiting the generality of the
preceding disclaimer) every effort has been made to check drug dosages;
however, it is still possible that errors have been missed. Furthermore,
dosage schedules are constantly being revised and new side effects
recognised. For these reasons the reader is strongly urged to consult the
drug companies' printed instructions before administering any of the drugs
recommended in this book.

British Library Cataloguing in Publication Data
A catalogue record for this book is available from the British Library

Library of Congress Cataloging-in-Publication Data
A catalog record for this book is available from the Library of Congress

ISBN 0 340 74230 5 (hb)

1 2 3 4 5 6 7 8 9 10

Commissioning Editor: Joanna Koster
Project Editor: Sarah de Souza
Production Editor: Wendy Rooke
Production Controller: Priya Gohil

Typeset by Phoenix Photosetting, Chatham, Kent
Printed in Suffolk by St Edmundsbury Press, and bound by MPG Books Ltd

What do you think about this book? Or any other Arnold title?
Please send your comments to feedback.arnold@hodder.co.uk

To my parents, Charles and Mary Ellen

Contents

Contributors

Cindy L Amundsen MD
Assistant Professor, Duke University Medical Center, Department of Obstetrics and Gynecology, Durham, NC 27710, USA

Tamara G Bavendam MD
Associate Professor of Surgery/Urology; Director, Center for Pelvic Floor Disorders, MCP Hahnemann University School of Medicine, 3300 Henry Avenue, Philadelphia, PA 19129, USA

R Duane Cespedes MD
Chief, Female Urology, and Urodynamics, Department of Urology/MMKU, Wilford Hall Medical Center, 2200 Bergguist Drive, Suite 1, Lackland AFB, TX 78236-5300, USA

Anita Chen MD
Consultant, Mayo Clinic, Jacksonville, FL, USA

Renee Edwards MD
Assistant Professor, Department of Obstetrics and Gynecology, Section of Urogynecology and Reconstructive Pelvic Surgery, Rush Medical College, 1725 W Harrison Street, Chicago, IL 60612-3873, USA

J Andrew Fantl MD, FACOG
Clinical Professor of Obstetrics and Gynecology, Women's Gynecologic Care, PC, 496 Nesconset Highway, Smithtown, New York, 11787, USA

Dee E Fenner MD
Director, Obstetrics and Gynecology Residency Program; Associate Professor, Rush-Presbyterican-St. Luke's Hospital, 1653 W. Congress Parkway, Chicago, IL 60612, USA

Robert L Harris MD, FACOG
Assistant Professor and Director, Section of Urogynecology and Reconstructive Pelvic Surgery, Department of Obstetrics and Gynecology, University of Mississippi Medical Center, 2500 North State Street, Jackson, MI 39216, USA

Marie-Andrée Harvey MD, FRCSC
Clinical and Research Fellow in Urogynecology, Department of Obstetrics and Gynecology, ASB 1st–3rd Floor, Brigham and Women's Hospital, 75 Francis Street, Boston, MA 02115, USA

Nicolette S Horbach MD
Associate Clinical Professor, George Washington University, Washington DC, Woodburn Rd, Annandale, VA 22003, USA

Mickey M Karram MD
Associate Director, Department of Obstetrics and Gynecology; Director,
Division of Urogynecology and Reconstructive Pelvic Surgery, Good Samaritan
Hospital, Seton Center, 375 Dixmyth Avenue, Cincinnati, OH 45220; and
Associate Professor of Obstetrics and Gynecology, University of Cincinnati,
Cincinnati, OH, USA

Neeraj Kohli MD
Division of Urogynecology and Reconstructive Pelvic Surgery, Mount Auburn
Hospital/Harvard Medical School, 300, Mount Auburn Street, Suite 302,
Cambridge, MA 02138, USA

Abner P Korn MD
Director of Gynecology, San Francisco General Hospital; Associate Clinical
Professor of Obstetrics, Gynecology and Reproductive Sciences, University of
California, San Francisco, 1001 Portero Avenue, San Francisco, CA 94110,
USA

Delbert J Kwan MD
Attending Urologist, Beche Medical Center, 1307 Savannah Road, Lewes, DE
19958, USA

Karl M Luber MD, FACOG
Director, Section of Urogynecology and Pelvic Reconstructive Surgery, San
Diego Medical Center, Southern California Permanente Medical Group:
Assistant Clinical Professor, University of California, San Diego, CA 92120,
USA

Michael E Mayo MBBS, FRCS
Professor of Urology, Department of Urology, University of Washington, Box
356510, Seattle, WA 98195, USA

Edward J McGuire MD
Professor and Director, Department of Surgery, Division of Urology, University
of Texas-Health Sciences Center, 6431 Fannin, Houston, TX 77030, USA

Mary T McLennan MD, FACOG
Assistant Professor, Director Urogynecology, Division of Urogynecology and
Reconstructive Pelvic Surgery, Department of Obstetrics and Gynecology, St.
Louis University, 6420 Clayton Road, St. Louis, MO 63117, USA

Ash Monga MRCOG
Consultant Gynaecologist, Subspecialist in Urogynaecology, Princess Anne
Hospital, Coxford Road, Southampton, SO16 5YA, UK

Ingrid Nygaard MD
Associate Professor, Department of Obstetrics and Gynecology; Head, General
Women's Health Division, University of Iowa College of Medicine, 2BT GN
Iowa City, IA 52242, USA

William A Peters III MD, FACS, FACOG
Clinical Professor of Obstetrics and Gynecology, University of Washington,
1101 Madison, Suite 1500, Seattle, WA 98104, USA

Stephanie Powell MD
Resident Physician, Department of Obstetrics and Gynecology, University of
Iowa College of Medicine, 2BT GH Iowa City, IA 52242, USA

Joseph Schaffer MD, FACOG
Assistant Professor, Director of Urogynecology and Reconstructive Pelvic
Surgery, University of Texas Southwestern Medical Center, Parkland Memorial
Hospital, 5323 Harry Hines Boulevard, Dallas, TX 75235-9032, USA

Steven E Speights MD
Fellow, Urogynecology and Reconstructive Pelvic Surgery, L4100 Women's
Hospital, 1500 E. Medical Center Dr., University of Michigan, Ann Arbor, MI
48109-0276, USA

Stuart Stanton
Professor of Pelvic Reconstruction and Urogynaecology, Urogynaecology Unit,
St George's Hospital Medical School, Cranmer Terrace, London, SW17 0RE,
UK

James P Theofrastous MD, FACOG
Clinical Associate Professor, UNC Chapel Hill School of Medicine; Director of
Urogynecology and Reconstructive Pelvic Surgery, Mountain Area Health and
Education Center, Department of Obstetrics and Gynecology, 60 Livingston
Street, Asheville, NC 28801-4400, USA

Sandra R Valaitis MD, FACOG
Assistant Professor, Director of Urogynecology, University of Chicago
Hospital, 5841 S. Maryland Avenue, MC 2050 Chicago, IL 60637, USA

Eboo Versi MD, PhD, MRCOG
Associate Professor of Obstetrics/Gynecology/Reproductive Biology; Chief,
Division of Urogynecology, Brigham and Women's Hospital, ASB 1st–3rd
Floor, Harvard Medical School, 75 Francis Street, Boston, MA 02115, USA

L Lewis Wall MD, D Phil
Director, Division of Gynecology, Urogynecology and Reconstructive Pelvic
Surgery, Department of Obstetrics and Gynecology, Cedars-Sinai Medical
Center, 8700 Beverly Blvd., Los Angeles, CA 90048, USA

Raul Yordan-Jovet MD, Lt Col, USAF, MC
Chief, Urogynecology and Reconstructive Pelvic Surgery, Department of
Obstetrics and Gynecology, Brooke Army Medical Center, 3851 Roger Brooke
Drive, Fort Sam Houston, San Antonio, TX 78234-6200, USA

Foreword

The subspecialty of urogynecology/reparative pelvic surgery is the latest subspecialty to be developed in obstetrics and gynecology. It has been developed in recognition of the need to train subspecialists to provide optimum care to women suffering from pelvic floor dysfunction and to stimulate meaningful research in this area. Although obstetricians and gynecologists traditionally care for women with pelvic floor dysfunction problems, it is hoped that emphasizing this aspect of the specialty of obstetrics and gynecology will enhance the skills of specialists in obstetrics and gynecology.

This book, *Urogynecology*, contributes greatly to the goal of bringing new knowledge in the field of urogynecology to the practitioner. With contributions by leaders in the field, it addresses the issues of structure and function of the urinary tract with consideration to all of the forces that influence micturition. In addition, it provides useful information on evaluating the patient with an incontinence problem, differentiating types of incontinence, and offering up-to-date management. Since pelvic floor dysfunction may also include the problem of anal incontinence, the book also includes information on this topic.

This book will be a useful addition to the reference library of all physicians dealing with patients suffering from pelvic floor dysfunction, including incontinence and prolapse.

Morton A. Stenchever, MD
Series Editor

Preface

Urinary incontinence affects 13 million Americans in community and institutional settings. Gains have been made in educating the public that successful treatments are available, and attempts made at reducing the embarrassment of seeking treatment. However, there are still barriers to individuals seeking help. Furthermore, once they seek help, they may face a practitioner with limited knowledge on the condition, as education on lower urinary tract disorders has often been neglected in medical training.

Another difficulty facing practitioners treating urinary incontinence is the vast array of diagnostic tests, procedures and operations available (some come and go or are modified every decade), the failure rate of various treatments and the limited knowledge we have on treating detrusor instability. Fortunately, urinary incontinence and pelvic floor dysfunction in the female are topics of growing interest for a number of medical disciplines. Research efforts are expanding and membership in related societies is growing, which brings hope for improvement in the care for women with incontinence.

The purpose of this book is to update the practitioner on the most current aspects of treating women with urinary incontinence and pelvic floor dysfunction. This includes the anatomy and physiology necessary for understanding these conditions, the newer and more complex testing available, and trends in medical therapy and surgical repairs. The chapters are written by a gynecologic oncologist, urogynecologists and urologists to reflect the multidisciplinary interest and views on these issues.

The prevalence of urinary incontinence increases with age. As the population ages, practitioners are going to see more women desiring treatment. Urinary incontinence can have a significant psychosocial impact on an individual, with possible social isolation and loss of self-esteem and independence. With predictions of lengthening life expectancy and a cohort of baby boomers aging in relatively good health, we are challenged to improve our understanding and treatment of incontinence. These women expect good quality of life in their later years, and we must offer treatments that improve their lifestyle.

I am indebted to, and especially wish to thank, the 28 contributors to this book who are dedicated to improving the quality of life for women with urinary incontinence and pelvic floor dysfunction. Special thanks to Dr Morton Stenchever at the University of Washington who guided and supported the entire project.

Gretchen M. Lentz, MD

PART I

EPIDEMIOLOGY OF INCONTINENCE

CHAPTER 1

Epidemiology and pathophysiology of urinary incontinence in women

ABNER P. KORN

Urinary incontinence is a common problem associated with significant morbidity. Tens of billions of dollars are spent each year to treat urinary incontinence in the United States. Despite this, only one-quarter of women with incontinence will seek medical attention.[1-3] Often, women consider urinary incontinence to be a normal part of aging. Furthermore, because of embarrassment and because many consider the condition to be untreatable, women may not report incontinence to health-care providers unless they are directly questioned. Unfortunately, the majority of primary care providers neither routinely questioned patients about urinary incontinence, nor could correctly estimate the proportion of incontinence cases which are curable.[4] This chapter considers the magnitude of the problem of urinary incontinence in women and some of its possible causes.

PREVALENCE AND INCIDENCE OF URINARY INCONTINENCE

Prevalence is the proportion of a population with a given condition at a point in time. The prevalence of urinary incontinence varies according to the population studied. A high prevalence of urinary incontinence exists in geriatric nursing-care facilities; Jewett and colleagues[5] reported 38% were incontinent, 20% used an indwelling catheter, and 11% had lower urinary tract symptoms without incontinence. Studies in noninstitutionalized women have been mostly performed in Europe and the United States but also in a few Asian countries and in Australia and New Zealand. Many of the studies sampled women in a single city or county; few are based on national sampling. A random sample of community-dwelling women would provide the best estimate of the magnitude of the problem of incontinence, while surveys of office-based practices would have much less generalizability. For this reason, the studies of community-dwelling women are most relevant for the purposes of this chapter. Surveys and interviews of community-dwelling (noninstitutionalized) women have shown a prevalence of any degree of incontinence ranging from 5% to 58%.[1,2,6–20] (Table 1-1). This wide range reflects different populations and methods. In particular, differences in studies relate to the following:

Table 1-1.   Prevalence of any urinary incontinence in community-dwelling women

Study (Ref.)	Site	Method	Ages	N_i/N_t	%	95%CI
Ju et al.[6]	Singapore	I	>65	23/484	5	3–7
Korn and Shiboski[7]	United States	I	≥55	768/9355	8	8–9
Koyano et al.[8]	Tokyo	Q	≥65	132/1345	10	8–12
Brocklehurst[9]	Great Britain	I	≥30	297/2124	14	13–16
Milsom et al.[10]	Göteborg	Q	46–86	1106/7459	15	14–16
Foldspang and Mommsen[11]	Aarhus	Q	30–59	450/2613	17	16–19
Molander et al.[12]	Göteborg	Q	≥65	677/4012	17	16–18
Campbell et al.[13]	Gisborne	I	>65	70/359	19	16–24
Mäkinen et al.[1]	Turku	Q	22–55	1056/5247	20	19–21
Kok et al.[14]	Amstelveen	Q	>60	164/719	24	20–26
Rekers et al.[2]	Zoetermeer	Q	35–80	316/1213	26	24–29
Hellström et al.[15]	Göteborg	I	85	191/551	35	31–39
Diokno et al.[16]	Washtenaw	I	>60	434/1150	38	35–41
Sommer et al.[17]	Denmark	Q	20–79	160/400	40	35–45
Vehkalahti and Kivelä[18]	Tampere	Q	84–85	103/250	41	35–48
Wetle et al.[13]	East Boston	I	>65	1038/2360	44	42–46
Yarnell and Voyle[20]	South Wales	I	>18	445/1000	45	41–48
Burgio et al.[3]	Pittsburgh	I	42–50	314/541	58	54–62

N_i, number incontinent; N_t, total number interviewed; CI, confidence interval; I, interview; Q, questionnaire.

1. *Population studied: a city, county or whole nation:* Wide variations in rates of incontinence occur in different geographic regions.[7]
2. *Study method: interview or survey:* Questionnaires may seem to offer the benefits of privacy and anonymity compared with a face-to-face interview. On the other hand, the latter could allow some flexibility in questioning about incontinence, which could lead to more accurate responses. For example, a questionnaire may ask about difficulty with control of urine. Some patients may not use these words to describe their incontinence but may understand terms such as "leaking" or "wetting clothing."[21]
3. *Sampling frame:* Studies include women attending a physician's office or a meeting of a geriatrics society. Such groups might be biased toward higher rates of incontinence than the general population.
4. *Questions asked of the study participants:* Questions about "control" of urination could better detect urge than stress incontinence.[21]
5. *Definition of incontinence:* Some variance among the studies could be due to the definition of urinary incontinence used. Most studies report the frequency or amount of incontinence and not whether it is perceived as

socially troubling to the woman. Certainly, daily incontinence seems more severe than infrequent incontinence. Nevertheless, a single large incontinence episode at the wrong time could be socially devastating, while frequent small losses could be of little concern.

Less variation exists among the estimates of the prevalence of daily incontinence; most studies show a prevalence of about 10% (range; 4–21%) in community-dwelling women. (Table 1-2).

Little is known about incontinence in minority racial and ethnic populations. Burgio and colleagues[3] noted a lower prevalence of urinary incontinence among black women aged 42–50 years than among whites. The National Health Interview Survey showed higher rates of urinary incontinence among Native Americans (24%: 95%CI: 11–40) than among white (8%: 95%CI: 7–9) or Asian Americans (3%: 95%CI: 0–11%).[7] But no significant difference emerged between the rate for African-Americans (11%: 95%CI: 9–13) and any other ethnic group.

Incidence is the probability of developing a given condition during a specified time period. The annual incidence of urinary incontinence ranges from 8% to 20%.[3,21] Remission rates may be about 13%.[21]

Table 1-2. Prevalence of daily urinary incontinence in community-dwelling women

Study (Ref.)	Site	Method	Ages	N_i/N_t	%	95%CI
Campbell et al.[13]	Gisborne	I	>65	16/359	4	3–7
Mäkinen et al.[1]	Turku	Q	25–55	182/5247	4	3–4
Korn and Shiboski[7]	United States	I	≥55	426/9355	5	4–5
Diokno et al.[16]	Washtenaw	I	>60	60/1150	5	4–7
Yarnell and Voyle[20]	South Wales	I	>18	49/1000	5	4–6
Rekers et al.[2]	Zoetermeer	Q	35–80	72/1213	6	5–7
Burgio et al.[3]	Pittsburgh	I	42–50	37/541	7	5–9
Molander et al.[12]	Göteborg	Q	≥65	376/4012	9	8–10
Wetle et al.[19]	East Boston	I	>65	208/2360	9	8–10
Kok et al.[14]	Amstelveen	Q	>60	96/719	13	11–16
Hellström et al.[15]	Göteborg	I	85	92/551	17	14–20
Vehkalahti and Kivelä[18]	Tampere	Q	84–85	53/250	21	16–27

N_i, number incontinent; N_t, total number interviewed; CI, confidence interval; I, interview; Q, questionnaire.

RISK FACTORS FOR URINARY INCONTINENCE

Several risk factors increase the likelihood of incontinence. Some factors are consistent, while others are inconsistent and may depend on the characteristics of the population studied. Many of these reports present associations that are uncontrolled and especially subject to confounding. Few attempt to control for known confounders by using methods such as multivariate analysis. For example, urinary incontinence may be associated with older age, but this does not prove that aging causes incontinence. Other factors, also associated with aging, such as medical illnesses, impaired mobility, and so on, may confound association of incontinence and old age.

Urinary incontinence increases with increasing age.[2,7,8,10,12,19,22] Poor health and chronic, debilitating medical conditions are consistently associated with incontinence.[7,19,22] Especially pertinent are chronic cough, and history of stroke.[15,19,20] Other conditions associated with incontinence are childhood bedwetting,[11] depression,[19] fecal incontinence,[19] and obesity or increased body mass index.[3,22,23] The relationship with parity is not consistent.[3,11,18,22,24,25] Hysterectomy is inconsistently associated with incontinence.[3,22,26] Nygaard and coworkers[27] have reported a high rate of incontinence among female athletes. Tobacco smoking has an inconsistent association with incontinence.[3,28]

Few if any of these studies addressed minority populations. Some evidence shows that risk factors for urinary incontinence in a black, inner-city population may differ from those discussed above. Peacock and coworkers[29] have noted no correlation between age, parity, and obesity with urinary incontinence in a black population. In this study and another by Bump[30] detrusor instability incontinence was more common in African-Americans than in whites.

What can be learned from the epidemiologic studies of incontinence? First, this condition is common yet generally not reported to health-care providers. Second, certain groups are at high risk for incontinence: the elderly, those with debilitating medical conditions, residents of nursing homes, and those who have chronic elevations in intraabdominal pressure, such as chronic coughers and, possibly, tobacco smokers. Third, knowledge about risk factors for urinary incontinence is incomplete, especially in minority populations.

PATHOPHYSIOLOGY

Storage and excretion of urine requires a complex interaction of the sympathetic and parasympathetic nervous systems. In addition, continence requires normal function of smooth and striated muscles, epithelial surfaces, fascia, and ligaments.

Incontinence can be due to fistulae (vesicovaginal, uterovesical, ureterovaginal, etc.). In developed countries these are usually the consequence of prior operations or are related to malignancy. In underdeveloped countries these usually follow obstetrical injuries.

The acronym DIAPPERS describes transient causes of urinary incontinence.[31]

D delirium
I infection (urinary tract infection)
A atrophic urethritis/vaginitis
P pharmaceuticals
P psychological
E excessive urine output—excessive intake, diuretics, mobilization of edema
R restricted mobility
S stool impaction

Other causes of urinary incontinence include abnormalities of detrusor or urethral sphincter function.

Overactive Detrusor Function

The normal detrusor muscle is quiescent with bladder filling. At a volume of about 200 ml most women will feel an urge to urinate. The bladder will usually accommodate about 400 ml before a strong urge to urinate occurs. When the detrusor contracts during filling of the bladder at low bladder volumes (and it cannot be inhibited) urge-associated incontinence occurs. Typically women with this condition complain of urgency with subsequent incontinence of a large volume of urine. When documented by urodynamics in the absence of neurologic disease the condition is detrusor instability. When neurologic disease is present, detrusor hyperreflexia is the preferred term. Lesions in the cerebral cortex may produce an uninhibited neurogenic bladder.[32] Patients with this condition sense urgency but cannot inhibit detrusor contractions. By contrast, patients with spinal cord lesions do not sense the urge to void. They have a reflex neurogenic bladder.

The etiology of detrusor instability is unknown. While the normal detrusor muscle contracts in response to acetylcholine, the detrusor in women with urge incontinence seems to respond to other neurotransmitters as well. Thus, treatment with anticholinergics is not effective in all women with this condition. Urge incontinence becomes more common with increasing age and often accompanies stress incontinence (termed *mixed incontinence*).[20] Mixed incontinence may be more common in African-Americans than in white women.[29,30] As noted above, detrusor hyperreflexia may be the result of interruption of descending inhibitory nerves which suppress detrusor contractions. Thus, conditions such as spinal cord trauma, multiple sclerosis, stroke, Parkinson's disease, and tumors may lead to overactive detrusor. These conditions may interfere with central or peripheral nerve function or both. Detrusor overactivity follows operations to correct stress incontinence in about 10% to 20% of cases.[33] Irritative conditions such as carcinoma *in situ* of the bladder may produce urge incontinence in some elderly women.

Underactive Detrusor Function

Patients with "overflow incontinence" may present with a variety of symptoms, including stress leakage, intermittent dribbling of small amounts of urine, or frequency. Overflow incontinence can result from chronic urinary tract infection or overdistention of the bladder, which can damage stretch receptors in the bladder wall. Other conditions that damage neurologic control of the bladder include those listed above (for overactive detrusor) and diabetes mellitus. Many commonly used drugs can inhibit detrusor contractions, including anticholinergics, phenothiazines, antidepressants, narcotics, calcium channel blockers, and antihistamines. An underactive detrusor is common following radical pelvic surgery.

Overactive Urethral Function

Urethral obstruction is rare in women in the absence of prior surgery to control urinary incontinence. It can occur with kinking of the urethra related to very large cystoceles. The symptoms will usually be incomplete emptying.

Underactive Urethral Function

Stress incontinence is the loss of urine related to increases in intraabdominal pressure. In the normal state such pressure increases impact on the urethra and compress it directly or are reflected by the anterior vaginal wall. When the anterior vaginal wall is damaged, the urethra is not supported on its inferior aspect and is outside the abdominal zone of pressure. Incontinence can result when intraabdominal pressure increases are transmitted to the bladder and not the urethra. Stress incontinence may also result from loss of muscular support of the urethra. Typically, women who have stress incontinence complain of leakage of small amounts of urine with walking, coughing, laughing, bouncing, and so on. Most stress incontinence results from damage to the anterior vaginal wall during childbirth or due to chronic increased intraabdominal pressures such as in smokers, obese women, and those who have occupations requiring heavy lifting.[23,27]

Childbirth may damage the pelvic floor fascial supports and may also injure the pudendal nerve. Damage to the pudendal nerve may result in stress incontinence, since the levator ani muscles also support the inferior aspect of the urethra.[34]

Age-related weakening of the supporting structures of the urethra may lead to stress incontinence. The urethral epithelium is estrogen-sensitive (as is the vaginal epithelium). Alpha-adrenergic receptors in the urethra increase in the presence of estrogen. Lack of estrogen may decrease thickness of the urethral epithelium, which results in a "leaky seal." Estrogen supplementation may help, but no urodynamic effect of estrogen replacement occurs in postmenopausal women who have stress incontinence.[35,36] Since the urethral sphincter has alpha-adrenergic innervation, alpha-adrenergic blocking drugs (commonly used to treat hypertension) may precipitate stress incontinence.

Incontinence with the Valsalva maneuver can occur in women who have overflow incontinence or in those who have intrinsic sphincteric deficiency. Most commonly this occurs after prior surgical procedures that have scarred or denervated the urethra.[37] Intrinsic sphincteric deficiency usually results in severe incontinence.

Urethral diverticula may result in incontinence of small amounts of urine, which may be positional or may resemble stress incontinence. Women may complain of dribbling small amounts of urine after voiding normally.

Finally, some women have instability of their urethral sphincter, which may cause occasional leakage of urine resembling stress incontinence. Varying degrees of obstructed voiding may occur with this condition.

In conclusion, urinary incontinence in women is a common condition that causes great suffering and expense. A variety of risk factors exist, but little is known about prevention of this condition. Since incontinence is treatable in most cases, and women may be reluctant to complain of this problem, health-care providers should question their patients about incontinence. If ignored, incontinence can cause unnecessary deterioration in the quality of life.

REFERENCES

1. Mäkinen JI, Grönroos M, Kiilholma PJA, Tenho TT, Erkkola RU. The prevalence of urinary incontinence in a randomized population of 5247 adult Finnish women. *Int Urogynecol J* 1992; **3**: 110–113.
2. Rekers H, Drogendijk AC, Valkenburg HA, Riphagen F. The menopause, urinary incontinence and other symptoms of the genitourinary tract. *Maturitas* 1992; **15**: 101–111.
3. Burgio KL, Matthews KA, Engel BT. Prevalence, incidence and correlates of urinary incontinence in healthy, middle-aged women. *J Urol* 1991; **146**: 1255–1259.
4. MMWR. Knowledge, attitudes and practices of physicians regarding urinary incontinence in persons aged ≥65 years: Massachusetts and Oklahoma 1993. *MMWR* 1995; **44**: 747–749.
5. Jewett MAS, Fernie GR, Holliday PJ, Pim ME. Urinary dysfunction in a geriatric long-term care population: Prevalence and patterns. *J Am Geriatr Soc* 1981; **29**: 211–214.
6. Ju CC, Swan LK, Merriman A, Choon TE, Viegas O. Urinary incontinence among the elderly people of Singapore. *Age Ageing* 1991; **20**: 262–266.
7. Korn AP, Shiboski S. Prevalence and correlates of urinary incontinence in community dwelling women age 55 and older. Data from the National Health Interview Survey. *Int Urogynecol J* 1994; **6**: 278.
8. Koyano W, Shibata H, Haga H, Suyama Y. Prevalence and outcome of low ADL and incontinence among the elderly: Five years follow-up in a Japanese urban community. *Arch Gerontol Geriatr* 1986; **5**: 197–206.
9. Brocklehurst JC. Urinary incontinence in the community-analysis of a MORI poll. *BMJ* 1993; **306**: 832–834.
10. Milsom I, Ekelund P, Mollander U, Arvidsson L, Areskoug B. The influence of age, parity, oral contraception, hysterectomy and menopause in the prevalence of urinary incontinence in women. *J Urol* 1993; **149**: 1459–1462.
11. Foldspang A, Mommsen S. Adult female urinary incontinence and childhood bed-wetting. *Urology* 1994; **152**: 85–88.
12. Molander U, Milsom I, Ekelund P, Mellström D. An epidemiological study of urinary incontinence and related urogenital symptoms in elderly women. *Maturitas* 1990; **12**: 51–60.
13. Campbell AJ, Reinken J, McCosh L. Incontinence in the elderly: Prevalence and prognosis. *Age Ageing* 1985; **14**: 65–70.
14. Kok ALM, Voorhorst FJ, Burger CW, Van Houten P, Kenemans P, Janssens J. Urinary and faecal incontinence in community-residing elderly women. *Age Ageing* 1992; **21**: 211–215.

15. Hellström L, Ekelund P, Milsom I, Mellström D. The prevalence of urinary incontinence and the use of incontinence aids in 85 year old men and women. *Age Ageing* 1990; **19**: 383–389.
16. Diokno AC, Brock BM, Brown MB, Herzog AR. Prevalence of urinary incontinence and other urological symptoms in the noninstitutionalized elderly. *J Urol* 1986; **136**: 1022–1025.
17. Sommer P, Bauer T, Nielsen KK, et al. Voiding patterns and prevalence of incontinence in women. *Br J Urol* 1990; **66**: 12–15.
18. Vehkalahti I, Kivelä S. Urinary incontinence and its correlates in old age. *Gerontology* 1985; **31**: 391–396.
19. Wetle T, Scherr P, Branch LG, et al. Difficulty holding urine among older persons in a geographically defined community: Prevalence and correlates. *J Am Geriatr Soc* 1995; **43**: 349–355.
20. Yarnell JWG, Voyle GJ. The prevalence and severity of urinary incontinence in women. *J Epidemiol Community Health* 1981; **35**: 71–74.
21. Herzog AR, Fultz NH. Prevalence and incidence of urinary incontinence in community dwelling populations. *J Am Gerontol Soc* 1990; **38**: 273–281.
22. Brown JS, Seeley DG, Fong J, Black D, Ensrud KE, Grady D. Urinary incontinence in older women: Who is at risk? *Obstet Gynecol* 1996; **87**: 715–721.
23. Dwyer PL, Lee ETC, Hay DM. Obesity and urinary incontinence in women. *Br J Obstet Gynaecol* 1988; **95**: 91–96.
24. Foldspang A, Mommsen S, Lam GW, Elving L. Parity as a correlate of urinary incontinence prevalence. *J Epidemiol Community Health* 1992; **46**: 595–600.
25. Thomas TM, Plymat KR, Blannin J, Meade TW. Prevalence of urinary incontinence. *BMJ* 1980; **281**: 1243–1245.
26. Iosif CS, Békássy Z, Rydhström H. Prevalence of urinary incontinence in middle-aged women. *Int J Gynecol Obstet* 1988; **26**: 255–259.
27. Nygaard I, DeLancey JO, Arnsdorf L, Murphy E. Exercise and incontinence. *Obstet Gynecol* 1990; **75**: 848–851.
28. Bump RC, McClish DK. Cigarette smoking and urinary incontinence in women. *Am J Obstet Gynecol* 1992; **167**: 1213–1218.
29. Peacock LM, Wiskind AK, Wall LW. Clinical features of urinary incontinence and urogenital prolapse in a black inner-city population. *Am J Obstet Gynecol* 1994; **171**: 1464–1471.
30. Bump RC. Racial comparisons and contrasts in urinary incontinence and pelvic organ prolapse. *Obstet Gynecol* 1993; **81**: 421–425.
31. Resnick NM. Urinary incontinence. *Lancet* 1995; **346**: 94–99.
32. Lapides J. The Lapides Classification. In: Gillenwater JY, Grayhack JT, Howards SS, Duckett JW (eds). *Adult and Pediatric Urology*. Chicago: Year Book Medical Publishers, 1987; 882–883.
33. Langer R, Ron-El R, Newman M, Herman A, Caspi E. Detrusor instability following colposuspension for urinary stress incontinence. *Br J Obstet Gynaecol* 1988; **95**: 607–610.
34. Smith A, Hosker G, Warell D. The role of pudendal nerve damage in the etiology of stress urinary incontinence in women. *Br J Obstet Gynaecol* 1989; **96**: 29–32.
35. Fantl JA, Cardozo L, McClish DK. Estrogen therapy in the management of urinary incontinence in postmenopausal women: A meta-analysis. [First report of the Hormones and Urogenital Therapy Committee.] *Obstet Gynecol* 1994; **83**: 12–18.
36. Fantl JA, Wyman JF, Anderson RL, Matt DW, Bump RC. Postmenopausal urinary incontinence: Comparison between estrogen-supplemented and non-estrogen-supplemented women. *Obstet Gynecol* 1988; **71**: 823–828.
37. Horbach NS, Ostergard DR. Predicting intrinsic urethral sphincter dysfunction in women with stress urinary incontinence. *Obstet Gynecol* 1994; **84**: 188–192.

PART II

LOWER URINARY TRACT STRUCTURE AND FUNCTION

CHAPTER 2

Anatomy of female pelvic support and continence

WILLIAM A. PETERS III

The assumption of erect posture and the large cranium of a human fetus lead to problems in the support of the pelvic viscera that are unique to the human female. The primary support is provided by the paired levator ani muscles, which together are termed the *pelvic sling*.[1] The pelvic viscera are invested by a dense fibrous tissue (endopelvic fascia), which coalesces laterally as fibrous bands or ligaments that attach to the pelvic floor muscles.[2-8] Continence of the urinary and fecal system is dependent on many of the same structures that support the pelvic viscera and an organ-specific sphincter system.[9-14]

The pelvis is comprised of four distinct bones: the left and right innominate, the sacrum, and the coccyx.[8] Each innominate bone is formed by fusion of the ileum, ischium, and pubis. The obturator foramen goes directly through the innominate bone and is covered on its internal surface by the obturator membrane, which is the origin of the obturator muscle. The obturator muscle passes posterior and lateral to the ischial spine, through the lesser sciatic foramen, and inserts on the greater trochanter. The obturator muscle is covered medially by the obturator fascia, through which all the supporting structures of the pelvic organs are attached to the bony pelvis.

PELVIC FLOOR MUSCLES

The pelvic floor consists of three separate components of the levator ani muscle: the pubococcygeus, the iliococcygeus, and the coccygeus (also called the ischiococcygeus) muscles.[3,8,15] The *pubococcygeus muscles* arise on the undersurface of the pubis, circle the pelvic viscera, and insert posterior to the rectum in the central tendon of the levator ani (anococcygeal raphe or levator plate). The *iliococcygeus muscles* make up the largest portion of the levator ani. They arise from a tendon lying on the medial surface of the obturator internus muscle known as the arcus tendineous levator ani (also called the "white line" in some old anatomic texts) (Figure 2-1). The arcus tendineous levator ani is a linear thickening of obturator fascia extending from the ischial spine to the posterior lateral pubis. The iliococcygeus muscles insert into the central tendon of the

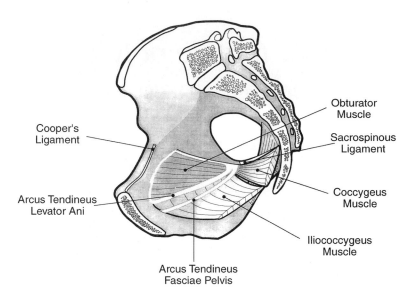

Figure 2-1.   Right pelvic sidewall showing attachment of iliococcygeus muscle to obturator fascia and attachment of the pelvic fascia to the iliococcygeus muscle.

levator ani (anococcygeal raphe) posterior to the rectum (Figure 2-2).[3] The *coccygeus muscles* arise from the sacrospinous ligament and insert into the coccyx. Since the coccyx is internal and fixed, this muscle has no function in humans and does not contribute to the support of the pelvic viscera, but rather, it is represented by dense fibrous tissue, with an overlying fascial membrane. The *puborectalis muscles* appear anatomically as the most caudal and medial portion of the pubococcygeus muscles, but function separately from the remainder of the pelvic floor muscles.[9] Two different types of skeletal muscle are present in the levator ani muscles:[17] *Slow-twitch fibers* provide baseline tone in the pelvic floor and support the viscera during normal activity, and *fast-twitch fibers* are reflexly contracted during a Valsalva maneuver or during a sudden increase in intra-abdominal pressure, such as a cough or sneeze. Contraction of the fast-twich fibers of the levator ani muscles elevates the pelvic viscera and closes the vaginal introitus. After passing through the levator ani muscles, the vagina and rectum curve posteriorly and assume a near-horizontal orientation (Figure 2-3).[1,4,15] When there is an increase in intraabdominal pressure,[19] the rectum and vagina are rotated more posteriorly over the central tendon of the levator ani as the levator ani muscles contract, elevating the central tendon of the levator ani and closing the genital hiatus. As long as the pelvic floor muscles are intact with normal neurologic function, the visceral attachments to the pelvic sidewall are protected from stretch injury.

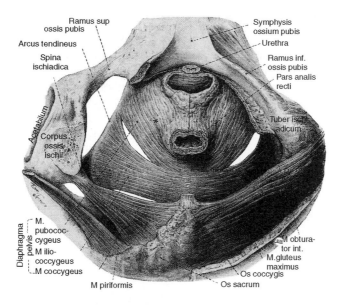

Figure 2-2. Anatomy of the pelvic floor. The asterisk marks the puborectalis portion of the pubococcygeus muscle. (From DeLancey JOL. Anatomy of the female pelvis. In: Rock JA, Thompson JD (eds). *TeLinde's Operative Gynecology*, 8th ed. Philadelphia: JB Lippincott, 1998; 63–93, with permission.)

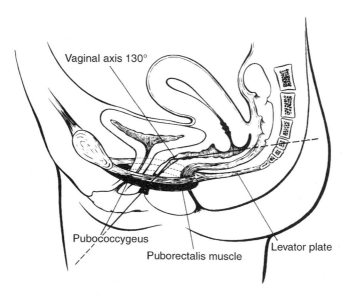

Figure 2-3. Normal axis of lower and upper vagina, which meet in a 130° angle. The upper one-third of vagina rests on the levator plate in a horizontal plane that passes through the third and fourth sacral vertebra. The posterior vaginal fornix is the deepest part of the vagina. (From reference 18, with permission.)

PELVIC BLOOD VESSELS

Knowledge of the anatomy of the major blood vessels of the pelvis is important, since the fibroareolar tissue investing the blood vessels (as they pass to the viscera) comprises the ligaments that provide lateral support. The *common iliac artery* bifurcates near the level of the pelvic brim, while the *common iliac vein* bifurcates 4–5 cm below the brim. The *external iliac artery and vein* pass directly to the femoral canal without significant pelvic branches. The *internal iliac (or hypogastric) vessels* divide into an anterior division, which is primarily visceral, and a posterior division, which is primarily somatic. The *uterine, vaginal, and superior and inferior vesicle arteries* all originate from the anterior division of the hypogastric artery, while the *middle hemorrhoidal artery* most frequently arises from a branch of the posterior hypogastric. All branches are invested with the fibroareolar tissue arising from the arcus tendineous fasciae pelvis and pass medially as the respective ligaments.[6,7]

VISCERAL FASCIA AND LIGAMENTS

The term "fascia" is quite controversial and loosely employed. The only true fascia in the pelvis are the membranes overlying the levator ani, piriformis, and obturator internus muscles.[2] However, many other structures have been called "fascia" in descriptions of surgical anatomy. *Sheets of fibroareolar tissue*, with some intermixed smooth muscle, follow the main blood supply from the pelvic sidewalls to the pelvic viscera; in essence, these sheets represent a retroperitoneal mesentery. As the sheets pass medially, they attach separately to the urinary, genital, and lower intestinal tract (Figure 2-4)[3,6,7] and form the "ligaments" that provide lateral attachment for the pelvic viscera; these are termed *endopelvic or pubocervical fascia* (Figure 2-5). In the classic anatomic descriptions of Uhlenhuth,[6,7] these fascia were referred to as the *hypogastric wings*. The ligaments, or wings, divide the pelvic retroperitoneum into the avascular spaces used in surgical exposure of the retroperitoneum. These ligaments all invest laterally on the iliococcygeus muscle (Figure 2-6). The point at which the structures coalesce forms a thick fibrous band passing on the iliococcygeus muscle and fascia, between the ischial spine and the inferior pubic tubercle. This point of attachment has been termed the "horizontal ground bundle," the "white line", and, more recently, the *arcus tendineous fasciae pelvis* (Figures 2-1, 2-6 and 2-7). A great deal of confusion has previously been encountered because this structure is so close in location to the *arcus tendineous levator ani*, which has also been termed the "white line".

The ligaments vary in their thickness and strength. The lateral support of the genital tract is thicker and better defined than that for the urinary or intestinal tract. The bladder and urethra are attached by the inferior hypogastric wing (or lateral bladder ligament), a fibroareolar band that contains the inferior vesicle

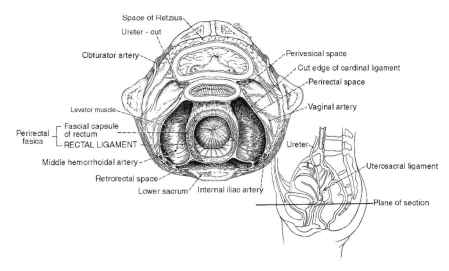

Figure 2-4. Transverse section viewed from above showing the lateral attachments of the pelvic viscera to the levator ani muscles. Note division of retroperitoneum into potential spaces by the lateral ligaments. (From Peters WA, Thornton WN. Surgical anatomy of the perirectal fascia: A gynecologic perspective. *Obstet Gynecol Surv* 1987; **42**: 605–611, with permission.)

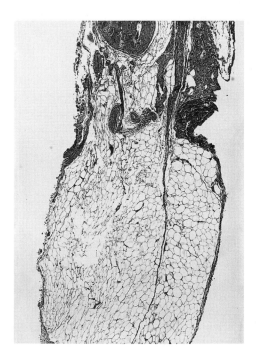

Figure 2-5. Sagittal histologic section of transverse rectal ligament showing fibroareolar tissue and branches of the middle hemorrhoidal vessels. This is a representative of the histologic composition of all the lateral fascial attachments of the pelvic viscera. (From Peters WA, Thornton WN. Surgical anatomy of the perirectal fascia: A gynecologic perspective. *Obstet Gynecol Surv* 1987; **42**: 605–611, with permission.)

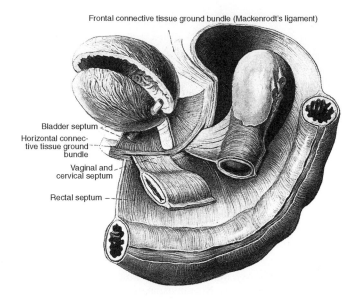

Frontal connective tissue ground bundle (Mackenrodt's ligament)

Bladder septum

Horizontal connective tissue ground bundle

Vaginal and cervical septum

Rectal septum

Figure 2-6. Schematic drawing illustrating the separate perivascular sheets investing the urinary genital and intestinal tracts. (From reference 3, with permission.)

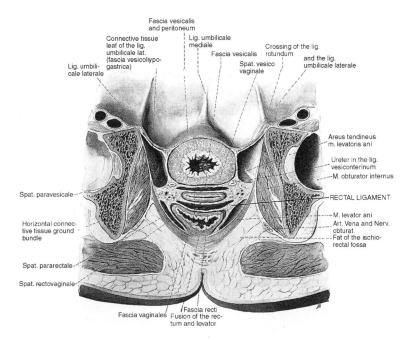

Fascia vesicalis and peritoneum

Connective tissue leaf of the lig. umbilicale lat. (fascia vesicoliypogastrica)

Lig. umbilicale mediale

Fascia vesicalis

Crossing of the lig. rotundum

and the lig. umbilicale laterale

Lig. umbilicale laterale

Spat. vesico vaginale

Areus tendineus m. levatoris ani

Ureter in the lig. vesiconterinum

M. obturator internus

Spat. paravesicale

RECTAL LIGAMENT

Horizontal connective tissue ground bundle

M. levator ani

Art. Vena and Nerv. obturat.

Fat of the ischio-rectal fossa

Spat. pararectale

Spat. rectovaginale

Fascia vaginales

Fascia recti
Fusion of the rectum and levator

Figure 2-7. Transverse section viewed from below at the level of the upper vagina showing a common attachment of the lateral ligaments to the arcus tendineous fasciae pelvis (horizontal ground bundle). (From reference 3, with permission.)

artery and its corresponding venous plexus.[7] The superior hypogastric wing (or superior bladder ligament) contains the superior vesicle artery and venous plexus. The superior hypogastric wing is the weakest and least defined of the ligaments. This ligament is divided before mobilizing the bladder for a psoas hitch. Thickening of the inferior hypogastric wing (lateral bladder ligament) at the proximal urethra and the bladder neck was previously described as having direct attachments to the symphysis and was called the *pubourethral ligament*. In actuality, this portion of the lateral bladder ligament attaches the proximal urethra and bladder neck to the arcus tendineous fasciae pelvis just posterior to the pubic tubercle (Figure 2-8). This segment of the fascial support also contains the smoothest muscle fibers of any of the visceral ligaments, and is termed the pubourethral muscle by DeLancey.[20]

The lateral attachments of the cervix and vagina have been called *parametrium, paracolpos, transverse cervical ligaments, Mackenrodt's ligaments, and cardinal ligaments*.[3–7,21] They begin at the level of the cervix and continue uninterrupted all the way to the level of the introitus where there is a direct fusion of the endopelvic fascia investing the vagina to the levator fascia. The uterine and vaginal arteries and the corresponding venous plexus pass within these ligaments. The ureter passes directly through the cardinal ligament ~2 cm lateral to the cervix at the level of the internal cervical os and its location is critical in performing total hysterectomy (Figure 2-4).

The *uterosacral ligaments* have been erroneously shown in some texts as being a separate structure. They are, in fact, the posteriormost portion of the cardinal ligaments, coming off at the level of the cervix and uppermost vagina. They do not insert on the sacrum, but rather insert into the posterior arcus tendineous fasciae pelvis. Traction on the uterus during hysterectomy either

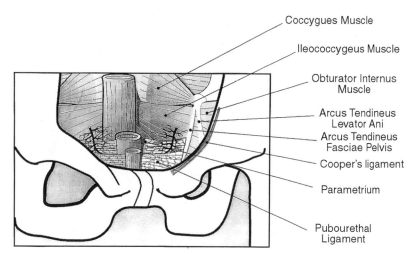

Coccygues Muscle

Ileococcygeus Muscle

Obturator Internus Muscle

Arcus Tendineus Levator Ani

Arcus Tendineus Fasciae Pelvis

Cooper's ligament

Parametrium

Pubourethal Ligament

Figure 2-8. Cross section of proximal urethra and midvagina showing lateral attachments to the arcus tendineous fasciae pelvis.

from above or below, gives a somewhat distorted impression as to the prominence and course of this portion of the cardinal ligament. The rectum is attached to the levator fascia by the *transverse rectal ligaments* (presacral branch of the hypogastric wing), which includes the middle hemorrhoidal vessels.

Debate raged for many years over the relative importance of the pelvic floor muscles and the lateral ligaments to the support of the pelvic viscera.[1,4,15] It is now generally accepted that the pelvic floor muscles are the primary support structures of the pelvic viscera, but the importance of the lateral attachments is also appreciated. There is variation among women in their susceptibility to prolapse with injury to the pelvic floor muscles. Clearly, there are women in whom the fibroareolar ligaments undergo hypertrophy and provide adequate support to the pelvic viscera despite defects in the pelvic floor.

RETROPERITONEAL SPACES

Above the levator ani muscles, the pelvic retroperitoneum is divided into avascular spaces by the visceral attachments previously described (Figure 2-9). The *space of Retzius* is employed in many urogynecologic procedures and should be thoroughly familiar to all surgeons operating for incontinence. Anteriorly, the two pubic bones are fused by the fibrocartilage of the symphysis. Cooper's ligament, a thick band of periosteum on the superomedial pubic ramus (Figure 2-8), is also known as the iliopectineal line and represents the origin of the pectineus muscles. Cooper's ligament is used as an anchor point in retro-pubic urethropexies as well as in the repair of femoral hernias. Laterally, the space of Retzius is defined by the obturator internus muscle and that portion of the levator ani muscle that lies anterior to the arcus tendineous fasciae pelvis. A rich venous plexus invests the anterior wall of the bladder and urethra, and

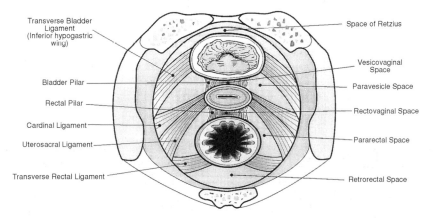

Figure 2-9.   Schematic drawing showing the division of the pelvis by the lateral fascial attachments of the viscera to the levator ani muscles.

passes laterally in the transverse urethral and bladder ligaments. Unless a surgical dissection is carried out, the vaginal and urinary attachments to the arcus tendineous fasciae pelvis are fused. The transverse bladder and urethral ligaments (along with the bladder and urethra themselves) from the posterior boundary of the space of Retzius.

If the space of Retzius is bluntly developed during a surgical procedure, the attachments to the arcus tendineous fasciae pelvis can be exposed. With a vaginal dissection, if there has been avulsion or tear in the perivaginal attachment, a finger can be directly passed into the space of Retzius. When performing needle suspension procedures, the lateral urethral and bladder ligaments (inferior hypogastric wing) are penetrated with blunt dissection to enter the space of Retzius. The neurovascular bundle to the urethra is contained in these ligaments, and some degree of injury with deinnervation occurs when they are penetrated.

During an abdominal approach, it is possible to create a space between the lateral bladder ligament and the cardinal ligament called the *paravesical space*, which is developed during radical hysterectomy or radical cystectomy. The *pararectal space*, which lies posterior to the cardinal ligament and anterior to the transverse rectal ligament, is frequently opened during abdominal surgery to identify the ureter and to free it from attachments to the adnexa, uterosacral ligament, or cul-de-sac. The pararectal space is also approached during transvaginal reconstructive surgery to reach the sacrospinous ligament or coccygeus fascia. The *presacral (retrorectal) space*, which is posterior to the transverse rectal ligament, must be created during resection of the rectosigmoid or during an abdominal sacral colpopexy.

Between the bladder and vagina there is also a potential space, the *vesico-vaginal space*, which, laterally, is bounded by an attachment between the "fascia" of the vagina and that of the bladder, and contains an anastomotic venous plexus known as Santorini's venous plexus. This thickening at the lateral bladder base is usually referred to as the "bladder pillar". Similarly, there is a potential space between the rectum and vagina known as the *rectovaginal space* with the lateral boundary containing fibrous bands containing a venous plexus and referred to as the "rectal pillar". Some illustrations have erroneously labeled the rectal pillar as the utcrosacral ligament. These rectal and bladder pillars are the frequent site of troublesome bleeding during both abdominal and vaginal surgeries.

SPHINCTERS OF PELVIC VISCERA

Each of the visceral systems (urinary, genital, and gastrointestinal) has a separate sphincter system.[9–14] The integration of structure and function are best understood for the *rectal sphincter*. The smooth muscle *internal* rectal sphincter is a continuation of the rectal smooth muscle and provides a baseline tone. The *external* rectal sphincter is a voluntary skeletal muscle and has separate superficial, medial, and deep segments. The separations are not surgically apparent. The smooth muscle in the vaginal wall could be considered as an analogous internal sphincter, although it has only a weak resting tone. The bulbocavernosus muscles are analogous to the primary skeletal sphincter of the vagina. The urethra has both an involuntary *smooth muscle sphincter*, which provides resting tone, as well as a *skeletal muscle sphincter*, which provides resting tone and some degree of voluntary bladder control.[12-14] The specifics of rectal and urinary sphincter function are described in detail in Chapters 3 and 19.

The puborectalis muscles are of great functional significance in rectal and urinary sphincter function.[9-13] Anatomically, these blend into the undersurface of the pubococcygeus muscles (Figure 2-2). The puborectalis muscles receive innervation directly from the sacral nerve plexus, which provides them some degree of protection from deinnervation injuries that occur following pudendal nerve stretch in childbirth. Shafrik[9-11] has examined in depth the role of the puborectalis muscles in urinary and fecal incontinence. The puborectalis muscles serve as a secondary sphincter system for the urinary, genital, and fecal tracts. In addition to the separate secondary sphincteric function of the puborectalis muscles, all the organ-specific sphincters are laterally attached by fibrous bands to the puborectalis muscles (Figure 2-10). The interaction of the smooth muscle sphincter, external sphincter, and puborectalis muscle is best understood in defecation, where the puborectalis muscles act in opposition to the iliococcygeus and pubococcygeus muscles. As long as the puborectalis muscles are intact, a patient with a severe injury to the pudendal nerve and/or external rectal sphincter will retain continence for solid stool but not flatus or liquid stool. The goal of Kegel exercises is to strengthen the puborectalis muscles, and, although their exact contribution to urinary continence is difficult to prove, there is undoubtedly a significant component. Plication or midline reefing of the puborectalis muscles is performed posteriorly to the rectum by colorectal surgeons in patients with idiopathic or neurogenic incontinence (Park's retrorectal levatorplasty).

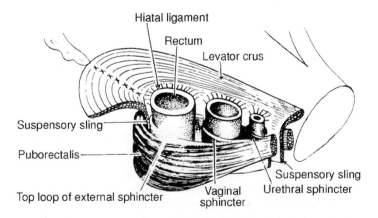

Figure 2-10.   Relationship of the primary organ-specific sphincters to the puborectalis muscles (secondary sphincter). (From Shafik A. A new concept of the anal sphincter mechanism and the physiology of defecation: VIII. Levator hiatus and tunnel anatomy and function. *Dis Colon Rectum* 1979: **22**: 539, with permission.)

Gynecologists routinely plicate the puborectalis muscles anterior to the rectum during posterior colpoperineorrhaphy and to support a rectal sphincteroplasty. Many anecdotal experiences have been reported where a patient has had restoration of urinary continence with plication of the puborectalis muscles without any coexisting surgical procedure to support the bladder neck. Variation in the plication of the puborectalis muscles anterior to the rectum may explain the wide variance of success that different surgeons have reported in the vaginal approaches to stress urinary incontinence.

PELVIC FLOOR INNERVATION

The *pudendal nerve branches* provide sensory and motor innervation to the inferior levator ani muscles, the external urethral and rectal sphincters, and the superficial perineal muscles.[22] The external urethral sphincter and the levator muscles also receive innervation on the superior side directly from the *sacral nerve plexus* (S3–S5). The puborectalis muscles obtain their primary innervation from the sacral nerve plexus (S3–S4) but, in some patients, also receive secondary innervation from branches of the pudendal nerve. Thus, the external rectal sphincter is the only striated muscle involved in continence that receives its innervation solely from the pudendal nerve. The internal anal sphincter receives sympathetic and parasympathetic fibers from the *presacral plexus* and *splanchnic nerves.*[22]

SUMMARY

The pelvic viscera are supported by the levator ani muscles and by ligaments formed by the fibroareolar tissue, which invests the pelvic vasculature. Each organ system has a primary sphincter with both a smooth muscle and skeletal muscle component. The puborectalis muscle provides a common secondary sphincter for each visceral system.

REFERENCES

1. Berglas B, Rubin IC. Study of the supportive structures of the uterus by levator myography. *Surg Gynecol Obstet* 1953; **97**: 677.
2. Berglas B, Rubin IC. Histologic study of the pelvic connective tissue. *Surg Gynecol Obstet* 1953; **97**: 277.
3. Peham HV, Amreich I. *Operative Gynecology.* [Translated by LK Ferguson]. Philadelphia: JB Lippincott 1934.
4. Porges RF, Porges JC, Blimick G. Mechanisms of uterine support and the pathogenesis of uterine prolapse. *Obstet Gynecol* 1960; **15**: 711.
5. Curtis AH, Anson BJ, Beaton LE. The anatomy of the subperitoneal tissues and ligamentous structures in relation to surgery of the female pelvic viscera. *Surg Gynecol Obstet* 1940; **70**: 643.

6. Uhlenhuth E. *Problems in the Anatomy of the Pelvis: An Atlas.* Philadelphia: JB Lippincott, 1953.
7. Uhlenhuth E, Day EC, Smith RD, Middleton ED. The visceral endopelvic fascia and the hypogastric sheath. *Surg Gynecol Obstet* 1948; **86**: 9.
8. Quimby WC. The anatomy and blood vessels of the pelvis. In: Meigs JV (ed). *Surgical Treatment of Cancer of the Cervix.* New York: Grune and Stratton 1954; 26–64.
9. Shafik A. A new concept of the anal sphincter mechanism and the physiology of defecation: II. Anatomy of the levator ani muscle with special reference to puborectalis. *Invest Urol* 1976; **13**: 175.
10. Shafik A. A new concept of the anal sphincter mechanism and the physiology of defecation: VIII. Levator hiatus and tunnel anatomy and function. *Dis Colon Rectum* 1979; **22**: 539.
11. Shafik A. Pelvic double sphincter control complex: theory of pelvic organ continence with clinical application. *Urol* 1984; **23**: 611.
12. DeLancey JOL. Structural aspects of the extrinsic continence mechanism. *Obstet Gynecol* 1988; **92**: 296.
13. Shafrik A. Micturation and urinary continence: new concepts. *Int Urogynecol J* 1992; **3**: 168.
14. DeLancey JOL. Anatomy and physiology of urinary continence. *Clin Obstet Gynecol* 1990; **33**: 298.
15. Halban J, Tandler J. The supporting apparatus of the uterus. [Translated by RF Porges and JC Porges] *Obstet Gynecol* 1960; **15**: 790.
16. DeLancey JOL. Anatomy of the female pelvis. In: Rock JA, Thompson JD (eds). *TeLinde's Operative Gynecology*, 8th ed. Philadelphia: JB Lippincott, 1997; 63–93.
17. Koelbl H, Strassegger H, Riss PA, Gruber H. Morphologic and functional aspects of pelvic floor muscles in patients with pelvic relaxation and genuine stress incontinence. *Obstet Gynecol* 1989; **74**: 789.
18. Thompson JD. Malposition of the uterus. In: Thompson JD, Rock JA (eds). *TeLinde's Operative Gynecology* 7th ed, Philadelphia: JB Lippincott, 1992; 832.
19. Peters WA, Thornton WN. Surgical anatomy of the perirectal fascia: A gynecologic perspective. *Obstet Gynecol Surv* 1987; **42**: 605.
20. DeLancey JOL, Starr RA. Histology of the connection between the vagina and levator ani muscles. *J Reprod Med* 1990; **35**: 765.
21. Rawge RL, Woodburne RT. The gross and microscopic anatomy of the transverse cervical ligaments. *Am J Obstet Gynecol* 1964; **90**: 460.
22. Snooks SJ, Swash M. The innervation of the muscles of continence. *Ann R Coll Surg Eng* 1986; **68**: 45.

CHAPTER 3

Physiology of the lower urinary tract and the mechanism of continence

JOSEPH SCHAFFER AND J. ANDREW FANTL ———————————

The lower urinary tract is composed of a group of interrelated structures whose function is the storage and timely evacuation of urine. While this would appear to be a relatively simple process, in fact, lower urinary tract function is highly complex and under the control of both of anatomic factors and an intricate system of reflexes located in the central and peripheral nervous systems. A full understanding of this system is still to be elucidated. Our current knowledge has been derived mostly from animal data and extrapolated to humans. However, a basic knowledge of anatomy and neurophysiology is vital to understanding lower urinary tract function and dysfunction. This chapter reviews the physiology of the lower urinary tract and the mechanism of continence with emphasis on clinically significant factors.

OVERVIEW OF LOWER URINARY TRACT PHYSIOLOGY

The lower urinary tract is composed of the bladder and urethra, and their supportive structures. The bladder acts as a low-pressure reservoir, while the urethra acts as a sphincter. During the storage phase the bladder fills without sensation or detrusor contractions and with minimal increases in detrusor pressure despite wide fluctuations in intravesical and intraabdominal pressure (Figure 3-1). The increase in volume without a significant increase in pressure is due to the passive elastic and viscoelastic properties of the smooth muscle and connective tissue of the bladder wall and is known as the process of *accommodation*.[1] Normal storage also depends on the ability of the urethra to function as a closed valve during bladder filling. The maintenance of continence during the storage phase can occur only if urethral resistance or pressure is always greater than intravesical pressure.

Under normal conditions, the voiding phase begins when the bladder reaches a specific volume. Tension receptors relay a sense of fullness to the central nervous system, and, at the appropriate time and place, voluntary micturition is

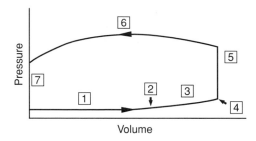

Figure 3-1. The bladder cycle represented as a pressure–volume loop: *1* accommodation: a gradual increase in bladder volume without a significant rise in detrusor pressure; *2* first sensation of fullness; *3* cortical suppression of the micturition reflex; *4* voluntary initiation of voiding; *5* isometric pressure rise as detrusor contraction begins before the bladder neck is fully open and the pelvic floor is fully relaxed; *6* sustained detrusor contraction resulting in complete bladder emptying; *7* detrusor relaxation. (From reference 2, with permission of Professor Stuart Stanton.)

initiated. For normal evacuation to occur there must be a volitionally controlled, coordinated decrease in urethral resistance with a concomitant increase in intravesical pressure.

OVERVIEW OF THE NERVOUS SYSTEM

The lower urinary tract is controlled by a series of complex neuronal pathways that connect the cerebral cortex to the midbrain, spinal cord, bladder, urethra, and pelvic floor. These pathways allow for reflex subconscious control and voluntary cortical control of the lower urinary tract. The system includes multiple reflexes involving the peripheral and central nervous systems. Lesions anywhere along these pathways can lead to disorders of storage and/or evacuation.

The nervous system comprises two major divisions: the central nervous system, which includes the brain and spinal cord, and the peripheral nervous system, which is composed of 12 pairs of cranial nerves, 31 pairs of spinal nerves, and their corresponding ganglia. Sensory nerves that supply information to the central nervous system are known as afferent, and those that convey information from the central nervous system to the end-organs are known as efferent.

The peripheral nervous system is further divided into autonomic and somatic components. The autonomic system which directs unconscious and involuntary function, receives sensory input and mediates smooth muscle, cardiac muscle, and gland function through visceral afferent and efferent nerves. The primary sensory system of the lower urinary tract is in the autonomic system, which is further divided into the sympathetic and parasympathetic system.[3] The sympathetic system controls urine storage, while the parasympathetic system controls bladder emptying: however, both are intimately related at the central and peripheral levels.

The somatic system controls skeletal muscle activity through sensory information relayed to the central nervous system, leading to both voluntary and reflex muscle activity. Two sets of neurons direct somatic motor activity in the pelvis: upper motor neurons, whose cell bodies lie in the cortex and brainstem, and lower motor neurons, whose cell bodies are in the ventral horns of sacral spinal cord segments S2–S4. Several of the important reflexes that influence urine storage and evacuation work through somatic reflex pathways.

PERIPHERAL NERVOUS SYSTEM

Neuroanatomy and Physiology

The autonomic efferent (motor) system functions through the use of a series of two-neuron chains: Preganglionic neurons have cell bodies in the intermediolateral cell column of the brain or spinal cord and their axons synapse at autonomic ganglia located outside the spinal cord. The postganglionic neuron then conveys impulses directly to the end-organ.

Sympathetic Division

The sympathetic division is derived from nerve fibers of the thoracolumbar spinal cord arising from T1–L2. Of these, T11–L2 innervate the lower urinary tract. After leaving the spinal cord, the nerves synapse at the sympathetic chain ganglia, then join the presacral nerve, and become the right and left hypogastric nerves (Figure 3-2). These nerves then form the pelvic plexus at the base of the hypogastric artery in conjunction with parasympathetic nerves S2–S4. Subsequently, nerves from this plexus diverge to innervate the upper vagina, bladder, proximal urethra, and lower ureter. The pelvic plexus has a wide distribution and is difficult to visualize, making it a site highly susceptible to injury during gynecologic surgery.

During the storage phase the sympathetic system exerts major control over the bladder and urethra through stimulation of end-organ beta-adrenergic and alpha-adrenergic receptors. Beta-adrenergic receptors are prominent in the detrusor, while alpha-adrenergic receptors are dominant in the muscle of the trigone and urethra (Figure 3-3). Beta-adrenergic receptors respond to low doses of the neurotransmitter norepinephrine and produce detrusor smooth muscle relaxation. Alpha-adrenergic receptors are stimulated by high doses of norepinephrine and cause muscle contraction at the bladder base and urethra. Therefore sympathetic discharge during the storage phase promotes continence by relaxation of the bladder and contraction of the proximal urethra. Inhibition of sympathetic stimulation during the voiding phase leads to relaxation of the smooth muscle of the trigone and urethra, open bladder neck, and subsequent passage of urine.

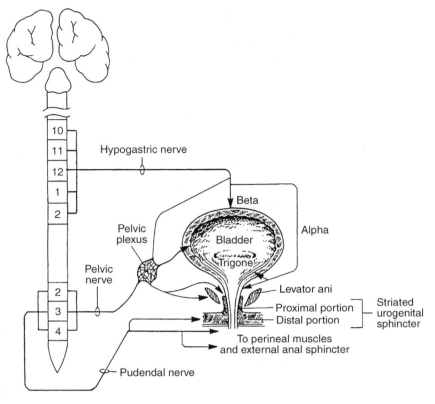

Figure 3-2.   Peripheral innervation of the female lower urinary tract. (From reference 4, with permission.)

Parasympathetic Division

The parasympathetic division is derived from the sacral spinal cord segments S2–S4. Preganglionic fibers arise in the intermediolateral gray matter, exit the cord at the ventral roots, and become the pelvic nerve. The pelvic nerve then joins the pelvic plexus and finally innervates the detrusor muscle. Parasympathetic preganglionic fibers synapse at ganglia within the bladder wall. Thus, these ganglia are quite vulnerable to end-organ diseases such as occur with stretch injury, infection, or fibrosis. It is likely that disorders of bladder contractility are at least partially due to injury at the level of the ganglia located within the bladder wall.

Acetylcholine regulates synaptic transmission at the parasympathetic ganglia within the bladder wall, therefore the postsynaptic receptor is cholinergic. The ganglia then send short postganglionic axons directly to the detrusor smooth muscle, which responds to the release of acetylcholine by contracting.

Storage phase activity is modulated by both the sympathetic and parasympathetic systems. The voiding phase, however, is mostly controlled by

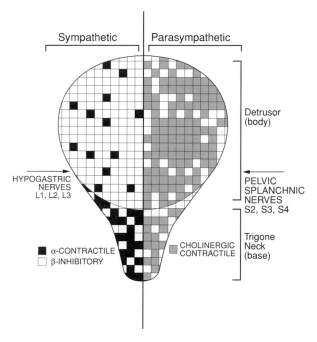

Figure 3-3. Distribution of cholinergic and adrenergic receptors in the bladder and urethra. (From reference 5, Fig. 2-23, with permission.)

parasympathetic activity. Cholinergic contractile receptors are predominate within the detrusor muscle (Figure 3-3) and parasympathetic stimulation of these receptors leads to a coordinated contraction of the muscle and subsequent bladder emptying.

Somatic System

The somatic portion of the peripheral nervous system is responsible for activity of voluntary muscle, which, in the lower urinary tract, includes the skeletal muscles of the urethra and pelvic floor.

The system works through a series of segmental skeletal reflex arcs, which are modulated by information from the central nervous system (Figure 3-4). Stretch receptors (muscle spindles) at the end-organs convey information through afferent neurons whose cell bodies are in the dorsal root ganglion. The information is then passed through small interneurons within the spinal cord to the efferent neuron. The axons of the efferent motor neuron then travel directly to the motor endplate on skeletal muscle. These reflex arcs may consist of a sensory and a motor limb, or they may be more complex with several interneurons between the two limbs. Reflex arcs are modulated through inputs from higher centers in the central nervous system.

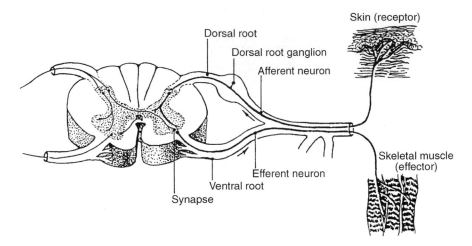

Figure 3-4. The somatic reflex arc. Somatic reflex arcs consist of a sensory and a motor limb. Stretch receptors at end-organs convey information to the spinal cord through somatic afferent neurons. The information is then passed through small interneurons to the efferent neuron. The axons of the efferent neuron travel directly to the motor endplate on skeletal muscle. (From reference 6, permission sought.)

The pudendal nerve provides the major somatic input to the lower urinary tract. The efferent portion arises from motor neurons whose cell bodies are in the anterior horn of sacral spinal cord segments S2–S4 (Onuf's nucleus). After exiting the cord, S2–S4 neurons become the pudendal nerve. The nerve then passes between the coccygeus and piriformis muscles, exits the pelvis through the greater sciatic foramen, passes around the ischial spine, and reenters the pelvis through the lesser sciatic foramen (Figure 3-5). The nerve then travels with the pudendal vessels along the internal surface of the obturator internus muscle through Alcock's canal, the tunnel formed by the splitting of the obturator fascia. Because the nerve is fixed at this point, it is believed to be the site of mechanical stretch injury that occurs to the pudendal nerve during vaginal childbirth or pelvic organ prolapse. After existing Alcock's canal, the pudendal nerve splits into three branches: *1)* the dorsal nerve of the clitoris; *2)* the perineal nerve, which innervates the striated urethral sphincter, anterior levator ani, and superficial perineal muscles; and *3)* the inferior hemorrhoidal nerve, which supplies the striated external anal sphincter.

The pudendal nerve innervates the distal periurethral skeletal muscles (compressor urethrae and urethrovaginal sphincter). Evidence suggests that the proximal component (sphincter urethrae) may be innervated by somatic efferent branches of the pelvic nerve.[8] This double innervation has clinical implications; a patient with pudendal neuropathy will have an impaired ability to use the distal periurethral muscles as a reserve or backup continence mechanism, however, an intact pelvic nerve may still maintain continence under nonstressful conditions.

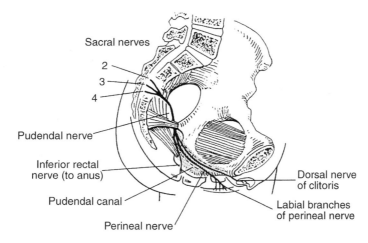

Sacral nerves
2
3
4

Pudendal nerve

Inferior rectal
nerve (to anus)

Pudendal canal

Perineal nerve

Dorsal nerve
of clitoris

Labial branches
of perineal nerve

Figure 3-5. Course and branches of the pudendal nerve in the female pelvis. Shaded area represents a section of nerve that is sometimes damaged in childbirth. (From reference 7, with permission.)

Skeletal muscle is composed of slow- and fast-twitch fibers. Slow-twitch muscle is resistant to fatigue and provides baseline tone. Fast-twitch muscle can be rapidly activated to provide an almost instantaneous augmentation of muscle contraction. The striated urethral sphincter is composed of ~65% slow-twitch fibers and 35% of the fast-twitch type. Therefore, a baseline constant tone is present, which can be augmented by activation of fast-twitch fibers in stress situations where urethral pressure needs to be rapidly increased.

During the storage phase, somatic stimulation to the pelvic floor and striated urethral sphincter muscles provides the constant muscle tone necessary to keep intraurethral pressure greater than intravesical pressure. Urodynamic studies have shown that urethral pressure increases as the bladder fills and with sudden increases in intravesical and intraabdominal pressure.[9] Somatic reflex arcs respond to intravesical pressure increases by contracting the striated urethral muscles.

Sensory Innervation of the Lower Urinary Tract

Sensation within the bladder is transmitted to the central nervous system through sensory afferent fibers of two types: *1*) proprioceptive nerve endings residing in collagen bundles that respond to tension and convey a sense of bladder distention; *2*) free nerve endings in the bladder mucosa and submucosa that are responsible for transmission of temperature, pain, and irritation. Sensors exist in both the trigone and the bladder body. Studies in the cat suggest that sensors for bladder distention are distributed evenly throughout all regions of the bladder, while sensors for pain, conscious touch, and distention are most dense in the trigone.[10,11] This would explain the frequency and urgency caused by intrinsic trigonal lesions and extrinsic compressing lesions such as uterine fibroids.

Detrusor afferent nerve fibers run along the same autonomic pathways as the efferent. Afferent nerve fibers have been demonstrated in the pelvic, hypogastric, and pudendal nerves.[12] Pelvic afferent nerves from the detrusor muscle ascend to S2–S4 spinal segments. Other detrusor afferent nerves may travel with the hypogastric nerve (T11–L2), which explains why some patients with thoracic lesions can still sense bladder distention.[9]

Urethral sensation is transmitted through afferent nerves, which relay information regarding pain, temperature, urethral distention, and passage of urine. Urethral smooth and striated muscle afferent nerve fibers travel in the pudendal nerve and terminate at the dorsal sacral cord, S2–S4.

CENTRAL NERVOUS SYSTEM

Autonomic and somatic peripheral activity within the lower urinary tract are ultimately under the control of the central nervous system (CNS). In general, the baseline activity of the CNS during bladder filling is inhibitory. The cerebral cortex and midbrain respond to increasing volume by triggering an increase in subconscious tonic inhibition of detrusor contraction and augmenting urethral muscle contraction. Lesions of the CNS therefore tend to result in detrusor hyperactivity. CNS activity during the evacuation phase directs detrusor contraction and urethral relaxation, leading to voluntary voiding.

The major area of detrusor innervation within the brain, that is, cortical control of the detrusor muscle, is the supermedial portion of the frontal lobes and the genu of the corpus callosum, known as the pyramidal detrusor area. Axons originating in this region travel in the corticobulbar tract through the basal ganglia and terminate in the pontine mesencephalic reticular formation on the detrusor motor nuclei of the nucleus lateralis dorsalis; this area is designated as the *pontine micturition center*.

Micturition was previously felt to be controlled in the sacral spinal cord; however, current evidence suggests that coordination of voiding occurs mostly in the pontine micturition center with support from the area of the sacral spinal cord known as the *sacral micturition center*.[13] The detrusor motor nuclei in the pons receive impulses from afferent neurons that are suppressive, from the basal ganglia; sensory, from stretch receptors in the detrusor muscle; and coordinating, from the cerebellum. Efferent neurons from detrusor motor nuclei then travel to detrusor motor neurons in the intermediolateral cell column, T10–L1 and S2–S4, facilitating the appropriate response. When the pathways between the pontine and sacral micturition centers are intact, micturition is achieved by activation of the micturition reflex, resulting in detrusor contraction, opening of the bladder neck and urethra, and relaxation of striated urethral musculature.

The sacral micturition center has been proposed to be the site where reflex activity involving the bladder, urethra, and pelvic floor is mediated. Anatomically, this site is the conus medullaris, which includes the S1–S5 cord segments.[14] Because of the disparity in the length of the spinal cord and vertebral column, the conus medullaris is located at the T11–L1 vertebral level, and the autonomic detrusor motor nuclei and the somatic pudendal motor nuclei lie within. Also this area of the cord has a complex web of collateral neurons that allow for central nervous system modulation of reflex activity. Injury above the sacral micturition center may result in detrusor hyperreflexia, in which the bladder functions solely by reflex activity, without volitional control, and in detrusor areflexia.

Several authors have hypothesized a series of spinal reflex arcs involved in bladder storage and micturition, which are mediated through the sacral micturition center (Table 3-1). Although several of these theoretical reflex arcs have been demonstrated in experimental animals, literature review does not show consistent agreement regarding the significance in humans.[15–17]

Table 3-1.   Proposed reflexes

Reflexes	*Actions*
Bladder storage reflexes	
Sympathetic detrusor to detrusor	Inhibits detrusor in response to increased detrusor
Detrusor–urethral stimulating	Increased detrusor tension stimulates urethral smooth muscle
Perineal–detrusor inhibition	Inhibits detrusor in response to perineal sphincter muscles
Urethrosphincter guarding	Contracts external striated sphincter in response to trigone tension
Micturition initiation reflexes	
Perineodetrusor facilitative	Decreasing pelvic floor muscle tone; stimulates detrusor
Detrusor–detrusor facilitative	Increased detrusor tension; stimulates detrusor
Reflexes to maintain micturition	
Detrusor urethral inhibiting	Detrusor to segmental inhibition of urethral smooth muscle
Detrusor sphincter inhibiting	Detrusor to segmental inhibition of external striated sphincter
Urethrodetrusor facilitative	Proximal urethra segmental reflex to stimulate detrusor
Urethrobulbar detrusor facilitative	Proximal urethra reflex to stimulate detrusor via brainstem
Urethrosphincteric inhibiting	Urethra to external striated sphincter; segmental reflex
Micturition cessation reflex	Pelvic floor afferent fibers to brainstem to inhibit detrusor

Periurethral striated muscle activity is modulated by the pudendal cerebral cortex area. Afferent and efferent somatic axons travel between the pudendal nuclei in the ventromedial portion of the ventral gray matter of S1–S3 and the central vertex of the pudendal cerebral cortex area and thus allow for voluntary and reflex control of the periurethral striated muscle. Voluntary cessation of voiding usually occurs with contraction of these muscles and thereby tests the integrity of these pathways, and the reflex contraction of slow- and fast-twitch fibers, which occurs with bladder filling and sudden increases in intravesical pressure, also test these pathways.

Neurologic lesions have variable effects on the micturition reflex, depending on the level of the lesion. Lesions that interrupt the pontine–sacral pathway lead to loss of central control, thereby causing uncoordinated voiding and detrusor sphincter dyssynergia. Lesions above the pons abolish inhibitory input, causing detrusor contraction, involuntary voiding, and incontinence. Patients with Parkinson's disease lack dopamine, the neurotransmitter at the basal ganglia, and studies suggest that, because the basal ganglia have a suppressive effect on the detrusor, these patients frequently suffer from incontinence secondary to detrusor hyperreflexia.

STORAGE PHASE

The unique compliance of the bladder allows it to function as a low-pressure, high-compliance organ that adapts to increasing volume with minimal increase in pressure. Compliance is a mathematical term defined as the change in volume divided by the change in pressure ($C = \Delta V/\Delta P$). It represents the mathematical expression of the phenomenon of accommodation.[18] Elastin, collagen, and smooth muscle contribute to appropriate compliance. The normal bladder has high compliance: large changes in volume produce minimal changes in pressure. An abnormal bladder with low compliance, the so-called "stiff" bladder, might occur after radiation therapy where the intrinsic viscoelastic properties are damaged. Reduction in compliance also occurs with aging.[19]

During the storage phase the bladder fills with urine at physiologic rates of ~20–100 ml/h. As the bladder fills, the walls stretch and it assumes a spherical shape. The thickness of the bladder wall decreases and individual muscle bundles reorganize and increase their length. Because the ureter is fixed to the superficial trigone, its intramural portion is stretched, making the lumen narrower and more resistant to flow, which prevents vesicoureteral reflux.

As the bladder fills, stretch receptors in the detrusor wall initiate afferent signals in the pelvic nerve, which stimulate the pontine micturition center. Detrusor contractility is inhibited by activation of the spinal sympathetic reflex, which receives impulses from the afferent pelvic splanchnic nerves and the efferent hypogastric nerve. Three sympathetic responses to afferent pelvic nerve firing associated with increasing volume have been demonstrated experimentally: *1*) beta-adrenergic receptor-mediated relaxation of the detrusor musculature; *2*) alpha-adrenergic receptor-mediated increase in urethral smooth muscle activity and urethral pressure; and *3*) inhibition of ganglionic transmission in the pelvic ganglia, which inhibits both sacral parasympathetic outflow to the bladder and detrusor contraction.[16]

Initially, central inhibitory signals overcome the reflex to void and detrusor contraction does not occur. With increased filling the urge to void increases, but contraction is still inhibited until either voluntary voiding occurs or a critical volume is reached. When this critical volume is reached, it is more difficult to suppress micturition. The normal functional bladder capacity of 400–600 ml is well below the volume at which inhibition is overcome.

In addition to reflex stimulation of smooth muscle during bladder filling, stimulation of the striated external sphincter occurs as a result of increased somatic efferent (pelvic and pudendal) nerve activity. Periurethral striated muscle activity, in turn, leads to a reflex inhibition of the detrusor muscle through inhibition of preganglionic detrusor motor neurons in the intermediolateral cell columns of the sacral spinal cord, which would explain the clinical observation that pelvic floor exercises are sometimes effective in the treatment of detrusor instability.

VOIDING PHASE

Voiding is a voluntary act involving reflex-coordinated relaxation of the urethra and sustained contraction of the bladder until emptying is complete. In the appropriate social situation, when a sensation of bladder fullness is felt, the micturition reflex is initiated. The micturition reflex pathway travels through the sacral micturition center and is modulated at the pontine micturition center. Voluntary control of the micturition occurs through the connection of the frontal cerebral cortex and the pons. Voluntary control of the external urethral sphincter occurs through the corticospinal pathway connecting the frontal cortex with the pudendal nucleus in the ventral horn of the sacral spinal cord.

Voiding is initiated voluntarily or by reflex when the critical volume is reached and inhibition is no longer possible. As the bladder fills, afferent pelvic nerve signals ascend in the cord to the pontine micturition center. Cortical signals act on the pontine center causing efferent neurons to inhibit pudendal nerve firing, relaxing the pelvic floor and external striated sphincter, and stimulating parasympathetic fibers S2–S4, causing detrusor contraction. During voiding, inhibition of sympathetic efferent neurons contributes to opening of the bladder neck. Furthermore, the bladder neck is opened by contraction of smooth muscle fibers, which are a continuation of the detrusor muscle. Loss of pelvic floor contraction cause the trigone and urethrovesical junction to drop caudally, facilitating funneling of the bladder neck.

Urodynamically, the micturition reflex begins with a sudden and complete relaxation of the striated muscles of the pelvic floor and a decrease in urethral pressure. Seconds later, intravesical pressure increases due to a contraction of the detrusor muscle. Descent and funneling of the bladder neck occur and flow begins. It should be noted that some women void simply with a decrease in urethral pressure and without a detrusor contraction.[20] In addition, some women have been noted to void primarily through Valsalva efforts. It is also likely that the mechanism may vary within the same individual, depending on variables such as volume or physical and environmental circumstances.

Brainstem modulation of the micturition reflex allows for a detrusor contraction long enough to completely empty the bladder. With voluntary termination of voiding ("stop test"), the striated muscles of the urethra and pelvic floor are contracted, intraurethral pressure increased, and the urethra emptied of urine. The detrusor muscle is reflexly inhibited and detrusor pressure returns to normal.

MECHANISM OF CONTINENCE

During the storage phase the urethra and bladder neck function as a closed valve, always maintaining urine within the bladder except during periods of voluntary voiding. The maintenance of continence therefore depends on urethral resistance always being greater than intravesical pressure. In addition to the neurophysiologic controls of the sphincter mechanism discussed above, anatomic factors contribute to the proper functioning of the urethral sphincter mechanism. It should be kept in mind that the mechanisms of continence are still incompletely understood and remain a subject of continued debate.

ANATOMY

Trigone and Bladder Neck

The trigone and bladder neck play an important role in the mechanism of continence. Trigonal and detrusor smooth muscle extend into the bladder neck and proximal urethra, and this anatomic configuration allows for opening of the bladder neck, which occurs during detrusor contraction and voiding. Closure of the bladder neck during bladder filling occurs in response to sympathetic stimulation of the alpha-adrenergic contractile receptors within the trigone. Bladder neck closure appears to be a factor in the maintenance of continence.

Urethra

The urethra is a muscular tube, 3–4 cm long and 6 mm diameter, embedded in the anterior vaginal wall. The urethral wall is composed of epithelium, a rich submucosal vascular plexus, and the urethral musculature (Figure 3-6). The vascular plexus lies between the smooth muscle and mucosa. The musculature is composed of a longitudinal layer of smooth muscle, a circular layer of smooth muscle, and the striated urogenital sphincter muscle.

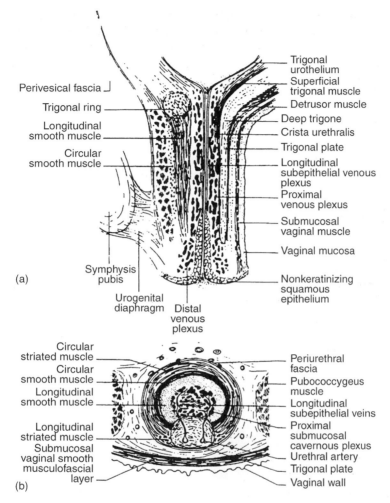

Perivesical fascia ⌐

Trigonal ring

Longitudinal
smooth muscle

Circular
smooth muscle

Symphysis
pubis

(a)

Urogenital
diaphragm Distal
venous
plexus

Trigonal
urothelium

Superficial
trigonal muscle

Detrusor muscle

Deep trigone

Crista urethralis

Trigonal plate

Longitudinal
subepithelial venous
plexus

Proximal
venous plexus

Submucosal
vaginal muscle

Vaginal mucosa

Nonkeratinizing
squamous
epithelium

Circular
striated muscle

Circular
smooth muscle

Longitudinal
smooth muscle

Longitudinal
striated muscle

Submucosal
vaginal smooth
musculofascial
layer

(b)

Periurethral
fascia

Pubococcygeus
muscle

Longitudinal
subepithelial veins

Proximal
submucosal
cavernous plexus

Urethral artery

Trigonal plate

Vaginal wall

Figure 3-6. Anatomy of the urethra: (a) sagittal section; (b) cross section. (From reference 21, with permission.)

The urethra is a potential lumen, open only during voiding and in abnormal conditions. The mucosal surfaces are normally apposed, creating a watertight seal. The urethral stratified epithelium is estrogen-sensitive. Premenopausal mucosa is thick and soft, allowing for compression and sealing. Estrogen deprivation may lead to atrophy, less pliability, poor apposition of the mucosal surfaces, and, therefore, decreased urethral pressure.[22] The role of estrogen in the continence mechanism is, however, still unclear.

The submucosal arteriovenous vascular plexus is believed to be an important part of the continence mechanism. It contributes to urethral closure by engorging with blood, thereby compressing the mucosal surfaces and creating the mucosal seal. Studies by Raz and colleagues[23] demonstrated a one-third reduction in urethral pressure after clamping the urethral blood supply in female dogs. In four women undergoing radical pelvic surgery Rud and coworkers[24] showed that clamping of the common iliac arteries resulted in a 31% decline in intraurethral pressure. These data support the concept of the vascular plexus providing ~30% of urethral closure pressure at rest. Estrogen deprivation at this level may contribute to decreased vascularity, less engorgement of the vascular plexus, and a less effective mucosal seal.

The urethral smooth muscle consists of circular and longitudinal layers. This muscle is contiguous with the muscle of the detrusor. It is suggested that contraction of the longitudinal muscle acts to shorten and widen the urethra during micturition. The circular muscle contributes to urethral closure pressure by providing a constant resting tone. Additionally, the trigonal smooth muscle extends into the proximal urethra and forms a ring around the urethral lumen (Figure 3-6).

The striated urogenital sphincter muscle consists of the sphincter urethrae, the urethrovaginal sphincter, and the compressor urethrae (Figure 3-7). The

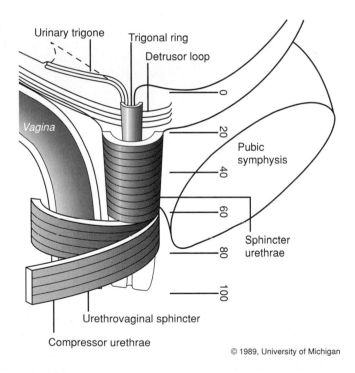

© 1989, University of Michigan

Figure 3-7. Diagrammatic representation showing the component parts of the internal and external sphincteric mechanisms and their locations. The sphincter urethrae, urethrovaginal sphincter, and compressor urethrae are all parts of the striated urogenital sphincter muscle. (From Wall LL, Norton PA, DeLancey JOL. *Practical Urogynecology.* Baltimore, MD: Williams and Wilkins, 1993; 17, with permission.)

sphincter urethrae comprises 20% to 60% of the length of the urethra with the urethrovaginal sphincter and compressor urethrae occupying the next 20% of the urethral length.[26] The urethrovaginal sphincter originates in the vaginal wall and the compressor urethrae at the urogenital diaphragm near the ischiopubic ramus. These muscles function as a single group and are mostly composed of slow-twitch fibers providing for the maintenance of a constant resting tone.[27] The fast-twitch fibers are able to contract quickly when urethral pressure needs to be augmented such as during abrupt increases in intraabdominal pressure.

The internal or proximal sphincter mechanism is comprised of the urethral, trigonal, and detrusor smooth muscle in the region of the bladder neck. The external or distal sphincter mechanism is represented by the striated urogenital sphincter muscles and the smooth muscle of the distal urethra. It is believed that under normal circumstances the internal sphincter is responsible for the maintenance of bladder neck closure. The external sphincter may be thought of as a reserve continence mechanism that can both consciously and reflexively keep the urethra closed. The striated muscle of the external sphincter is contracted voluntarily both to interrupt urine stream and when a sense of urgency is felt but the social situation is inappropriate for voiding. It is contracted reflexively during increases in intraabdominal pressure when urethral resistance needs to be augmented. Additionally, in the group of continent women who have a resting open bladder neck, the external sphincter supplies the necessary urethral pressure to prevent leakage.

Urethral Support

Our understanding of urethral support mechanisms and their role in continence has undergone significant revision over the past few years. Traditionally, support of the proximal urethra and bladder base was felt to be due to the attachment of the pubourethral ligaments to the inferior surface of the pubic bone. Support of the distal urethra was felt to be due to its interaction with the urogenital diaphragm. Stress incontinence was postulated as being secondary to defects in the pubourethral ligament.[28–31]

Recent work by Delancey[32,33] suggests a different mechanism of support. Anatomic studies show the urethra is embedded in the anterior vaginal wall. The urethra and vagina, along with the other pelvic structures, are surrounded by a web of connective tissue known collectively as endopelvic fascia. The proximal urethra has two lateral supports: *1*) the attachment of the endopelvic fascia (pubocervical fascia), which connects the periurethral tissues and the anterior vaginal wall to the arcus tendineus fasciae pelvis, and if this attachment is disrupted, a paravaginal defect occurs;[34] *2*) a muscular attachment also connects the periurethral endopelvic fascia to the medial portion of the levator ani muscle (Figure 3-8), which keeps the bladder neck in a retropubic position due to the constant resting tone of the levator ani. Relaxation of the pelvic floor at the onset of micturition causes the bladder neck to rotate downward, facilitating

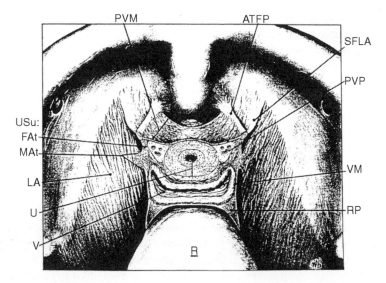

Figure 3-8. Cross section of the urethra (*U*), vagina (*V*), arcus tendineus fasciae pelvis (*ATFP*), and superior fascia of levator ani (*SFLA*) just below the vesical neck (drawn from cadaver dissection). Pubovesical muscles (*PVM*) lie anterior to urethra and anterior and superior to paraurethral vascular plexus (*PVP*). The urethral supports (*USu*) ("the pubourethral ligaments") attach the vagina and vaginal surface of the urethra to the levator ani muscles (MAt, muscular attachment) and to the superior fascia of the levator ani (FAt, fascial attachment), *R*, rectum; *RP*, rectal pillar; *VM*, vaginal wall muscularis.

voiding. Likewise, intraabdominal pressure increases cause a reflex contraction of the levator muscles, thereby maintaining the urethra in an intraabdominal position.

Historically, the pressure transmission theory has been used to explain anatomic stress incontinence:[36] with normal urethral support, increases in intraabdominal pressure are transmitted equally to the bladder and urethra, therefore, intraurethral pressure remains greater than intraabdominal pressure and continence is maintained. With weakened urethral support, hypermobility develops, causing the bladder neck to be displaced outside the abdominal cavity (Figure 3-9); as such, increases in intraabdominal pressure are not equally transmitted to the urethra and incontinence develops.

It is likely that weakened urethral support contributes to the development of anatomic stress incontinence, evidenced by the fact that correction of urethral hypermobility in patients with simple genuine stress incontinence is very successful in correcting incontinence. However, experimental evidence does not support urethral hypermobility as the only factor in anatomic stress incontinence, proof of which lies in the fact that continent women often demonstrate urethral hypermobility.[37]

Deficient pressure transmission alone does not explain the experimental findings regarding the behavior of the urethra during stress. Studies of urethral

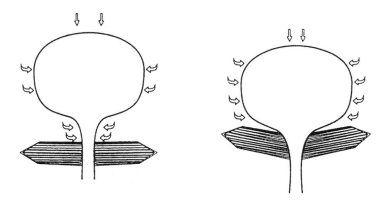

Figure 3-9. Pressure transmission theory of genuine stress incontinence. Left: A normal anatomic relationship with equal transmission of intraabdominal pressure to the bladder and proximal urethra. Right: Weakened urethral support such that there is descent of the bladder neck and proximal urethra outside of the abdominal cavity. This leads to poor transmission of intraabdominal pressure to the urethra and the subsequent development of stress incontinence. (From Chancellor MB, Blaivas JG. Physiology of the lower urinary tract. In: Kursh ED, McGuire EJ (eds). *Female Urology*, Philadelphia: JB Lippincott, 1994, with permission.)

pressure during cough reveal pressure elevations highest in the distal urethra.[32] If intraabdominal transmission of pressure were the only factor involved in continence one would expect to see pressure rises greatest in the proximal urethra. In addition, pressure rises in the urethra during cough are often higher than those seen in the bladder, resulting in a pressure transmission ratio >100%, which suggests that forces other than passive pressure transmission are at work. These forces most likely consist of reflex contractions of the striated muscles of the levator ani and external sphincter mechanism. This theory is further supported by the finding that urethral pressure rises before bladder pressure in response to intraabdominal stress.[38]

Recent work by Delancey[33] suggests that the anterior vaginal wall functions as a hammock against which the urethra is compressed during increases in intraabdominal pressure. The lateral attachments of the vagina to the arcus tendineus fasciae act as supporting structures, which, when disrupted, lead to loss of urethral compression and closure and thus incontinence.

It is clear that many factors affect urethral closure and are therefore implicated in the development of genuine stress incontinence, including the internal urethral sphincter mechanism, transmission of pressure from the abdomen to the bladder and urethra, supporting structures of the urethra and vagina, and contractility and tone of the external urethral sphincter mechanism and the pelvic floor muscles. Derangements in any of these areas can contribute to the development of genuine stress incontinence. These factors are difficult to measure and there is significant variation within the same individual.

SUMMARY

The bladder and urethra, and their supportive structures, should be viewed as a functional unit whose purpose is the storage and voluntary evacuation of urine. Continence of urine represents the capability of retaining urine in the bladder and emptying it when socially acceptable. This ability requires normal anatomy and physiology and adequate neuromuscular control, as well as the acquisition of behavior. Such behavior is learned during early childhood and is usually referred to as "toilet training". The maintenance of continence therefore implies a balance between physiology and behavior. When pathologic processes develop, affecting either physiology or behavior, it is likely that a reserve or compensatory function is called upon to overcome insufficiencies.[40] The failure to be able to compensate for insufficiencies may result in urinary incontinence or other lower urinary tract syndromes. This hypothesis is not yet objectively proven; however, it represents a reasonable framework for the understanding of incontinence and the therapeutic interventions designed to manage it.

REFERENCES

1. McGuire EJ. Physiology of the lower urinary tract. *Am J Kidney Dis* 1983; **2**: 402–408.
2. Torrens MJ. Neurophysiology. In: Stanton SL (ed). *Clinical Gynecologic Urology*. St. Louis, MO: CV Mosby, 1984.
3. Van Arsdalen, Wein AJ. Physiology of micturition and continence. In: Krane RJ, Siroky MB (eds). *Clinical Neurourology*, 2nd ed. Boston: Little, Brown, 1991.
4. Benson JT, Walters MD. Neurophysiology of the lower urinary tract. In: Walters MD, Karram MM (eds). *Clinical Gynecology*. St. Louis, MO: CV Mosby, 1993; 117–128.
5. Rohmer TJ Jr. In: Hinman F (ed). *Benign Prostatic Hypertrophy*. New York: Springer-Verlag, 1983; 361–372.
6. April EW. The nervous system. In: *Anatomy*. New York: Wiley, 1984; 38–42.
7. Walters MD, Newton ER. Pathophysiology and obstetrics issues of genuine stress incontinence. In: Walters MD, Karram MM (eds). *Clinical Urogynecology*. St. Louis, MO: CV Mosby, 1993; 157–162.
8. Benson JT. Pelvic floor neuropathy. In: Benson JT (ed). *Female Pelvic Floor Disorders*. New York: WW Norton, 1992.
9. Weidner AC, Versi E. Physiology of micturition. In: Ostergard DR, Bent AE (eds). *Urogynecology and Urodynamics*, 4th ed. Baltimore: Williams and Wilkins, 1996.
10. Fletcher TF, Bradley WE. Neuroanatomy of the bladder-urethra. *J Urol* 1978; **119**: 153.
11. Benson JT. Neurophysiologic control of lower urinary tract. *Obstet Gynecol Clin North Am* 1989; **16**: 733–752.
12. Kuru M. Nervous control of micturition. *Physiol Rev* 1965; **45**: 425.
13. Chancellor MB, Blaivas JG. Physiology of the lower urinary tract. In: Kursh ED, McGuire EJ (eds). *Female Urology*. Philadelphia: JB Lippincott, 1994.
14. Benson JT. Clinical application of electrodiagnostic studies of female pelvic floor neuropathy. *Int Urogynecol J* 1990; **1**: 164–167.
15. Mahoney DT, Laberte RO, Blais DJ. Integral storage and voiding reflexes: Neurophysiologic concept of continence and micturition. *Urology* 1977; **10**: 95–106.

16. Benson JT, Walters MD. Neurophysiology of the lower urinary tract. In: Walters MD, Karram MM (eds). *Clinical Urogynecology*. St. Louis, MO: Mosby-Year Book, 1993.
17. DeGroat WC. Neuroanatomy and neurophysiology: innervation of the lower urinary tract. In: Raz S (ed). *Female Urology*. Philadelphia: WB Saunders, 1996.
18. Fantl JA, Miller DA. Physiology of micturition. In: Benson JT (ed). *Female Pelvic Floor Disorders*. New York: WW Norton, 1992.
19. Fantl JA. The lower urinary tract in women: Effect of aging and menopause on continence. *Exp Gerontol* 1994; **29**: 417–422.
20. Tanagho EA, Miller ER. Initiation of voiding. *Br J Urol* 1970; **42**: 175.
21. Asmussen M, Miller ER. *Clinical Gynecologic Urology*. Oxford: Blackwell, 1983.
22. Schaffer J, Fantl JA. Urogenital effects of the menopause. *Baillieres Clin Obstet Gynaecol* 1996; **10**: 401–417.
23. Raz S, Caine M, Ziegler M. The vascular component in the production of intraurethral pressure. *J Urol* 1972; **108**: 93–96.
24. Rud T, Andersson KE, Asmussen M, et al. Factors maintaining the intraurethral pressure in women. *Invest Urol* 1980; **17**: 343.
25. Wall LL, Norton PA, DeLancey JOL. *Practical Urogynecology*. Baltimore, MD: Williams and Wilkins, 1993; 17.
26. DeLancey JOL. Correlative study of paraurethral anatomy. *Obstet Gynecol* 1986; **68**: 91–97.
27. Wall LL, Norton PA, DeLancey JOL. Pelvic anatomy and the physiology of the lower urinary tract. In: *Practical Urogynecology*. Baltimore, MD: Williams and Wilkins, 1993.
28. Walters MD. Mechanisms of continence and voiding, with International Continence Society classification of dysfunction. *Obstet Gynecol Clin North Am* 1989; **16**: 773–785.
29. Krantz KE. The anatomy of the urethra and anterior vaginal wall. *Am J Obstet Gynecol* 1951; **62**: 374.
30. Milley PS, Nichols DH. The relationship between the pubo-urethral ligaments and the urogenital diaphragm in the human female. *Anat Rec* 1971; **170**: 281.
31. Zacharin RF. The suspensory mechanism of the female urethra. *J Anat* 1963; **97**: 423.
32. DeLancey JOL. Structural aspects of the extrinsic continence mechanism. *Obstet Gynecol* 1988; **72**: 296–301.
33. DeLancey JOL. Structural support of the urethra as it relates to stress urinary incontinence: The hammock hypothesis. *Am J Obstet Gynecol* 1994; **170**: 1713–1723.
34. Richardson AC, Edmonds PB, Williams NL. Treatment of stress urinary incontinence due to paravaginal fascial defect. *Obstet Gynecol* 1981; **57**: 357–362.
35. DeLancey JOL. *Neurourol Urodyn* 1989; **8**: 53–63.
36. Enhorning G. Simultaneous recording of intravesical and intraurethral pressure. *Acta Chir Scand* 1961; **267(Suppl)**: 1–6.
37. Wise BG, Khullar V, Cardozo LD. Bladder neck movement during pelvic floor contraction and intravaginal electrical stimulation in women with and without genuine stress incontinence. *Neurourol Urodyn* 1992; **11**: 309.
38. Constantinou CE, Govan DE. Spatial distribution and timing of transmitted and reflexly generated urethral pressures in healthy women. *J Urol* 1982; **127**: 964.
39. Fantl JA. Genuine stress incontinence. In: Sciarra JJ (ed). *Gynecology and Obstetrics*, Vol 1. Philadelphia: JB Lippincott, 1990.

PART III

EVALUATION

CHAPTER 4

Urodynamics in the evaluation of the incontinent female patient

DELBERT J. KWAN AND TAMARA G. BAVENDAM ————————

An incontinence evaluation begins with a complete history and physical examination, which will provide a list of possible etiologic factors, an impression as to the type(s) of incontinence, and the impact of urinary incontinence on the person's life. An assessment of the dynamics of lower urinary tract function (urodynamics) during the storage and emptying phases will be necessary in some women to diagnose the specific lower urinary tract dysfunction and delineate a treatment plan. Proper utilization of urodynamic testing depends on a good understanding of its indications, techniques, and limitations.

This chapter briefly reviews the general anatomy and physiology of the lower urinary tract as well as the initial assessment of the incontinent female patient. It focuses on the different types of urodynamic studies available: "eyeball" urodynamics, single-channel cystometry, and multichannel videourodynamics. Guidelines will be presented on the indications, value, and limitations of each type of urodynamic study. In addition, the current limited role of urethral pressure profiles will be discussed.

OVERVIEW OF URINARY TRACT FUNCTION

Urinary continence is the result of normal bladder and urethral function as well as the support and function of the pelvic floor support. Urine storage (continence) results when intraurethral pressure continually exceeds intravesical pressure. The bladder is able to hold urine as long as the intravesical pressure remains low and the outlet is continuously competent. Voluntary complete emptying of the bladder is a product of a coordinated urethral smooth muscle and skeletal muscle relaxation and an adequate, sustained detrusor muscle contraction. Involuntary escape of urine (incontinence) is common and may result from functional or anatomic changes in any or all these elements.

The bladder wall is composed of urothelium, smooth muscle (detrusor muscle), and connective tissue.[1] The urothelium consists of cuboidal-shaped transitional cells that are able to accommodate bladder filling by changing shape. At capacity volumes, the cells are stretched and flattened.[2] The adult female urethra is a 3- to 4-cm muscular tube composed mainly of smooth muscle. Located at the level of the midurethra and fanning out proximally and distally along the urethra are the voluntary striated muscle urethral sphincter and the pelvic floor muscles. Normally, the bladder and proximal urethra are held in an intraabdominal position by the combination of good muscular (levator ani, especially pubococcygeus) and fascial (endopelvic fascia) support.

The lower urinary tract is controlled by both parasympathetic and sympathetic nerves.[3] The parasympathetic nerves originate in the sacral spinal cord segments S2–S4. Stimulation of pelvic parasympathetic nerves causes the detrusor muscle to contract.[3] The sympathetic fibers originate from thoracolumbar segments (T10–L2) of the spinal cord. The sympathetic system includes alpha- and beta-adrenergic components. The beta fibers terminate primarily in the detrusor muscle, while the alpha fibers terminate primarily in the bladder neck and urethra. Alpha-adrenergic stimulation contracts the bladder neck and urethra and relaxes the detrusor.[3] The pudendal nerve (S2–S4) provides motor innervation to the striated urethral sphincter and sensory innervation to the perineum and anal canal.[4]

Sensation of bladder fullness "urge" passes to S2–S4 levels of the spinal cord via the pelvic parasympathetic nerves, while sensations of pain, touch, temperature, and "distention" are carried along sympathetic fibers.[3] Micturition is initiated by the voluntary relaxation of the external sphincter and pelvic floor muscles. Urethral pressure falls, the bladder neck opens, an immediate detrusor contraction occurs, and urine flows across an unobstructed bladder neck and urethra until the bladder is completely emptied.[5]

INITIAL ASSESSMENT

Evaluation of the incontinent patient begins with a detailed account of the patient's symptoms. Women will commonly describe leakage associated with activity (stress incontinence), being unable to get to the bathroom in time (urge incontinence), just suddenly finding themselves wet (spontaneous or unaware incontinence), constant sense of wetness (continuous incontinence), leakage after urination (postvoid dribbling), or wetting their bedding or external protection while sleeping (nocturnal enuresis). The description of when the leakage occurs can be the same even though the underlying causes for the leakage may be different (e.g., spontaneous incontinence may be secondary to an involuntary detrusor contraction with impaired bladder sensation: no urge is perceived with the involuntary contraction, or intrinsic urethral deficiency, where the activity that precipitated the leakage is so minimal, it is not perceived as an activity).

Urinary incontinence may result from detrusor or sphincteric dysfunction as well as extraurethral sources.[6–10] The detrusor may be overactive or may be hypocontractile. Sphincteric incompetence may be due to intrinsic sphincteric deficiency or to anatomic malposition of an intact sphincteric unit. Multiple

Table 4-1.   Urinary incontinence: diagnosis and predisposing conditions

Diagnosis	*Predisposing condition(s)*
Impaired detrusor contractility	Neurogenic Prior urethral, bladder, or pelvic surgery Myogenic secondary to overdistention injury
Detrusor overactivity	Idiopathic Neurogenic Outlet obstruction Bladder cancer Urinary tract infection
Urethral hypermobility	Pelvic floor relaxation secondary to trauma or denervation
Intrinsic urethral deficiency	Atrophic vaginitis/urethritis Idiopathic Neurogenic Prior urethral/bladder/pelvic surgery
Extraurethral incontinence	Ectopic ureter Urinary-vaginal fistula from trauma
Postvoid dribbling	Urethral diverticulum Vaginal pooling of urine

factors may predispose to detrusor, sphincteric, and extraurethral abnormalities (Table 4-1).[6–10]

URODYNAMICS

Urodynamics is the evaluation of the storage and emptying functions of the lower urinary tract—the bladder and the outlet. It is not one specific test, but rather a series of tests that yield useful information regarding the dynamics of lower urinary tract function. A simple residual urine measurement is one measure of bladder function. Other tests that are a part of urodynamic evaluation include uroflowmetry, cystometry, and cystourethrogram. Each test may be performed separately or together as the complete study. Information yielded from a urodynamic study is valid only if the urodynamic abnormalities identified during the study are consistent with the symptoms reported by the patient.

Many factors in patients' histories suggest a urodynamic evaluation would be appropriate before beginning empirical treatment:

1. Recurrent or refractory urinary tract infection
2. Urinary retention
3. Previously failed antiincontinence surgery
4. Changes in voiding function following head, neck, or back surgery
5. Failure to improve voiding difficulties with conservative management

6. For legal purposes: documentation of function following genitourinary or nerve damage potentially caused by a motor vehicle accident, surgery, or work-related injuries
7. Acute onset of incontinence
8. Secondary enuresis that occurred after a period of time free of enuresis

Uroflowmetry

Uroflowmetry measures the urinary flow rate. The urine flowometry represents the coordination between detrusor function, bladder neck, and urethral and pelvic floor relaxation. An average urine flow rate can be performed with a stop-watch—measuring the time it takes to urinate—and a container to measure the voided volume. The average flow is determined by dividing the volume voided by the time (milliliters per second). Studies obtained with electronic equipment yield printed computerized calculations include the total voiding time (including interruptions), total flow time, time to maximum flow, voided volume, and maximum or peak urinary flow rate, as well as the average urinary flow rate. The graph of the "pattern" of the urine flow also provides useful clinical information.

The patient is instructed to arrive with a full bladder. The uroflowmeter should be placed in a private toilet to provide familiar surroundings for voiding. After voiding, the postvoid residual (PVR) volume should be measured. PVRs can be measured noninvasively with an ultrasonic bladder scan or by in/out catheterization. Little or no PVR remains after normal voiding. Common factors that can adversely affect uroflowmetry results include: *1*) patient voided just before arrival (low bladder volume), *2*) patient has an overdistended bladder, and *3*) patient is inhibited by the surroundings.

The normal voided volume is >150–200 ml. Voided volumes are influenced by detrusor instability and conditions that affect bladder capacity.[11,12] Normal peak urinary flow rates for women[13] are

Women <50 years old: >25 ml/s
Women >50 years old: >18 ml/s

Women tend to have higher urinary flow rates than men because normal urethral resistance is less than in the male urethra. Women with genuine stress urinary incontinence often have high urinary flow rates due to even lower urethral resistance.

A flow curve should rise steeply with the average urinary flow approximately half the maximum urinary flow. The overall configuration of a normal uroflow curve is bell-shaped (Figure 4-1). Essential to uroflowmetry is the patient's account (or that of an observer) of any coughing, sneezing, or straining during voiding. In addition, the patient should state whether the void closely resembled that of a typical void at home. These questions establish the accuracy of the recorded uroflow pattern and avoid the interpretation of an isolated occurrence in the testing environment as "usual" for the patient.

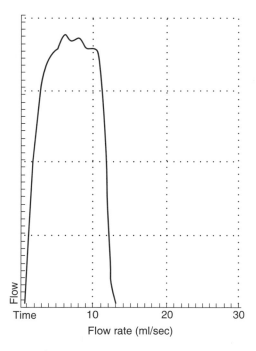

Figure 4-1. Normal uroflow curve.

Maximum urinary flow rate provides an objective measure of outlet obstruction. Except for low (<150 ml) and high (>500 ml) voided volumes, there is an almost linear relationship between maximum urinary flow rate and voided volume.[14] Inadequate bladder contractility or increased bladder outlet resistance can result in:[15]

1. Urinary flow rates less than 15 ml/s in women
2. Less than normal voided volumes
3. Increased voiding time
4. Increased PVR

Rarely, normal uroflowmetry can occur in the presence of outflow obstruction if high-pressure detrusor contractions have developed which are sufficient to overcome the "obstruction".

The usual patient response to a decreased urinary force of stream is to contract the abdominal muscles (i.e., strain or perform the Valsalva maneuver). The abdominal muscles fatigue and cannot maintain continuous urinary flow. In Figure 4-2, the maximum urinary flow rate and the average urinary flow rate appear normal. However, this uroflow curve actually represents the inability of the computerized scan to distinguish between the true maximum urinary flow rate and the surge produced by the Valsalva maneuver. Urinary flow rate can be significantly augmented by Valsalva (Figure 4-3).

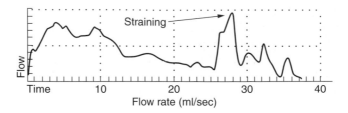

Figure 4-2.   Effect of straining on urinary flow rate.

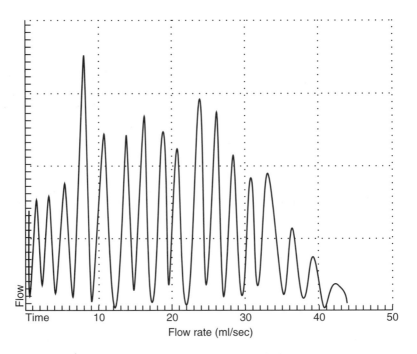

Figure 4-3.   Uroflow augmented by Valsalva maneuver.

Cystometry

"Eyeball" or Bedside Cystometry

"Eyeball" cystometry is performed without special electronic equipment. A Foley catheter is inserted and the PVR is measured. A 60-ml catheter tip syringe with the plunger removed is connected to the Foley catheter and held straight up from the patient. Water or saline is poured through the open end of the syringe. The fluid meniscus in the syringe represents the intravesical pressure. This is recorded as centimeters above the pubic symphysis. Changes in intravesical pressure are noted as rises and falls in the level of the fluid meniscus. This test can be completed in the supine, sitting, or standing positions.

During bladder filling, the patient is instructed to try not to void or to inhibit voiding—in other words, "just relax", report what sensations they are perceiving and let whatever is going to happen, happen. The patient should report first bladder sensation, normal urge to void, and strong urge to void.[16] The bladder capacity should be noted as well as any changes in intravesical pressure. A change in pressure may be due to a detrusor contraction, an increase in abdominal pressure, or low bladder wall compliance. Any sudden rise in pressure accompanied by an urge to void or by urethral leakage of fluid is an involuntary detrusor contraction.[16] If no change in pressure occurs, the catheter is withdrawn and the patient is asked to cough or strain in the supine or standing positions to evaluate for incontinence secondary to intraabdominal pressure changes.

Eyeball cystometry is inexpensive and easy to perform. It is indicated for patients with uncomplicated stress urinary incontinence with evidence of pelvic floor relaxation who have not undergone prior antiincontinence procedures. It can be used to evaluate patients who elect conservative therapy: to establish residual urine and volumes of sensation and urgency. A person who reports spontaneous incontinence, may be found on this study to have an involuntary contraction (observed rise in the water meniscus) without having any awareness of urge. However, eyeball cystometry does not provide sufficient anatomic and functional information upon which surgical decisions are based. Confounding factors such as abdominal straining, rapid rate of bladder filling, and inability to evaluate detrusor contractility during voiding can lead to misdiagnosis. Therefore, eyeball cystometry alone is not adequate for patients who are considering surgery as a treatment option.

Single-Channel Cystometry

Single-channel cystometry consists of filling the bladder at a predetermined rate measuring pressure (intravesical as opposed to true detrusor), electronically obtaining a graph of the measured pressures during filling. During filling, volumes are recorded at initial sensation, normal urge, urgency and maximum bladder capacity.

As the bladder fills, intravesical pressure (phase 1) increases slightly as a result of the detrusor response to the stretch of the initial filling (Figure 4-4). Beyond this initial response, there is no further increase in pressure with continued filling. Since pressure (phase 2) remains constant, it is the wall tension and volume that stimulate the bladder mechanoreceptors. At capacity and during initial voiding, pressure (phase 3) increases due to a detrusor contraction. In reality, the phase 1 and phase 3 pressure rises are often not observed during bladder filling; the intravesical pressure remains constant until a voluntary or involuntary detrusor contraction develops.

Bladder capacity is 400–600 ml in normal women. Problems arise with the following clinical situations:

1. Decreased capacity with increased bladder pressures that can occur with inflammation or fibrosis.

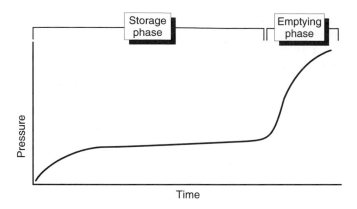

Figure 4-4. Bladder pressure during filling and emptying.

2. Increased capacity with decreased bladder pressures found in the flaccid or areflexic bladder, which may predispose to overflow incontinence; sensation may be normal or decreased.

Once bladder capacity is reached, the patient is asked to void. At the peak of the voluntary detrusor contraction, the patient is asked to inhibit voiding. The isometric detrusor pressure is measured with the closure of the bladder outlet. In normal individuals, the detrusor contraction should cease and intravesical pressure should decrease with voluntary contraction of the bladder outlet. However, in patients with involuntary, uninhibited detrusor contractions, a rise in intravesical pressure occurs without the specific instruction to void. Patients may or may not be able to inhibit the involuntary detrusor contraction with voluntary contraction of the outlet. The request to stop voiding (or leaking) is also a good way of assessing whether the patient has the ability to localize and contract the pelvic floor.

Changes observed on the intravesical pressure tracing may reflect a phasic detrusor contraction (voluntary or involuntary), abdominal straining or low bladder wall compliance. Since the intraabdominal pressure is not recorded with single channel cystometry, it is important to be aware of its potential to be a confounding factor with observed increases in intravesical pressure. Visual inspection and palpation can reveal abdominal straining.

Compliance is defined as change in bladder volume/change in bladder pressure. Normal compliance is >10. Poor compliance (<10) is commonly associated with prolonged catheter drainage, chronic urinary tract infection, interstitial cystitis, chemotherapy, neurogenic conditions, obstructive uropathy, and prior pelvic, bladder, or urethral surgery.[17]

Findings noted on single-channel cystometry may be correlated with the results of a cystourethrogram. The appearance and position of the bladder, bladder neck, and urethra at rest and with the Valsalva maneuver can provide important anatomic information. In order to obtain an informative cystourethrogram, it is important to discuss with the radiology technologists the particular views and patient maneuvers (e.g., cough, strain, interrupt stream, stand) that are desired.

The limitations of single-channel cystometry are similar to those of bedside cystometry. In practice, bedside cystometry usually provides as much information about sensation, compliance and presence or absence of involuntary detrusor contractions as single-channel cystometry without the additional equipment cost. Since a filling study does not provide information about voiding function, a uroflowometry can be a useful adjunct to a single channel cystometrogram or a bedside cystometry. Unlike single-channel cystometry, the information gained from uroflowmetry cannot be obtained from another source.

Multichannel Videourodynamics

Multichannel videourodynamics offers the most comprehensive means to evaluate voiding dysfunction and incontinence. It permits the synchronous measurement of pelvic floor activity, intravesical pressure, intraabdominal pressure, subtracted true detrusor pressure, uroflow curve, and cystourethrogram (Figure 4-5).

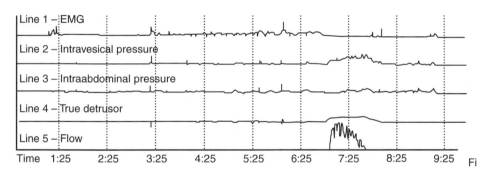

Figure 4-5. Multichannel urodynamic tracing.

Multichannel Urodynamic Procedure

1. A noninvasive uroflow is performed.
2. The bladder is catheterized to record the amount of residual urine.
3. A small-caliber dual-lumen catheter (5–7 Fr) or microtip catheter is inserted into the bladder so that the urethra is not obstructed and voiding can occur around the catheter. (For simultaneous urethral pressure measurements, a triple-lumen catheter may be used.)
4. The catheter is connected at its infusion port to contrast medium which has been stored at room temperature. The remaining port is attached to a pressure transducer to record intravesical pressure or total bladder pressure (Figure 4-5, line 2).

5. Rectal or intravaginal pressures are regarded as suitable measures of intra-abdominal pressure. An inflatable pressure catheter or microtip transducers are placed in the rectum or vagina (Figure 4-5, line 3).
6. True detrusor pressure may be calculated as total bladder pressure minus intraabdominal pressure (Figure 4-5, line 4 = line 2 − line 3).
7. Periurethral wires, perianal patches or a intraanal sponge can be used to measure pelvic floor muscle activity (Figure 4-5, line 1).
8. All the manometer lines are secured to with tape to the thigh, flushed with water, and zeroed.
9. The patient is asked to cough to assess the correct functioning of the pressure recording apparatus. Both the intravesical and rectal pressures should rise.
10. The bladder is filled with radiographic contrast under low pressure (45 cm above pubic symphysis) at 50–80 ml/min. The patient is instructed not to inhibit or to attempt voiding.
11. The patient is asked to report: first sensation of bladder filling, normal urge to void, strong urge to void, and true urgency. Capacity is reached when the patient cannot tolerate any more filling (usually 400–600 ml).
12. If detrusor contractions are noted before volitional voiding, the patient is asked whether or not she feels an associated urge or is aware of leakage.
13. At 200–250 ml of filling or at half bladder capacity, the patient is asked to cough or to strain. The intraabdominal pressure at the time of leakage is the abdominal or Valsalva leak point pressure (VLPP). The VLPP may be assessed sitting or standing. The advantage to the standing position is that it is the position in which leakage frequently occurs.
14. Periodically, the patient is asked to cough or strain to look for evidence of activity-induced detrusor contractions and leakage (and to monitor the fluoroscopic appearance and position of the bladder, bladder neck, and urethra).
15. The patient is allowed to void into a uroflowometer (Figure 4-5, line 5). During voiding, the intravesical and intraabdominal pressures are monitored allowing determination of the true detrusor pressure (subtracted pressure) as well as the shape of the uroflow curve.

The goal of the multichannel study is to reproduce the circumstances of urinary leakage in a laboratory setting. Simultaneously correlating the objective data with clinical symptoms is necessary to develop a treatment plan.

Electromyography–Pelvic Floor Activity

The sphincter electromyography (EMG) assesses the overall activity of the external urethral sphincter and the external anal sphincter, as well as the general activity of the pelvic floor, and the integrity of the external pudendal nerve. Normally, there is a gradual increase in activity with bladder filling. A marked increase in EMG activity is observed with coughing, the Valsalva maneuver, and pelvic muscle contractions to voluntarily stop voiding. This is known as the urethrovesical reflex whereby contraction of the external urethral sphincter inhibits detrusor contraction. Conversely, electromyographic activity of the external urethral sphincter and pelvic floor musculature virtually ceases during a voluntary voiding detrusor contraction (Figure 5, line 1).

Intraabdominal Pressure

Abdominal pressure is increased with coughing, the Valsalva maneuver, or when straining is used to initiate or to augment voiding (Figure 4-6). VLPP is a urodynamic recording of an increase in intraabdominal pressure which is required to overcome urethral resistance and results in urinary leakage. The patient is filled to a predetermined bladder volume and then is asked to strain, or if no urinary leakage occurs, to cough. The intraabdominal pressure at the time of leakage is recorded.

Currently, there is no standardized method for performing a VLPP. Typically, the patient is placed upright, the bladder is filled with 200–250 ml of contrast, and the patient is asked to perform a Valsalva maneuver. Removing the urethral catheter decreases resistance to leakage. If fluoroscopy is not available, the lithotomy position provides the advantage of direct observation of the urethral

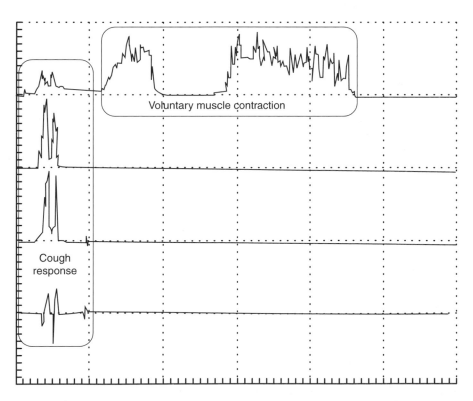

Figure 4-6. Pelvic muscle response to cough and voluntary contraction.

meatus for leakage. Direct visualization for leakage may be difficult in the standing position; inspection of pads for leakage may be useful in this situation.

If no leakage occurs at VLPP >100 cmH$_2$O, the sphincter is considered competent. Patients with low VLPP (<60 cmH$_2$O) with little or no urethral mobility are candidates for periurethral injection agents (e.g., collagen, autologous fat).[17] Those with low VLPP and urethral mobility are best suited for sling procedures. Patients with higher VLPP (>100 cmH$_2$O) and hypermobility may require a bladder neck suspension or stabilization procedure.[17] VLPP between 60 and 100 cmH$_2$O are in the "gray zone" and require thoughtful correlation of the history, physical examination and urodynamic findings to decide the optimal treatment.

Detrusor Activity

As previously described, micturition is initiated by the voluntary relaxation of the external sphincter followed by an immediate voluntary detrusor contraction. If the contraction is sufficient to sustain emptying, normal voiding occurs. Detrusor muscle contractions, whether voluntary or involuntary, lead to increased bladder pressures. Voluntary contractions usually increase the intravesical pressure above that of the bladder outlet pressure, which allows urination to occur. Involuntary contractions may or may not result in urine leakage. If the bladder pressure produced by the involuntary detrusor contraction is greater than that of the bladder outlet pressure, the patient will experience urine loss. An involuntary bladder contraction may be inhibited if the urethrovesical reflex is intact. Contraction of the external urethral sphincter and pelvic muscle floor muscles would inhibit the involuntary detrusor contraction and prevent leakage.

Cystometrograms do not reliably diagnose the presence of involuntary detrusor contractions. Up to 40% of patients with stress urinary incontinence and involuntary detrusor contractions do not develop the involuntary detrusor contraction during a cystometrogram.[18] Treatment in these instances is based upon a history consistent with urinary urgency and/or urge-related leakage of urine. The presence of detrusor instability and stress urinary incontinence in patients with urethral hypermobility should not preclude surgery. In the majority of these patients, the detrusor instability resolves after suspension surgery.[9]

It is important to remember that urodynamics is an artificial way of assessing clinical information. The presence of a physician or a well-trained urodynamic nurse who is familiar with the patient's history and physical examination at the time of the study is crucial in interpreting information.

Voiding Cystourethrogram

Radiographic evaluation of the lower urinary tract may be performed separately or simultaneously with cystometry. The bladder is filled with a contrast medium with the patient in the sitting and upright positions. It is not uncommon for radiologists to perform supine studies unless they are specifically requested in the standing position. Most radiology suites are usually not equipped with tables that allow studies to be performed in the sitting position. A voiding cystourethro-gram (VCUG) that can only be performed in the supine position because of logistical reasons (limitations of equipment) is generally a waste of time and energy (for making surgical decisions about incontinence treatment), unless the patient has a significant spinal cord injury and the bladder activity is entirely involuntary. Bladder sensation, bladder neck competence, and capacity can all be assessed during the course of the examination. Films are taken in the antero-posterior (AP) and lateral positions with the patient relaxed and then with cough-ing and straining.

Normally, the bladder base rests above the superior margin of the pubic bone on the AP view. Straining pushes the well-supported bladder downward minimally and not beyond the inferior border of the pubic bone. A bladder that rests or descends below the inferior margin of the pubis with straining indicates weakened pelvic support.

Normally, the urethra and bladder base should be at a right angle, which is maintained with cough and Valsalva. The urethral axis (the measured angle between the urethra and a vertical line) is normally less than 30 degrees. With pelvic floor relaxation, the urethral axis increases and the angle between the urethra and bladder base posteriorly (posterior urethral angle) widens.

The bladder neck should be closed at rest even with a full bladder. Funneling of the bladder neck at rest indicates bladder neck incompetence. When associated with a sense of urge, detrusor instability may be present. Up to 50% of normal, continent women demonstrate slight funneling or beaking of the bladder neck during straining with no evidence of detrusor contractions.[19] The significance of an opened bladder neck during cystography is best interpreted with simultaneous bladder pressure measurements. An open bladder neck may be due to involuntary bladder contractions, trauma, surgery, neurologic damage, low bladder compliance, anterior vaginal wall prolapse, and radiation damage.[18]

Sphincteric (anatomic) weakness is suggested by a widened urethral axis, competent bladder neck and rest with loss of urine during cough or Valsalva. Intrinsic urethral dysfunction (type III incontinence) is suggested by passive leakage around the catheter at low bladder volumes with the patient at rest or with minimal activity. In many women, this information along with a complete history and physical examination may be sufficient to make a correct diagnosis and design a therapeutic plan without requiring multichannel urodynamic evaluation.

Summary of Multichannel Videourodynamics

Filling Phase

1. *Bladder residual:* volume of urine noted after voiding when urethral testing catheter is placed.

2. *Rate of bladder filling:* determined by neurologic history: if patient has neurologic disorder or is suspicious for having a neurologic lesion, rate of bladder filling is set at 40–50 ml/min. If patient is neurologically intact, rate of bladder filling is set at 70–80 ml/min.

3. *Intact temperature sensation:* warm or cool depending on whether the fluid is warmed or at room temperature.

4. *Volume at first urge:* volume at which patient notes sensation of bladder fullness and urge to urinate. Sensory urgency is suggested if volume at first urge is <150 ml. Decreased sensation is suspected if first urge does not occur by 250–300 ml.

5. *Bladder capacity* (when full or when involuntary contraction occurs): volume at which patient feels she can no longer tolerate filling or the volume at which an involuntary detrusor contraction occurs in a patient with detrusor instability. May also be measured as voided volume plus residual urine volume.

6. *Bladder outline* (shape, diverticula—site and number): contour of bladder is viewed on fluoroscopy and noted for evidence of high pressure (trabeculation, diverticula, pear-shaped) or hypocontractile (large, smooth-walled). Bladder base position is noted at rest and with stress maneuvers (cough, strain).

7. *Bladder neck:* the appearance of the bladder is viewed on fluoroscopy. In the absence of denervation secondary to surgery, trauma, or neurologic disease, the bladder neck is closed at rest. It remains closed with stress maneuvers and positional changes. It funnels and opens as the patient begins a volitional void. The bladder neck remains open until the completion of a normal, coordinated void. The patient should be placed in the oblique position to view the urethral axis, which is measured at rest and with stress maneuvers (cough, strain).

8. *Valsalva leak point pressure:* (VLPP): at 200–250 ml of filling, the patient is asked to perform stress maneuvers (cough, strain) in the standing position. The urethral catheter may be removed to prevent irritant effect and "potential" obstruction. The rectal catheter is left in place to measure the intra-abdominal pressure at which leakage is noted. The VLPP should be recorded along with any evidence of hypermobility of the bladder base and urethra in order to arrive at a treatment plan.

9. *Bladder compliance:* the volume at bladder capacity divided by the detrusor pressure at capacity prior to voiding determines the compliance. A value >10 is considered normal.

10. *Presence or absence of detrusor instability:* any detrusor activity which occurs during filling and prior to volitional voiding is evidence of instability. When present, the patient should be queried whether she felt an urge associated with the contraction and the bladder neck should be viewed to see if remained competent or leakage occurred.

11. *Vesicoureteral reflux:* passive ureteral reflux occurring during filling is abnormal and indicates an incompetent ureterovesical junction. Ureteral

reflux is noted for grade and laterality. Further radiographic evaluation may be required to assess renal function and presence of renal scarring.

Voiding Phase

1. *Initiation of voiding:* with a normal void, EMG activity should decrease followed by a rise in detrusor pressure. No abdominal pressure rise should be recorded unless there is abdominal straining. Abdominal straining may be used to initiate a void, augment a void already in progress, or to complete a void.
2. *Standing:* changes in position during filling should not lead to detrusor pressure changes. In patients with detrusor instability, standing will unmask detrusor contractions.
3. *Uroflow curve:* the flow rate and shape of the curve should be reviewed in the same manner as an noninvasive uroflow. In some patients, the presence of the urethral catheter may result in mild obstruction and result in a diminution in flow rate with the invasive study versus noninvasive study.
4. *Voiding pressure:* the detrusor contraction should be noted for its magnitude and duration.
5. *Ability to interrupt stream:* the patient is asked to contract her pelvic muscles in the middle of her void. The isometric detrusor pressure is noted to establish inherent detrusor activity. In the presence of an intact urethrovesical reflex, the detrusor pressure will decrease.
6. *Activity of external urethral sphincter:* with a normal, coordinated void, EMG activity should decrease just prior to a detrusor contraction.
7. *Urethral appearance:* the contrast filled urethra during voiding is viewed to look for evidence of urethral diverticula, filling defects (tumor, stone), narrowing (stricture, sphincter dyssynergia), or extravasation (fistula).
8. *Voided volume/residual volume:* measurements are made to determine bladder capacity.
9. *Vesicoureteral reflux:* ureteral reflux during voiding indicates high voiding pressure in the presence of a marginally competent ureterovesical junction. Ureteral reflux is noted for grade and laterality. Further radiographic evaluation may be indicated to assess renal function and rule out renal scarring, and if suspected, ureteral ectopia.

Urethral Pressure Profile

The urethral pressure profile (UPP) is a graphic recording of the pressure along the length of the urethra obtained by means of a pressure-sensitive recording catheter, which is slowly and progressively withdrawn through the urethra. The resulting bell-shaped curve provides a measurement of the urethral closing pressure (intraurethral minus intravesical pressure) and the functional length of the urethra (the length of the urethra along which urethral pressure exceeds bladder pressure). The urethral closing pressure normally varies between 50 and

100 cmH$_2$O and the functional length between 3 and 5 cm. Urethral pressures <20 cmH$_2$O suggests intrinsic sphincteric deficiency.[17]

A normal continent woman responds to the stress of bladder filling, postural change, coughing, sneezing, or jolting by increasing the urethral closing pressure and urethral length. Abnormally high urethral closing pressures may be associated with voiding difficulties, hesitancy, and urinary retention.

Patients with intrinsic sphincteric deficiency have poor proximal urethral closure, which may be associated with low urethral closure pressures. It is difficult to measure proximal urethral pressures without fluoroscopic guidance. In addition, urethral closure pressures have not been shown to reliably correlate with any particular voiding symptom or any specific type of incontinence.[17] Multichannel videourodynamics with Valsalva leak point determination is a more accurate way of assessing intrinsic urethral function.

CONCLUSION

A careful history and physical examination can determine whether urodynamic testing is required. Multichannel videourodynamics provides functional and anatomic information and is recommended if a surgical procedure is contemplated. It is important to remember the symptoms which brought the patient to the physician and make sure that the treatment plan addresses the patient's symptoms. Ideally, the symptoms should be reproduced during the course of the urodynamic study, but this is not always possible. Be wary of artifacts and/or findings during the study which do not relate to the patient's complaints. Treatment plans will be the most successful when the balance between bladder storage (continence) and emptying (voiding) is kept in mind as treatment strategies are being planned. Women must be evaluated to determine the effect any treatment recommendation may have on both the storage and emptying phases of the lower urinary tract function. All discussions regarding treatment options need to include information about continence and ability to voluntarily urinate.

REFERENCES

1. Tanagho EA, Smith DR. The anatomy and function of the bladder neck. *Br J Urol* 1966; **38**: 54.
2. Gosling, JA. The structure of the female lower urinary tract and pelvic floor. *Urol Clin North Am* 1985; **12**: 207.
3. Gosling JA, Dixon DS. The structure and innervation of smooth muscle in the wall of the bladder neck and proximal urethra. *Br J Urol* 1975; **47**: 549.
4. Tanagho EA, Schmidt RA, de Araujo CG. Urinary striated sphincter: What is its nerve supply? *Urology* 1982; **20**: 415.
5. Tanagho EA. The anatomy and physiology of micturition. *Clin Obstet Gynecol* 1978; **5**: 3.
6. Diokno AC, Brock BM, Herzog AR, et al. Prevalence of urologic symptoms in the noninstitutionalized elderly. *J Urol* 1985; **133**: 179.

 7. Blaivas JG, Olsson CA. Stress incontinence: classification and surgical approach. *J Urol* 1988; **139**: 727.
 8. Blaivas JG. Sphincteric incontinence in the female: pathophysiology, classification, and choice of corrective surgical procedure. *AUA Update Ser* 1987; **25**: 1.
 9. McGuire EJ. Bladder instability in stress incontinence. *Neurourol Urodyn* 1988; **7**: 563.
10. Resnick NM. Initial evaluation of the incontinent patient. *J Am Geriatr Soc* 1990a; **38**: 311.
11. Abrams PH, Torrens M. Urine flow studies: symposium on clinical urodynamics. *Urol Clin North Am* 1979; **6**: 71.
12. McInerney PD. The practice of urodynamics. In: Mundy AR, Stephenson, TP, Wein, AJ (eds). *Urodynamics*, 2nd ed, London: Churchill Livingstone, 1994; 101–110.
13. Siroky MB, Olsson CA, Krane RJ. The flow rate nomogram: II. Clinical correlations. *J Urol* 1980; **123**: 208.
14. Susset JG, Picker P, Kretz M, et al. Critical evaluation of uroflowmeters and analysis of normal curves. *J Urol* 1973; **109**: 874.
15. Blaivas JG. Urodynamic testing. In: Raz S (ed). *Female Urology*. Philadelphia: WB Saunders, 1983; 79–103.
16. McGuire EJ. Urodynamic evaluation of stress incontinence. *Urol Clin North Am* 1995; **22**: 551.
17. McGuire EJ, Lytton B, Pepe V, et al. Stress incontinence. *Am J Obstet Gynecol* 1976; **47**: 255.
18. Stothers L, Chopra A, Raz S. Vaginal reconstructive surgery for female incontinence and anterior vaginal-wall prolapse. *Urol Clin North Am* 1995; **22**: 641.

CHAPTER 5

Neurophysiology of pelvic floor dysfunction

JAMES P. THEOFRASTOUS

Few areas in the field of urogynecology remain as poorly understood as the role of normal pelvic muscle tone and innervation in maintaining the normal support and function of the pelvic organs. While clinicians commonly recognize that women with symptoms of pelvic floor dysfunction may have poor pelvic muscle function on examination, the reason for this muscular atrophy and the relationships between neuromuscular compromise and urinary incontinence, pelvic organ prolapse, and fecal incontinence are uncertain. This chapter presents current concepts in pelvic muscle anatomy and innervation in normal and symptomatic women and outlines the role of neurophysiologic testing in the evaluation and treatment of conditions related to pelvic floor dysfunction.

EARLY OBSERVATIONS

Investigators have debated the etiology of pelvic organ prolapse and urinary incontinence for more than a century. Clinicians have recognized for several centuries that females with abnormal innervation to the pelvic musculature may demonstrate severe defects in pelvic support. Several reports in the eighteenth and nineteenth centuries noted congenital neonatal complete uterine prolapse in female infants born with various types of spinal dysraphism, such as spina bifida.[1-4] In the nineteenth century Halban performed elegant anatomic studies of pelvic muscle and fascial attachments and described the support of the female pelvis as "a system of strings to the pelvic wall . . . maintained in suspension, just as the weight of a spider is supported as it rests on its system of threads".[5]

A vigorous debate began at the turn of the century between supporters of Makenrodt, who advocated the primacy of fascial connections between the pelvic organs and the sidewall in maintaining pelvic support, and followers of Halban who proposed that the pelvic musculature rather than endopelvic fascia supported the pelvic viscera. The proponents of fascia as the primary basis of pelvic support argued that without the firm paravaginal connective tissue attachments, "the plastic viscera would slip through its lower opening like sand through an hour-glass, like fæcal masses from the rectum, and like the products of conception from the parturient canal".[6] Advocates of pelvic muscle as the primary basis of pelvic support countered that the strength of the connective tissue attachments was "too trifling to define" and they are prevented from becoming relaxed, not by any virtue of their own, but by the support that is given to them, as well as the pelvic viscera, by the tonically contracted and healthy muscle which lies beneath them".[5] In a postdarwinian fervor of comparative anatomy both sides proposed that the assumption of an erect posture and the loss of a prehensile tail in the evolution of our species resulted in either the hypertrophy or the atrophy of human pelvic musculature, depending on their bias.[6]

Over the subsequent decades much attention was focused on the anatomy of the pelvis and the neurophysiology of micturation, but the role of the pelvic neuromuscular structures in maintaining support and normal function of the pelvic structures remained difficult to study. With the development of neurophysiologic testing in the 1940s it became possible to assess the in vivo activity of skeletal muscle. Early investigators of pelvic muscle physiology noted that, in contrast to other striated muscles except the respiratory diaphragm, the pelvic muscles have continuous electrical activity that maintains tone at rest.[7–10] Reflex activity of the pelvic muscles increases during bladder filling, coughing, and anal stimulation, and muscle activity decreases or silences during voiding.[10–12] In 1962, Porter[7] noted that subjects with destruction of the dorsal horn ganglion cells (afferent) in tabes dorsalis had no resting pelvic muscle tone but normal voluntary activity, and he speculated that normal resting tone is contingent upon continuous afferent sensory impulses from visceral receptors and proprioceptors in and around the pelvic musculature. The importance of autonomic activity in maintaining pelvic muscle tone was further supported by observations of normal resting activity and the absence of voluntary activity in the pelvic floor muscles of patients with L3 paraplegia, and the absence of both voluntary and resting activity of the pelvic muscles of patients with conditions that destroy sensory and motor fibers and central reflex connections such as cauda equina.[7]

The fundamental concepts of the surgical treatment of urinary incontinence were formulated in the early 1900s by such pioneering gynecologic surgeons as White[13] and Kelly.[14] The central precept of most continence procedures since then is that restoration of normal pelvic anatomy by repair of defects in fascial attachments will result in normal function. In 1950, after observing that intensive pelvic muscle training often improved continence in parous women and in surgical failures, Kegel and Powell[15] speculated that urinary incontinence was due to a reversible neuromuscular injury rather than trauma to the pelvic support structures alone. Since that time, clinicians have employed various forms of nonsurgical and surgical therapy without a clear understanding of the role of normal pelvic neurophysiologic function in contributing to the underlying clinical condition or in predicting clinical response. Impediments to the delineation of the role of normal pelvic innervation and muscle function in maintaining normal urogenital and colorectal function have included a poor understanding and description of clinical symptoms, a lack of a consensus for describing pelvic support in a standardized fashion to enable meaningful communication between clinicians, difficulty in assessing the function of pelvic muscles in a reproducible and clinically relevant fashion, and an absence of long-term prospective studies of the natural history of pelvic floor dysfunction.

ANATOMY

In order to investigate the role of neuromuscular function in the maintenance of normal pelvic support and function it is important to understand the macroscopic and microscopicanatomy of the pelvic musculature. While composed primarily of striated muscle, the muscles of the pelvic diaphragm also contain smooth muscle and have unique functional attributes compared to musculature outside of the pelvis. The pelvic diaphragm consists of the puborectalis, pubococcygeus, and iliococcygeus muscles of the levator ani anterioriy and the coccygeus muscles posteriorly. The levator ani form a broad concave diaphragmatic floor upon which the pelvic viscera lie (Figure 5-1). While traditional anatomy describes these muscles as discrete entities, recent studies suggest that the boundaries between these muscles are indistinct and that a more general term such as "pubovisceralis" may be more functionally accurate.[17,18]

The major nerve supply to the pelvic musculature is via the pudendal nerve. The pudendal nerve arises from the second through fourth sacral rami and

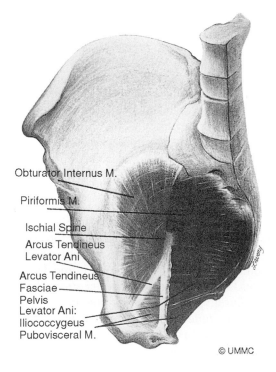

Figure 5-1. The pelvic musculature. The puborectalis and pubococcygeus muscles are grouped together as the "pubovisceralis." (From DeLancey JOL. Anatomy and biomechanics of genital prolapse. *Clin Obstet Gynecol* 1993; **36**: 905, with permission.)

Obturator Internus M.

Piriformis M.

Ischial Spine

Arcus Tendineus
Levator Ani

Arcus Tendineus
Fasciae
Pelvis
Levator Ani:
Iliococcygeus
Pubovisceral M.

© UMMC

provides most of the innervation to the pelvic musculature. The pudendal nerve passes inferior to the ischial spine, enters the pelvis through the lesser sciatic foramen, and courses through Alcock's, or the pudendal, canal to reach the pelvic muscles (Figure 5-2). A direct branch of the pudendal nerve supplies the levator ani and two distal branches, the inferior hemorrhoidal and the perineal nerves, supply the external anal sphincter and the striated urethral sphincter, respectively.[19–22] The perineal branch of the pudendal nerve innervates the periurethral striated muscle and provides the sensory innervation of the urethral mucosa. The urethra has an additional intrinsic (intramural) component of striated muscle which is supplied by somatic efferent fibers traveling in the pelvic nerves.[22] The intramural striated (external) sphincter is largely composed of slow-twitch fibers with tonic activity at rest. The periurethral striated muscle sphincter augments closure during stress and demonstrates reflex activity through alpha motor neurons in the conus medullaris (S2–S4) through sensory afferent neurons in the urethra, bladder, and pelvic floor. The inferior hemorrhoidal (or rectal) nerve innervates the external anal sphincter, the lining of the lower anal canal, and the perianal skin.

MOTOR UNIT

Striated muscle is organized at a microscopic level into functional motor units. A motor unit consists of a terminal branch of a somatic nerve originating from an anterior horn cell and a number of muscle fibers. Skeletal muscle contains two major divisions of muscle fibers with different rates of activation. Type I, or

A

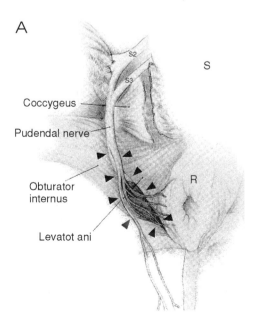

Coccygeus

Pudendal nerve

Obturator internus

Levatot ani

S2

S3

S

R

Figure 5-2.   The origin and course of the pudendal nerve. (From Juenmann KP, Lue TF, Schmidt RA, Tanagho EA. Clinical significance of sacral and pudendal nerve anatomy. *J Urol* 1988; **139**: 74–80, with permission.)

slow, fibers contract within 90 ms of nerve activation, have a primarily oxidative metabolism, and are fatigue-resistant. Type II, or fast, fibers contract within 36 ms of nerve activation, have a primarily glycolytic metabolism, and fatigue rapidly. Type I fibers in the pelvic musculature have tonic activity at rest. The pelvic muscles contain an increased ratio of type I to type II muscle fibers compared to extrapelvic musculature, which reflects the large role these muscles have in maintaining pelvic tone at rest.

When a terminal efferent nerve is stimulated all of the functional muscle fibers within the motor unit contract in unison and continue to fire as a unit as long as the nerve is stimulated. Most motor units contain 8–12 muscle fibers, which are 60–80 μm in diameter. Muscle fibers within a motor unit are dispersed throughout a region of the muscle, are interdigitated with muscle fibers from several other motor units, and are usually more than 300 μm apart. Type I motor units fire tonically at a rate of 6–10 Hz with a maximum rate of 18 to 20 Hz. Type II motor units fire in brief bursts at 10–25 Hz and have a maximum rate of 16–50 Hz. The frequency of motor unit firing normally increases with progressive voluntary effort.

HISTOLOGIC STUDIES

Histologic studies have provided indirect evidence that impaired support and function of the urogenital tract is associated with neuromuscular damage. In a study of women with pelvic organ prolapse and genuine stress urinary incontinence (GSI), women with striated muscle on biopsy had higher measures of urethral resistance on urodynamic testing[24] and a lower incidence of GSI compared to women without striated muscle on levator biopsy.[25] The presence of severe muscle atrophy in this study suggests an association between damage to the levator muscles and/or pudendal innervation and impairment of the continence mechanism.

Histologic examination of biopsies of the puborectalis and pubococcygeus muscles of women with stress urinary incontinence has revealed evidence of denervation with destruction of muscle fibers (Figure 5-3).[25,26] This has also been noted in biopsies of the external anal sphincter in patients with anorectal incontinence.[27] These studies demonstrate that women with various forms of pelvic floor dysfunction may have significant alterations in the structural arrangement of the pelvic floor musculature. These changes include alterations in the diameters and ratios of type I and type II muscle fibers, and increased pathologic appearing fibers with central nuclei.[5,28] Electron microscopy of the anal sphincter in patients with idiopathic anorectal incontinence has demonstrated gross alterations in muscle and nerve microanatomy.[29] While indicative of end-organ damage, these findings are nonspecific and do not differentiate between muscle atrophy secondary to denervation and direct muscle-damage. The differentiation between nerve and muscle mechanisms of injury at an histologic level is also hampered by the observation that chronic denervation may result in both

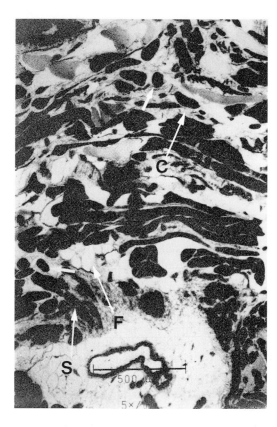

Figure 5-3. Pubococcygeus biopsy of a woman with pelvic organ prolapse and genuine stress incontinence demonstrating muscle fiber atrophy (*small arrows*) and wide endomysial clefts containing connective tissue (*C*), smooth muscle (*S*), and adipose (*F*). Calibration bar = 500 μm. (From reference 23, with permission.)

myopathic and neuropathic changes in muscle.[30] Furthermore, these histologic studies are limited by the discrete possibility of sampling error and the difficulty in performing longitudinal studies.

ELECTROPHYSIOLOGIC STUDIES

While histologic studies provide gross evidence that women with symptomatic pelvic organ prolapse may have nonspecific damage to the neuromuscular structures of the pelvis, these studies provide no information regarding the functional status of the remaining muscle. Electrophysiologic testing has the ability to assess nerve and muscle function *in vivo*. Unfortunately, most neurologists are neither well versed in pelvic neuromuscular anatomy nor skilled in examining these relatively inaccessible muscles, and most gynecologic investigators have little or no formal training in neurologic theory or testing. As a result, very little research in basic pelvic neurophysiology exists.

Over the last three decades considerable research has been directed toward understanding alterations in neuromuscular activity in women with symptomatic pelvic organ prolapse. Neurophysiologic testing techniques assess the status of nerve and muscle function by examining the conductivity of the efferent or afferent nerve supply or by examining the electrical activity of the muscle. The most common electrophysiologic techniques used to assess pelvic floor nerves and muscles are pudendal nerve terminal motor latency tests, single-fiber electromyography, and electromyographic motor unit action potential analysis. The roles of each of these tests in evaluating women with pelvic floor dysfunction is examined in the following sections.

Pudendal Nerve Terminal Motor Latency

Pudendal nerve terminal motor latency testing has been studied extensively in women with symptomatic pelvic organ prolapse over the last two decades. The purpose of this test is to determine the velocity of transmission along the pudendal nerve by applying an electrical stimulus along the axon and measuring the contraction of distal musculature. The time interval between stimulus and evoked response is termed the terminal motor latency and is measured in a few milliseconds. With nerve damage, the rate of depolarization along the nerve axon is slowed and the response is delayed. Most clinicians perform this test by stimulating the pudendal nerve transrectally at the level of the ischial spine and measuring contraction of the anal or urethral sphincter. The technique is relatively simple and involves minimal discomfort for the patient. The patient may have unilateral or bilateral nerve damage, and most testing is done bilaterally.[31–33]

When damage to the pudendal nerve is caused by stretch, direct trauma, or disease, conduction along the nerve is slowed (Figure 5-4). This may reflect diffuse disease within the nerve, as in the loss of fast-conducting axons or damage to Schwann cells, or local damage to the nerve at a more proximal site, resulting in distal loss of myelinated axons. Some evidence seems to indicate that fibrosis and tethering below the ischial spine as it passes through the pudendal canal can cause pudendal nerve damage. This theory is supported to some degree by preliminary observations that surgical neurolysis or "release" of the pudendal nerve is associated with some clinical improvement and partial normalization of crude electrophysiologic parameters;[34] but the reproducibility and long-term follow-up of this technique remain to be established.

Numerous studies have documented abnormal pudendal nerve conduction to the external anal and/or striated urethral sphincters of women with a variety of clinical conditions related to pelvic floor dysfunction, including stress urinary incontinence,[35–40] pelvic organ prolapse,[41,42] and fecal incontinence.[43,44] Furthermore, prospective studies of women after delivery[45–49] and pelvic surgery,[50–53] have implicated vaginal childbirth and vaginal surgery, respectively, as events that may damage the pudendal nerve. Snooks and Swash[54–56] have also observed delayed transmission of an electrical stimulation delivered transcutaneously over L1 and L4 to the urethral and anal sphincters and the pubococcygeus muscle in

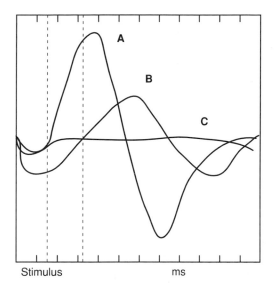

Figure 5-4. Pudendal nerve terminal motor latency recordings: *A*, before pudendal nerve damage; *B*, after pudendal nerve damage; *C*, control tracing without stimulation.

women with urinary and/or fecal incontinence, suggesting that damage to pelvic innervation may occur above or below the pelvic floor. These studies are summarized in Table 5-1. Further evidence that the prolongation of pudendal nerve conduction, which occurs immediately after delivery is at least partially reversible over 6–8 weeks,[45,47] suggests that alterations immediately following vaginal surgery may also be partially or completely reversible with time. The process of nerve repair after nerve damage involves myelination and subsequent coordination and stabilization of nerve transmission and muscle contraction. This repair process results in progressive increases in the efficiency and speed of nerve transmission.

Pudendal nerve transmission studies have been used extensively by colorectal and gynecologic clinicians in the investigation of patients with fecal incontinence. Recent studies have demonstrated a correlation between prolonged pudendal nerve conduction and other proposed markers of anorectal dysfunction, including reduced pressures on anal manometry, impaired anorectal excitatory reflexes during distention, and anatomic defects noted on anal sphincter ultrasound imaging.[57–59]

The clinical interpretation of alterations in pudendal nerve transmission is limited by the absence of a verified definitive link between gross changes in nerve conductivity and clinical symptoms or pelvic muscle function. While statistically significant, the clinical significance and natural history of these small alterations in nerve conduction are uncertain. Furthermore, clinical studies of the inter- and intraobserver reproducibility of pudendal conductivity have been limited.[60] While indicative of alterations in nerve function at a gross level,

Table 5-1.   Neurophysiologic tests and findings in women with pelvic floor dysfunction

Clinical test	Technical details	Findings in women with pelvic floor dysfunction
Pudendal nerve terminal motor latency	Stimulate nerve transrectally at ischial spine, record contraction of urethral or anal sphincter	Nerve conduction often delayed in women with pelvic organ prolapse, urinary incontinence, fecal incontinence, after vaginal delivery, after vaginal surgery
Single-fiber density	Intramuscular electrode records activity from muscle fibers of one motor unit	Fiber density often increased in women with pelvic organ prolapse, urinary incontinence, fecal incontinence, after vaginal delivery
Qualitative interference pattern analysis	Intramuscular electrode records summation of all motor units in recording area	Reduced interference pattern in women with urinary and fecal incontinence
Quantitative electromyography	Intramuscular electrode records configuration of individual motor unit action potentials	Action potential duration, amplitude and polyphasicity increased following vaginal delivery

demonstration of prolonged nerve transmission does not identify which specific axons within the nerve have been damaged, since only the fastest conducting axons are assessed, and the level of the damage is uncertain. Interpretation of pudendal nerve transmission is also hampered by the presence of confounding variables that have been proposed to affect nerve conduction, including age, hormonal status, perineal descent, and chronic constipation.[61–65] The findings of abnormal pudendal nerve transmission in asymptomatic women and normal nerve transmission in symptomatic women[63,66,67] challenges the sensitivity and specificity of this measure of pudendal neuropathy in women with symptoms related to pelvic organ prolapse.

Single-Fiber Density

A second neurophysiologic test for assessing the functional status of the neuromuscular unit is single-fiber density measurements of striated muscle. Single-fiber density recordings quantify the number of muscle fibers that compose a given motor unit and the stability of electrical transmission within the motor unit. In healthy muscle, single-fiber recordings generally record less than two muscle fibers discharging at a given time. Nerve damage with destruction of peripheral nerve fibers will result in atrophy and loss of the motor fibers supplied by that nerve fiber. In an attempt to preserve the denervated motor fibers, adjacent nerves will sprout collateral fibers to the affected motor fiber units over the next few months. The net result of this process of reinnervation is that depolarization of the nerve fibers that have sent new collateral sprouts will activate a greater number of motor units than before the repair process occurred (Figure 5.5). This is measured clinically by single-fiber electromyography as an increase in the fiber density of the muscle. Multiple studies have documented both prolongation of pudendal nerve terminal motor latency and increased anal sphincter muscle fiber density after vaginal delivery and in women with urinary incontinence, fecal incontinence, and/or pelvic organ prolapse.[28,35-40,44,49,63] Abnormal anal sphincter single-fiber density recordings have also been noted in asymptomatic elderly patients.[68,69]

The clinical utility of single-fiber density electromyography is largely limited by the high level of technical expertise necessary for performing the procedure and the complicated equipment required for data analysis. As with nerve transmission studies, the relationship between alterations in fiber density and clinical function is not established. It is even possible that the process of reinnervation with preservation of motor fibers and increased fiber density is a favorable marker of functional compensation following nerve damage. Women who do not

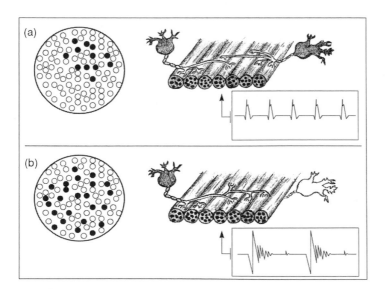

Figure 5-5. Reinervation following nerve damage. (a) Both neurons are intact. The muscle fibers that are innervated by the neuron on the left are shaded in the cross section, and normal EMG activity is present in the *inset*. (b) The neuron on the left has sprouted axons and preserved some motor fibers of the neuron on the right following neuron or nerve damage, resulting in increased fiber density and neuropathic EMG signals.

experience reinnervation with a coincident increase in fiber density following neuromuscular trauma may experience more pelvic floor dysfunction compared to women with evidence of pelvic muscle reinnervation due to a relative loss of motor fibers.

Motor Unit Action Potential Analysis

A third neurophysiologic method of evaluating whether alterations have occurred in pelvic floor neuromuscular function is the electromyographic (EMG) analysis of motor unit action potential configurations during muscle contraction. Striated muscle activity is assessed during electromyography by inserting a concentric or monopolar needle with a recording surface into a muscle and noting the electrical activity during insertion, at rest, and during voluntary contraction.[70] The needle records the electrical depolarization of adjacent muscle fibers within a certain area and displays this signal as an algebraic summation referred to as a motor unit action potential.[71,72]

The most simple method of EMG analysis of gross muscle activity is to assess the ability to increase muscle activity with progressive voluntary effort. During a normal, progressive, isometric, voluntary muscle contraction the number of motor units recruited and activated increases progressively with effort until the maximum contraction is obtained. The EMG needle records the discharge of the active motor units within the uptake area of the recording surface of the electrode and displays the summation of the electrical activity. A concentric needle electrode generally records from 10 to 15 motor fibers of a given motor unit.[73] When a nerve is damaged or diseased, the maximum number of motor units during a contraction is decreased, and the interference pattern is reduced or absent. A normal interference pattern is displayed on an EMG display as a progressively dense pattern of motor units and is recognized audibly as an increase in the volume and frequency of motor unit discharges and is referred to as a "full" interference pattern (Figure 5.6).

Experienced investigators can discriminate between neurologic and myopathic processes by the visual and audible patterns of motor unit discharges at rest and during contraction. Nerve damage leads to the loss of motor units through atrophy and fewer motor units are available for recruitment; thus the firing rate and interference pattern during muscle contraction is diminished. Muscle damage characteristically results in hyperexcitability of the motor units and rapid activation during contraction with an interference pattern which is full at abnormally low levels of contraction.

Many studies have noted alterations in pelvic muscle EMG activity in women with pelvic floor dysfunction. Porter[7] noted in 1962 that patients with fecal incontinence had reduced motor unit activity on concentric needle electromyography. In 1966, Parks and coworkers[74] noted similar abnormalities in women with perineal descent. In 1984, Fowler and colleagues[75] reported reduced interference patterns in the urethral sphincters of patients with urethral sphincter

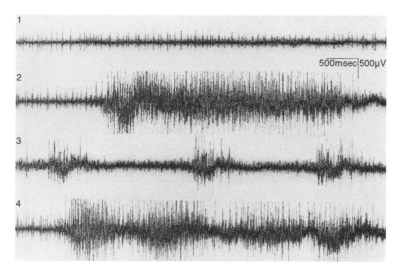

Figure 5-6. EMG of a normal urethral sphincter: *1*, tonic activity at rest; *2*, full interference pattern with voluntary contraction of the pelvic muscles; *3*, reflex activity during coughing; *4*, reflex activity during a digital rectal examination. (From Jesel M, Isch-Treussard C, Isch F. Electromyography of striated muscle of anal and urethral sphincters. In: Desmedt JE (ed). *New Development in Electromyography and Clinical Neurophysiology*, Vol 2. Basel: Karger, 1973: 406–420, with permission.)

dysfunction secondary to neurologic disorders. In a study of postpartum women, subjects with reduced pelvic muscle interference patterns had a higher prevalence of genuine stress incontinence.[45]

Gross alterations in anal sphincter EMG activity of patients with fecal incontinence have been documented and noted to correlate with other measures of anorectal function including pudendal nerve transmission, anal ultrasound, and anal manometry.[57,76] Electromyographic "mapping" of the external anal sphincter may be of prognostic importance in the preoperative evaluation of women with fecal incontinence. A woman with a sphincter disruption on examination or ultrasound imaging but with normal EMG activity of the remaining sphincter may have a better prognosis following sphincteroplasty compared to a woman with abnormal anal sphincter EMG activity with or without an anatomic defect.[77]

While evaluation of muscle activity by electromyography provides a gross assessment of motor unit function and some information as to the mechanism of injury in patients with dysfunction, a more sophisticated analysis of discrete motor unit activity can provide further information as to the functional status of the muscle and may help to identify the mechanism of injury. Most motor unit action potentials have a characteristic biphasic or triphasic configuration (Figure 5-7). The process of denervation with subsequent reinnervation results in characteristic alterations in the configuration, duration, and amplitude of the action potential that can be displayed and measured by sensitive recording

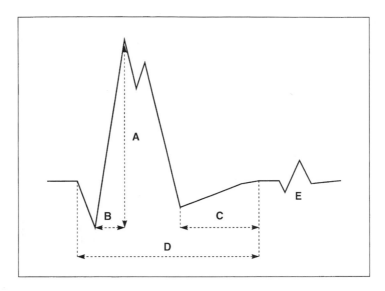

Figure 5-7.   Motor unit action potential: *A*, amplitude; *B*, rise time; *C*, terminal portion; *D*, duration; *E*, satellite component.

equipment. The process of reinnervation of muscle fibers by adjacent neuronal sprouting results in varying degrees of a loss of synchronization of muscle fiber discharge with delayed conduction in the nerve terminals or muscle fibers, dispersion of endplate location, and/or longer nerve terminals. These functional alterations following nerve damage with reinnervation create characteristic neuropathic patterns on EMG recordings, including increased duration and amplitude of the motor unit action potential, increased numbers of polyphasic potentials (≥5 phases) and late components referred to as satellite potentials, and abnormal discharges at rest including fibrillation potentials, positive sharp waves, and repetitive discharges. Myopathic alterations in EMG activity following muscle damage include reduced duration and amplitude of the motor unit action potential with increased activity of motor units at lower levels of stimulation (Figures 5-5 and 5-8).[78] Electromyographic alterations follow a characteristic pattern following nerve and muscle trauma and may take up to a year to stabilize.

Increases in anal sphincter motor unit action potential duration and increased numbers of polyphasic action potentials have been documented in women following vaginal delivery,[79] in women with genuine stress incontinence,[38] and in women with fecal incontinence.[80] In 1990, Allen and colleagues[45] noted increased motor unit action potential duration and polyphasicity in pubococcygeus recordings following their patients' first vaginal delivery. A 5-year follow-up evaluation of roughly half these women revealed a continued increase in action potential duration and polyphasicity without further deliveries.[81,82] This suggests that vaginal childbirth results in damage to the muscles of the pelvic

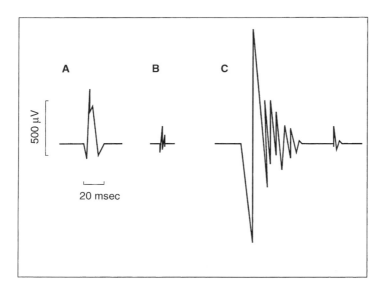

Figure 5-8. Electromyographic recordings in *A*, normal muscle; *B*, following muscle damage and, *C*, following nerve damage with reinnervation.

floor through nerve injury and that once initiated this is a self-perpetuating process. This study also noted that women with urinary incontinence had signifi-cantly increased action potential duration compared to continent vaginally parous women, providing an indirect link between pudendal nerve damage and genuine stress incontinence. These findings are summarized in Table 5-1. Similar alterations in muscle activity have been noted in neuropathic conditions outside the pelvis such as carpal tunnel syndrome which occur secondary to compression and damage of a large neuron.[83]

One of the major limitations of needle EMG studies is the discomfort involved in the placement of the electrodes. For some types of analysis it is necessary to insert the needle in several different areas in order to obtain a representative sample of the electrical activity within the muscle. In order to maximize the reliability of motor unit analysis it may be necessary to obtain recordings of up to 20 action potentials from each muscle.[84] The interpretation of action potential analysis is also limited by fact that the morphology of motor unit action potentials can be altered by factors such as temperature,[85] age,[86] and fatigue.[80]

Surface EMG techniques have the potential advantage of avoiding painful needle insertions while providing some information as to underlying muscle activity.[87] These recordings are frequently made using a vaginal plug with a circumferential recording surface and are used widely in pelvic muscle rehabili-tation to provide biofeedback during muscle contraction. While surface EMG recordings provide recordings of the gross muscle activity of the pelvic muscles the interpretation of this information is limited by the difficulty in obtaining a firm connection of the electrode plate to the vaginal epithelium, the limited recording range of the electrode (10–12 mm), the variable orientation between the electrode and the muscle fibers, the possibility of signal contamination from adjacent musculature, and the difficulty of the surface electrode to obtain an undistorted signal at maximum contraction efforts.[88–90]

Quantitative Electromyographic Analysis

Traditional electromyography is limited by the subjective nature of evaluating the auditory and visible patterns of action potentials during muscle activity. While skilled neurologists may accurately interpret EMG signals in a reproducible fashion, investigators with less experience in neurology are limited in their ability to obtain and analyze muscle activity in a meaningful fashion. The use of computer analysis of EMG signals has the potential advantage of applying objective criteria to the specific components of motor unit activity. With advanced developments in software it is now possible to analyze the microanatomy of motor unit action potentials in a reproducible fashion. Pertinent detailed components of the motor unit action potential include: the number of turns or changes in direction in the direction of the EMG signal, which is a reflection of polyphasicity; the ratio of the number of turns to mean amplitude; the number of small segments, which reflects polyphasicity; and activity, which is reflection of the fullness of the interference pattern.[91,92] Multiple studies have suggested that computerized quantitative interference pattern analysis has the potential to discriminate between neurologic and myopathic disorders.[93] These studies evaluate alterations in the interference pattern with progressive increases in the force of muscle contraction. Sophisticated software provides a quantitative display of the motor unit amplitude and polyphasicity at different levels of effort, and normal "envelopes" of activity for a given muscle provide a reference to diagnose neuropathic or myopathic dysfunction (Figure 5-9). To date this method of motor unit analysis has not been applied systematically to the pelvic musculature in either normal or symptomatic women, but it appears to have the potential to elucidate the relative contributions of nerve and muscle damage in women with pelvic floor dysfunction. The ability to discriminate between neurologic and muscular dysfunction would contribute to the understanding of the etiology of pelvic floor dysfunction and may aid clinicians in selecting appropriate surgical or nonsurgical therapy based on the likelihood of a favorable clinical response. A woman with severe myopathic alterations in her pelvic musculature may be less likely to respond to pelvic muscle exercises than a woman who has evidence of reinnervation and neuropathic changes.

FUTURE DIRECTIONS

The vast majority of clinical research into the neurophysiology of pelvic floor dysfunction to date has focused on the efferent, or motor, supply to the pelvic

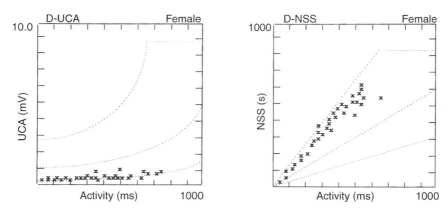

Figure 5-9. Quantitative EMG concentric needle interference pattern recordings from the pubococcygeus muscle of a multiparous woman with dual incontinence demonstrating findings suggestive of myopathy. D-UCA, deviation of upper centile amplitude; D-NSS, deviation of number of small segments.

musculature. While some research into the status of the sensory nerve supply has been described,[94] our comprehension of normal pelvic reflexes and sensation is extremely limited and the clinical interpretation of these reports is uncertain. Given that alterations in motor nerve conductivity have been documented in women with various types of pelvic floor dysfunction, it is logical to postulate that abnormalities in afferent nerve function may coexist. As electrophysiologic testing techniques for assessing pelvic sensory innervation are validated it may become possible to gain insight into the role of normal sensation of the pelvic viscera and musculature in maintaining urinary and fecal continence and pelvic tone and support.

SUMMARY

Women with symptomatic pelvic organ prolapse display numerous gross alterations in pelvic muscle and nerve morphology and many abnormalities on electrophysiologic testing. These findings are consistent with pudendal neuropathy with or without direct damage to the pelvic muscles; but the relative roles of each of these mechanisms of injury in creating anatomic and/or functional abnormalities are uncertain. Several precipitating events of neuro-muscular injury have been described including vaginal parity, aging, pelvic surgery, and chronic constipation; but the degree to which any of these factors is critical in producing symptoms in a particular woman is variable and may depend on other congenital or environmental influences.

The sensitivity, specificity, and reproducibility of most tests of nerve and muscle function are not established and the correlation between normal and abnormal test results and the presence or absence of clinical symptoms is often unclear. Pudendal nerve injury and pelvic muscle damage are dynamic processes which may be partially or completely reversed or compensated for with time. Neurophysiologic testing has the potential to shed light upon our understanding of the etiology of pelvic floor dysfunction and may provide information of prognostic importance in selecting therapeutic options for a symptomatic woman.

REFERENCES

1. Noyes IH. Uterine prolapse of associated with spina bifida in the newborn, with report of a case. *Am J Obstet Gynecol* 1927; **13**: 209–213.
2. Fraser RD. A case of genital prolapse in a newborn baby. *BMJ* 1961; **1**: 1011–1012.
3. Dixon RE, Acosta AA, Young RL. Penrose pessary management of neonatal genital prolapse. *Am J Obstet Gynecol* 1974; **119**: 855–857.
4. Lee FA, McComb JG. Brief clinical communication: Neurogenic perineal prolapse in neonates. *Radiology* 1983; **148**: 433–435.
5. Paramore RH. The supports-in-chief of the female pelvic viscera. *J Obstet Gynaecol Br Emp* 1908; **13**: 391–408.
6. Fothergill WE. The supports of the pelvic viscera: A review of some recent contributions to pelvic anatomy, with a clinical introduction. *J Obstet Gynaecol Br Emp* 1908; **13**: 18–28.
7. Porter NH. A physiological study of the pelvic floor in rectal prolapse. *Ann R Coll Surg Eng* 1962; **31**: 379–404.
8. Taverner D, Smiddy FG. An electromyographic study of the normal function of the external anal sphincter and pelvic diaphragm. *Dis Colon Rectum* 1959; **2**: 153–160.
9. Petersen, Franksson C, Danielson CO. Electromyographic study of the muscles of the pelvic floor and urethra in normal females. *Acta Obstet Gynecol Scand* 1955; **34**: 273–285.
10. Jesel M, Isch-Treussard C, Isch F. Electromyography of striated muscle of anal and urethral sphincters. In: Desmedt JE (ed). *New Development in Electromyography and Clinical Neurophysiology*, Vol 2. Basel: Karger, 1973: 406–420.
11. Floyd WF, Walls EW. Electromyography of the sphincter ani externus in man. *J Physiol* 1953; **122**: 599–609.
12. Deindl FM, Vodusek DB, Hesse U, Schuessler B. Activity patterns of pubococcygeal muscles in nulliparous continent women. *Br J Urol* 1993; **72**: 46–51.
13. White GR. Cystocele, a radical cure by suturing lateral sulci of vagina to white line of pelvic fascia. *JAMA* 1909; **53**: 1707–1711.
14. Kelly HA. Incontinence of urine in women. *Urol Cutan Rev* 1913; **17**: 291–293.
15. Kegel AH, Powell TO. The physiologic treatment of urinary stress incontinence. *J Urol* 1950; **63**: 808–814.
16. Delancey JOL. Anatomy and biomechanics of genital prolapse. *Clin Obstet Gynecol* 1993; **36**: 905.
17. Strohbehn K, Ellis JH, Strohbehn JA, DeLancey JOL. Magnetic resonance imaging of the levator ani with anatomic correlation. *Obstet Gynecol* 1996; **87**: 277–285.
18. Aronson MP, Bates SM, Jacoby AF, Chelmow D, Sant GR. Periurethral and paravaginal anatomy: An endovaginal magnetic resonance imaging study. *Am J Obstet Gynecol* 1995; **173**: 1702–1710.
19. Fearnsides EG. The innervation of the bladder and urethra: A review. *Brain* 1917; **40**: 150–187.
20. Tanagho EA, Schmidt RA, De Araujo CG. Urinary striated sphincter: What is its nerve supply? *Urology* 1982; **20**: 415–417.

21. Zvara P, Carrier S, Kour NW, Tanagho EA. The detailed neuroanatomy of the striated urethral sphincter. *Br J Urol* 1994; **74**: 182–187.
22. Juenmann KP, Lue TF, Schmidt RA, Tanagho EA. Clinical significance of sacral and pudendal nerve anatomy. *J Urol* 1988; **139**: 74–80.
23. Gosling JA. The structure of the female lower urinary tract and pelvic floor. *Urol Clin North Am* 1985; **12**: 207–214.
24. Koelbl H, Strassegger H, Riss PA, Gruber H. Morphologic and functional aspects of pelvic floor muscles in patients with pelvic relaxation and genuine stress incontinence. *Obstet Gynecol* 1989; **74**: 789–795.
25. Hanzal E, Berger E, Koelbl H. Levator ani muscle morphology and recurrent genuine stress incontinence. *Obstet Gynecol* 1993; **81**: 426–429.
26. Gilpin SA, Gosling JA, Smith ARB, Warrell DW. The pathogenesis of genitourinary prolapse and stress incontinence of urine: a histological and histochemical study. *Br J Obstet Gynaecol* 1989; **96**: 15–23.
27. Parks AG, Swash M, Urich H. Sphincter denervation in anorectal incontinence and rectal prolapse. *Gut* 1977; **18**: 656–665.
28. Henry MM, Parks AG, Swash M. The pelvic floor musculature in the descending perineum syndrome. *Br J Surg* 1982; **69**: 470–472.
29. Parks AG, Swash M, Urich H. Sphincter denervation in anorectal incontinence and rectal prolapse. *Gut* 1977; **18**: 656–665.
30. Drachman DB, Murphy SR, Nigam MP, Hills JR. "Myopathic" changes in chronically denervated muscle. *Arch Neurol* 1967; **16**: 14–24.
31. Lubowski DZ, Jones PN, Swash M, Henry MM. Asymmetrical pudendal nerve damage in pelvic floor disorders. *Colorect Dis* 1988; **3**: 158–160.
32. Cheong DM, Vaccaro CA, Salanga VD, Waxner SD, Phillips RC, Hanson MR. Electrodiagnostic evaluation of fecal incontinence. *Muscle Nerve* 1995; **18**: 612–619.
33. Vernava AM III, Longo WE, Daniel GL. Pudendal neuropathy and the importance of EMG evaluation of fecal incontinence. *Dis Colon Rectum* 1993; **36**: 23–27.
34. Shafik A. Pudendal canal decompression in the treatment of urinary stress incontinence. *Intl J Urogynecol* 1994; **2**: 215–220.
35. Snooks SJ, Barnes PRH, Swash M. Damage to the innervation of the voluntary anal and periurethral sphincter musculature in incontinence: an electrophysiological study. *J Neurol Neurosurg Psychiatry* 1984; **47**: 1269–1273.
36. Snooks SJ, Badenoch DF, Tiptaft RC, Swash M. Perineal nerve damage in genuine stress urinary incontinence: an electrophysiologic study. *Br J Urol* 1985; **57**: 422–426.
37. Anderson RS. A neurogenic element to urinary genuine stress incontinence. *Br J Obstet Gynaecol* 1984; **91**: 41–45.
38. Varma JS, Fidas A, Mclnnes, Smith AN, Chisholm GD. Neurophysiologic abnormalities in genuine female stress urinary incontinence. *Br J Obstet Gynaecol* 1988; **95**: 705–710.
39. Snooks SJ, Swash M. Abnormalities of the innervation of the urethral striated sphincter musculature in incontinence. *Br J Urol* 1984; **56**: 401–405.
40. Smith ARB, Hosker GL, Warrell DW. The role of pudendal nerve damage in the aetiology of genuine stress incontinence in women. *Br J Obstet Gynaecol* 1989; **96**: 29–32.
41. Beevors MA, Lubowski DZ, King DW, Carlton MA. Pudendal nerve function in women with symptomatic utero-vaginal prolapse. *Int J Colorectal Dis* 1990; **6**: 24–28.
42. Smith ARB, Hosker GL, Warrell DW. The role of partial deveration of the pelvic floor in the aetiology of genitourinary prolapse and stress incontinence of urine. *Br J Obstet Gynecol* 1989; **96**: 24–28.
43. Kiff ES, Swash M. Slowed conduction in the pudendal nerves in idiopathic (neurogenic) faecal incontinence. *Br J Surg* 1984; **71**: 614–616.

44. Snooks SJ, Henry MM, Swash M. Faecal incontinence due to external anal sphincter division in childbirth is associated with damage to the innervation of the pelvic floor musculature: A double pathology. *Br J Obstet Gynaecol* 1985; **92**: 824–828.
45. Allen RE, Hosker GL, Smith ARB, Warrell DW. Pelvic floor damage and childbirth: A neurophysiologic study. *Br J Obstet Gynaecol* 1990; **97**: 770–779.
46. Snooks SJ, Swash M, Setchell M, Henry MM. Injury to innervation of pelvic floor sphincter musculature in childbirth. *Lancet* **9/8** 1984: 547–550.
47. Snooks SJ, Swash M, Henry MM, Setchell M. Risk factors in childbirth causing damage to the pelvic floor innervation. *Int J Colorect Dis* 1986; **1**: 20–24.
48. Sultan AH, Kamm MA, Hudson CN, Chir M, Thomas JM, Bartram CI. Anal-sphincter disruption during vaginal delivery. *N Engl J Med* 1993; **329**: 1905–1911.
49. Sultan AH, Kamm MA, Hudson CN. Pudendal nerve damage during labour: Prospective study before and after childbirth. *Br J Obstet Gynaecol* 1994; **101**: 22–28.
50. Benson JT, McClellan E. The effect of vaginal dissection on the pudendal nerve. *Obstet Gynecol* 1993; **82**: 387–390.
51. Zivkovic F, Tamussino K, Ralph G, Scheid G, Auer-Grumbach M. Long-term effects of vaginal dissection on the innervation of the striated urethral sphincter. *Obstet Gynecol* 1996; **87**: 257–260.
52. Zivkovic F, Ralph G, Schied G, Tamussino K. Die neurourodynamischen Folgen der vaginalen Kontinenzchirurgie. [Neuro-urodynamic sequelae of vaginal continence surgery]. *Gynakol Geburtshilfl Rundsch* 1994; **34**: 27–28.
53. Laurberg S, Swash M, Henry MM. Effect of postanal repair on progress of neurogenic damage to the pelvic floor *Br J Surg* 1990; **77**: 519–522.
54. Snooks SJ, Swash M. Perineal nerve and transcutaneous spinal stimulation: new methods for investigation of the urethral striated sphincter musculature. *Br J Urol* 1984; **56**: 406–409.
55. Snooks SJ, Swash M. Abnormalities of the innervation of urethral striated sphincter musculature in incontinence. *Br J Urol* 1984; **56**: 401–405.
56. Percy JP, Neill ME, Swash M, Parks AG. Electrophysiologic study of motor nerve supply of pelvic floor. *Lancet* 1981; **1/3**: 16–17.
57. Aubert A, Mosnier H, Amarenco G, Contou JF, Gallot D, Guivarc'h M, Malafosse M. Incontinences anales post-chirurgicales ou traumatiques: Étude prospective de 40 malades explores par echographie endorectale et electromyographie. [Post-surgical or traumatic anal incontinences: Prospective study in 40 patients explored by endo-rectal ultrasonography and electromyography]. *Gastroenterol Clin Biol* 1995; **19**: 598–603.
58. Roig JV, Villoslada C, Lledo S, Solana A, Buch E, Alos R, Hinojosa J. Prevalence of pudendal neuropathy in fecal incontinence: Results of a prospective study. *Dis Colon Rectum* 1995; **38**: 952–958.
59. Sangwan YP, Coller JA, Barrett RC, Murray JJ, Roberts PL, Schoetz DJ Jr. Distal rectoanal excitatory reflex: A reliable index of pudendal neuropathy? *Dis Colon Rectum* 1995; **38**: 916–920.
60. Rogers J, Laurberg S, Misiewicz JJ, Henry MM, Swash M. Anorectal physiology validated: A repeatability study of the motor and sensory tests of anorectal function. *Br J Surg* 1989; **76**: 607–609.
61. Vaccaro CA, Cheong DM, Wexner SD, Nogueras JJ, Salanga VD, Hanson MR, Phillips RC. Pudendal neuropathy in evacuatory disorders. *Dis Colon Rectum* 1995; **38**: 166–171.
62. Barrett JA, Brocklehurst JC, Kiff ES, Ferguson G, Faragher EB. Anal function in geriatric patients with faecal incontinence. *Gut* 1989; **30**: 1244–1251.
63. Laurberg S, Swash M. Effects of aging on the anorectal sphincters and their innervation. *Dis Colon Rectum* 1989; **32**: 737–742.
64. Vaccaro CA, Cheong DM, Wexner SD, Salanga VD, Phillips RC, Hanson MR. Role of

pudendal nerve terminal motor latency assessment in constipated patients. *Dis Colon Rectum* 1994; **37**: 1250–1254.

65. Jameson JS, Chia YW, Kamm MA, Speakman CT, Chye YH, Henry MM. Effect of age, sex and parity on anorectal function. *Br J Surg* 1994; **81**: 1689–1692.

66. Jorge JM, Wexner SD, Ehrenpreis ED, Nogueras JJ, Jagelman DG. Does perineal descent correlate with pudendal neuropathy? *Dis Colon Rectum* 1993; **36**: 475–483.

67. Strijers RL, Felt-Bersma RJ, Visser SL, Meuwissen SG. Anal sphincter EMG in anorectal disorders. *Electromyogr Clin Neurophysiol* 1989; **29**: 405–408.

68. Laurberg S, Swash M. The effects of aging on the anorectal sphincters and their innervation. *Dis Colon Rectum* 1989; **32**: 737–742.

69. Bischoff C, Machetanz J, Conrad B. Is there an age-dependent continuous increase in the duration of the motor unit action potential? *Electroencephalogr Clin Neurophysiol* 1991; **81**: 304–311.

70. Nandekar SD, Sanders DB. Recording characteristics of monopolar EMG electrodes. *Muscle Nerve* 1991; **14**: 108–112.

71. Siroky MB. Electromyogrpahy: needle. In: Johnson EW (ed). *Practical Electromyography*, 2nd edn. Baltimore, MD: Williams & Wilkins, 1982: 93–102.

72. Aminoff MJ. Clinical electromyography. In: Aminoff MJ (ed). *Electrodiagnosis in Clinical Neurology*, 2nd edn New York: Churchill Livingstone, 1986: 231–263.

73. Jabre JF. Concentric macro electromyography. *Muscle Nerve* 1991; **14**: 820–825.

74. Parks AG, Porter NH, Hardcastle J. The syndrome of the descending perineum syndrome. *Proc R Soc Med* 1966; **59**: 477–482.

75. Fowler CJ, Kirby RS, Harrison MJG, Milroy EJG, Turner-Warwick R. Individual motor unit analysis in the diagnosis of disorders of urethral sphincter innervation. *J Neurol Neurosurg Psychiatry* 1984; **47**: 637–641.

76. Wexner SD, Marchetti F, Salanga VD, Corredor C, Jagelman DG. Neurophysiologic assessment of the anal sphincters. *Dis Colon Rectum* 1991; **34**: 606–612.

77. Felt-Bersma RJ, Cuesta MA, Koorevaar M, Strijers RL, Meuwissen SG, Dercksen EJ, Wesdorp RI. Anal endosonography: Relationship with anal manometry and neurophysiologic tests. *Dis Colon Rectum* 1992; **35**: 944–949.

78. Roth G. Repetitive discharge due to self-ephaptic excitation of a motor unit. *Electroencephalogr Clin Neurophysiol* 1994; **93**: 1–6.

79. Allen RE, Warrell DW. The role of pregnancy and childbirth in partial denervation of the pelvic floor. *Neurourol Urodyn* 1987; **6**: 183–184.

80. Celichowski J, Grottel K, Rakowska A. Changes in motor unit action potentials during the fatigue test. *Acta Neurobiol Exp Warsz* 1991; **51**: 145–155.

81. Allen RE, Hosker GL, Smith ARB, Warrell DW. The role of pregnancy and childbirth in partial denervation of the pelvic floor – an update. *Neurourol Urodyn* 1993; **12**: 237–239.

82. Mallett V, Hosker G, Smith ARB, Warrell D. Pelvic floor damage and childbirth: A neurophysiologic follow up study. *Neurourol Urodyn* 1994; **13**: 357–358.

83. Werner RA, Albers JW. Relation between needle electromyography and nerve conduction studies in patients with carpal tunnel syndrome. *Arch Phys Med Rehabil* 1995; **76**: 246–249.

84. Engstrom JW, Olney RK. Quantitative motor unit analysis: The effect of sample size. *Muscle Nerve* 1992; **15**: 277–281.

85. Bertram MF, Nishida T, Minieka MM, Janssen I, Levy CE. Effects of temperature on motor unit action potentials during isometric contraction. *Muscle Nerve* 1995; **18**: 1443–1446.

86. Soderberg GL, Duesterhaus M, Nelson RM. A comparison of motor unit behaviour in young and aged subjects. *Age Ageing* 1991; **20**: 8–15.

87. Thorp JM Jr, Bowes WA, Droegemueller W, Wicker H. Assessment of perineal floor function. Electromyography with acrylic plug surface electrodes in nulliparous women. *Obstet Gynecol* 1991; **78**: 89–92.

88. Wall LL, Massey JM. Comment on Thorp JM Jr, Bowes WA, Droegemueller W, Wicker H. Assessment of perineal floor function: Electromyography with acrylic plug surface electrodes in nulliparous women. *Obstet Gynecol* 1991; **78**: 1149–1151.
89. Fuglevand AJ, Winter DA, Patla AE, Stashuk D. Detection of motor unit action potentials with surface electrodes: Influence of electrode size and spacing. *Biol Cybern* 1992; **67**: 143–153.
90. Bhullar HK. Loudon GH, Fothergill JC, Jones NB. Selective noninvasive electrode to study myoelectric signals. *Med Biol Eng Comput* 1990; **28**: 581–586.
91. Nandedkar SD, Sanders DB, Stålberg EV. Automatic analysis of the electromyographic interference pattern. Part I: Development of quantitative features. *Muscle Nerve* 1986; **9**: 431–439.
92. Nandedkar SD, Sanders DB, Stålberg EV. Simulation and analysis of the electromyographic interference pattern in normal muscle. Part II: Activity, upper centile amplitude, and number of small segments. *Muscle Nerve* 1986; **9**: 486–490.
93. Nandedkar SD, Sanders DB, Stålberg EV. Automatic analysis of the electromyogrpahic interference pattern. Part II: Findings in control subjects and in some neuromuscular diseases. *Muscle Nerve* 1986; **9**: 491–500.
94. Shafik A. Levator-urethral reflex: a new reflex with clinical applications. *Urology* 1990; **36**: 93–96.

CHAPTER 6

Radiologic investigation of the pelvic floor with regard to anatomic defects and prolapse

RENEE EDWARDS AND DEE E. FENNER

Imaging of the female pelvic floor has emerged as an important addition to the armamentarium in the evaluation of patients with urinary incontinence and pelvic organ prolapse. Early efforts that concentrated primarily on the bladder and posterior urethrovesical angle have given way to modalities that attempt to assess the pelvis as a whole with the knowledge that pelvic floor dysfunction rarely occurs in isolated compartments. In the patient who presents with a singular complaint of urinary incontinence or a vaginal bulge, it becomes the clinician's responsibility to assess all anatomic and functional aspects of the pelvic floor, including the bladder, urethra, vaginal apex, and rectum, along with the connective tissue and muscles that maintain their support.

Radiologic investigation is an important adjunct to the clinician's physical examination of the patient. In the woman who has never had pelvic surgery, physical examination alone may provide a clear determination of the defects that exist. However, in the patient who has had prior pelvic surgery, one should expect that the physical forces affecting the pelvis and its connective tissue supports will have been altered by that previous intervention. Radiologic imaging such as dynamic cystoproctography then becomes a precise tool for outlining the various components of a patient's prolapse. This type of imaging is also appropriately applied to the patient whose physical examination is unclear, whether due to unusual anatomy, suboptimal straining during examination, or findings not consistent with the patient's history. More recently, magnetic resonance imaging has emerged as a viewing modality for the muscles and connective tissue that support the pelvis.

Imaging studies have also gone beyond simply viewing anatomy to address pelvic floor function. Cystourethrograms or ultrasound imaging may disclose anatomic correlates to impaired function, such as bladder neck funneling in the patient with an intrinsically deficient urethral sphincter observed on urodynamic testing. Ultrasound imaging has also been advocated as a means of evaluating urethral mobility and levator ani contractility. Dynamic proctograms, in addition to outlining anatomy, provide insight into levator ani and rectal function.

CYSTOURETHROGRAPHY

Cystourethrography was introduced in 1937 as a means of evaluating the bladder neck and urethra in patients with urinary incontinence.[1] Lateral bead-chain cysto-urethrograms were later popularized by many authors[2–4] as a radiologic method for diagnosing and classifying stress-type urinary incontinence. Green,[2] whose study is most often cited, described type I incontinence as loss of the posterior urethrovesical angle to >115°. Type II incontinence also included vertical incli-nation of the urethral axis. These angles were believed to relate to the severity of a patient's incontinence and were used to help direct surgical management. However, this classification has not proven useful in the management of patients with incontinence due to poor correlation with urodynamic parameters.[5] Cystourethrography also showed significant overlap between incontinent patients and normal multiparous controls.[6,7] Wall and colleagues[8] were unable to find any definitive position of the bladder neck on lateral bead-chain cystourethrography that was associated with surgical correction of stress urinary incontinence.

Currently, the main clinical applications of cystourethrography in patients with urinary incontinence and pelvic organ prolapse are for the diagnosis of bladder neck funneling and cystocele. The procedure is performed by having the patient empty her bladder spontaneously. A transurethral catheter is then placed, and, after the bladder has been completely emptied of urine, radiopaque contrast is instilled to a volume of ~300 ml. The patient is either returned to a sitting position on a radiolucent commode or requested to stand. Resting and straining views are obtained in the lateral position. The catheter is removed. The patient is asked to cough several times. Leakage of contrast through the urethra documents stress-type incontinence. The patient is then asked to void, and a postvoid film is obtained to document complete bladder emptying.

If at any time during the course of the radiologic study the bladder contracts spontaneously, detrusor instability will be documented. It should be remembered, however, that the contrast medium may serve as an irritant to the bladder and thus provide false positive results or cause contractions at a lower volume than clinically symptomatic.

Bladder neck funneling may be seen on rest or strain films and will be evident as a loss of the distinct junction between the bladder neck and urethra. (Figure 6-1). This may be radiographic evidence for intrinsic urethral sphincteric deficiency and should be interpreted in the context of the patient's history and urodynamic findings. Normal physiologic funneling will be present immediately prior to a spontaneous or unstable detrusor contraction as the urethra relaxes with voiding. Therefore, it is important to make the diagnosis of bladder neck funneling when the detrusor is otherwise relaxed.

A bladder base which lies at rest or strain below the level of the inferior border of the pubic symphysis is defined as a cystocele. The size of the cystocele is determined by the strain film as it represents the maximum excursion of the bladder. (Figure 6-2).

Some centers employ video cystourethrography as a real-time visual

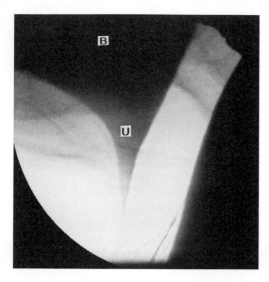

Figure 6-1. Bladder neck funneling. With the bladder filled to maximum capacity with contrast media, the bladder neck is noted to taper into the urethra. *B*, bladder; *U*, urethra.

evaluation of the bladder during multichannel urodynamic testing. Rather than sterile water, the bladder is filled with contrast media and the bladder, urethral and abdominal pressure transducers are placed as usual. This allows for documentation of detrusor instability both visually and via vesical transducers. Advocates of this testing also suggest that they can document urine leakage with stress incontinence more accurately as contrast is visualized the moment it enters the urethra from the bladder rather than relying on visual inspection of the external urethral meatus by the urodynamacist. This advantage must be weighed against the additional x-ray exposure to the patient as compared with urodynamics without fluoroscopic bladder imaging.

Voiding cystourethrograms are also used to evaluate many other conditions of the bladder and lower urinary tract. These include urethral diverticulum, urinary tract fistulas, vesicoureteral reflux, bladder stones, and tumors. Bladder diverticulum may also be identified.

DYNAMIC CYSTOPROCTOGRAPHY

Background

Defecography or dynamic proctography is an imaging technique that has been explored widely in the evaluation of anorectal function and anatomy, dating back to 1964.[9] However, its clinical usefulness as regards anorectal disorders has been questioned due to the wide range of "normal" findings seen even in asymptomatic subjects.[10–12]

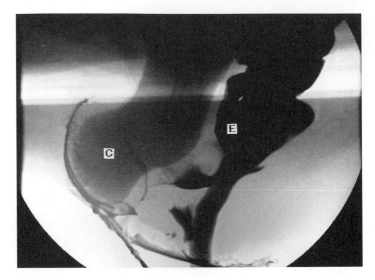

Figure 6-2.   Cystocele. The entire bladder is lying below the level of the inferior border of the pubic symphysis. This patient also has an enterocele. *C*, cystocele; *E*, enterocele.

The clinical utility of defecography has been expanded upon by the addition of bladder, small bowel, and vaginal opacification to outline pelvic support defects. Early work by Lash and Levin[13] revealed the importance of small bowel opacification in confirming the diagnosis of an enterocele. Further investigation first by Bethoux and colleagues[14] and subsequently by Lazarevski and colleagues[15] added the techniques of bladder and vaginal contrast media. This technique, referred to as dynamic fluoroscopic evaluation of the pelvic floor or dynamic cystoproctography has now been refined and reported upon by many authors.[16–18] The goal of this examination is to completely outline and define all pelvic floor hernial defects so that each may be addressed at the patient's operative setting.

Dynamic cystoproctography may be used as an adjunct to physical examination in any patient where it is desirable to image the sites and relative contributions of all pelvic organ hernias. This would include patients who have had prior pelvic surgery in whom the organs that comprise their prolapse may not be as predictable, patients with unusual vaginal prolapses or unclear physical examinations. Patients may not strain maximally during physical examination due to modesty or fear of leakage of bladder or bowel contents. Dynamic cystoproctography corrects for this problem by permitting full excursion of pelvic hernias during evacuation of contrast media. This imaging study is particularly useful in differentiating between the relative contribution of an enterocele as opposed to a rectocele in any given patient.

In those patients who complain of constipation, the usefulness of dynamic cystoproctography is further expanded upon by the addition of a transit study. A single commercially available capsule containing 24 radiopaque rings (Sitzmark™; Konsyl Pharmaceuticals, Fort Worth, TX) is ingested 5 days before the examination. This allows for a rough assessment of colonic motility[19] and investigates the possibility of "rectal trapping". Patients with symptomatic rectoceles frequently note a sensation of distal stool trapping or incomplete fecal emptying. They may additionally complain of needing to manually assist defecation with a hand in the vagina or on the perineal body to reduce a rectal bulge. The appearance of retained markers in the rectum confirms a clinically significant rectocele. However, markers distributed throughout the colon are more suggestive of a colonic motility disorder as the etiology of constipation[20] (Figure 6-3). Naturally, this would not be expected to resolve after the surgical reduction of a rectocele.

Technique

A prescription for a single Sitzmark (Konsyl Pharmaceuticals, Inc., Fort Worth, TX) capsule is given to the patient and she is requested to ingest this capsule 5

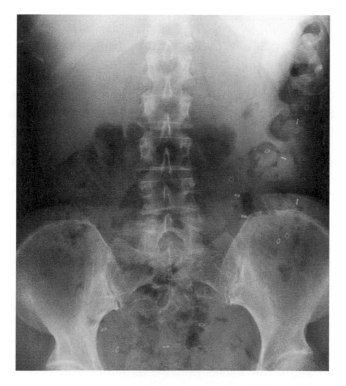

Figure 6-3. Abnormal colonic transit study. This patient ingested 24 radiopaque markers 5 days before this examination; 16 markers remain distributed through the descending colon and rectum, suggestive of a colonic motility disorder.

days before her scheduled examination, and she is further instructed not to use any laxatives or other bowel cathartics, as these would alter colonic transit time.

Upon arrival in the radiology department, a single AP view of the abdomen is obtained so that the number and location of retained markers can be evaluated. At least 80% of the markers should have been evacuated in the preceding days so that no more than five markers should be visible on the film.[19] The patient is then requested to drink two cups of dilute barium sulfate solution to opacify the small bowel. An additional AP view of the abdomen is obtained one hour later to confirm opacification.

The patient is then placed supine on the fluoroscopy table. After insertion of a 5 Fr transurethral catheter, the bladder is retrograde filled with ~300 ml of a commercially available water soluble contrast material. The patient is seated on a radiolucent commode and two lateral views of the pelvis are obtained. The first pictures the patient at rest and the second view is obtained with the patient straining. This evaluation is performed before filling the rectum with contrast material as this maneuver may artificially elevate the bladder base and create the appearance of bladder neck funneling.[16]

The patient is then returned to the supine position and the vagina is opacified with a barium powder that has been reconstituted to a thick paste. The rectum is filled with 30–50 ml of a high density barium suspension in a standard fashion. The patient is returned to the defecography commode. Lateral views are again obtained. The initial view is at rest and the patient is then requested to squeeze or voluntarily contract the pelvic floor. This allows for a functional assessment of the levator ani musculature as reflected by a "pulling up" of the pelvic floor or a measurable reduction in the anorectal angle (Figure 6-4). She is then asked to bear down maximally without releasing contrast material. This maneuver should result in relaxation of the pelvic floor musculature as manifested by a reduction in the anorectal angle.

The patient is then requested to empty all contrast material. The study is done with a digital photospot technique with three images per second recorded as a hard copy for later viewing. The entire study is videotaped so that dynamic films may be reviewed as necessary. The total radiation dose received is less than that of a lower GI evaluation. After the patient has emptied completely, an additional lateral view of the pelvis is obtained with the patient again straining maximally. This view typically reveals the maximum excursion of an enterocele. Because a bladder which has retained contrast material may impinge upon the full excursion of an enterocele by blocking its descent, if the patient is unable to empty her bladder in the x-ray suite, she is escorted to a washroom to void in private then returned to the suite for this final view (Figure 6-5).

This examination is well tolerated by patients, but it is imperative that it be performed by thoughtful personnel who respect the patient's privacy. The patient should be keep draped with a sheet from the waist down during the entire examination. Unnecessary personnel should not be allowed to wander in and out of the examination room and placement of all contrast material should be explained to the patient before its insertion. It is beneficial if the ordering physician briefly

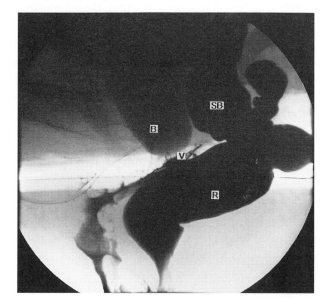

(a)

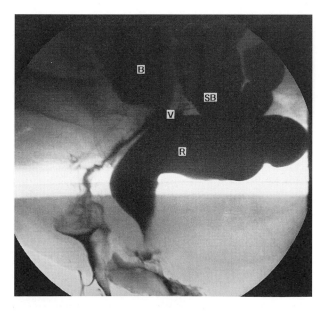

(b)

Figure 6-4. Levator ani function. (a): The patient's pelvic floor is at rest after filling the small bowel, bladder, vagina, and rectum with contrast material. (b): The patient has been asked to contract her pelvic floor. A functioning levator ani complex is demonstrated by a reduction in the anorectal angle. *B*, bladder; *V*, vagina; *SB*, small bowel; *R*, rectum.

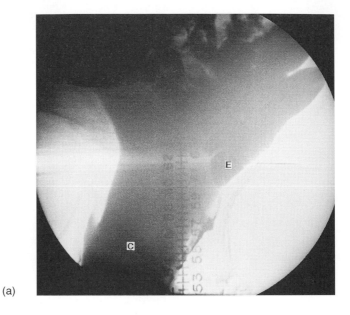

(a)

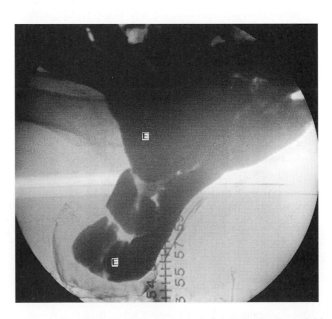

(b)

Figure 6-5. Enterocele "masked" by large cystocele. The full excursion of this patient's large enterocele, as seen in (b), was not appreciated until the large cystocele present in (a) was emptied. *C*, cystocele; *E*, enterocele.

explains the examination to the patient so that she knows what to expect when she arrives in the radiology department.

Evaluation of Defects; Anterior Wall

Information that may be obtained about the anterior vaginal wall from dynamic cystoproctography is much the same as that noted in cystourethrography. Bladder neck funneling, potentially suggestive of an incompetent urethral sphincter, may be seen on the views obtained after bladder opacification but before patient voiding. The existence and size of any cystocele is noted. Generally, a cystocele is thought to exist if the bladder extends below the level of the inferior border of the pubic symphysis. Measurements of the urethrovesical angle may be taken on the rest, squeeze and strain views if desired.

Vaginal Apex

Evaluation of the vaginal apex is one of the more useful components of the proctogram. Opacification of the small bowel helps to differentiate between simple uterine prolapse and true enterocele formation in the patient who presents with uterine descent on physical examination. In the woman who has previously undergone hysterectomy or other pelvic operative procedures, bowel opacification again aids in outlining the existence and extent of enterocele formation. This is particularly important as enteroceles have been missed on physical examination due to poor patient straining efforts or failure to evaluate patients in the standing position. They also may be mistaken for "high" rectoceles. At times an enterocele may be suspected on physical examination, but dynamic cystoproctography reveals apical bulging to consist entirely of a cystocele.

Another important finding when evaluating the vaginal apex or high posterior wall is the presence of a sigmoidocele. These are found in up to 5% of all dynamic proctograms,[21,22] and, on physical examination, may masquerade as an enterocele.

Currently, dynamic proctography is the only means of diagnosing a sigmoidocele, but they should be suspected in a patient with a history significant for constipation or difficult defecation and an enterocele on physical examination. A sigmoidocele is diagnosed when the leading edge of the sigmoid colon descends more than 4 cm below the pubococcygeal line (Figure 6-6). Clearly this is an important preoperative finding, as it may significantly alter a patient's operative plan and require the additional expertise of a colorectal surgeon.[22]

Posterior Wall

Evaluation of the posterior vaginal wall with defecography for a clinical diagnosis of rectocele is particularly useful when the patient complains of disordered

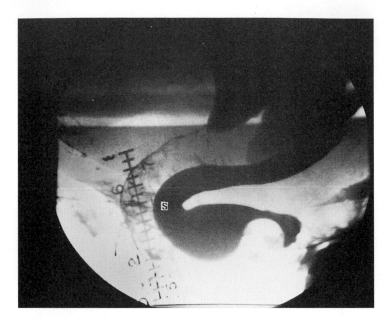

Figure 6-6.　Sigmoidocele. On physical examination, this patient had complete vault eversion. Dynamic cystoproctography revealed this prolapse to consist entirely of the proximal rectum and sigmoid colon. *S*, sigmoidocele.

defecation or needing to manually digitate to effect defecation. The appropriate diagnosis of a rectocele has long been a controversial area within gynecology as many nulliparous volunteers without defecatory complaints have been noted to have a rectocele upon flouroscopic examination.[10,12] Even the correct way to measure and diagnosis excursion of the anterior rectal wall when clearly viewed radiographically has varied among experts.[10,23,24]

Determining which rectoceles found on physical examination should undergo surgical repair may be aided by the radiographic findings coupled with the patient's history. Sitzmarkers retained in the distal rectum on the initial plain film of the abdomen suggest a significant rectocele as does barium retained at the conclusion of the proctogram (Figure 6-7). The clinician should be aware, however, that a large enterocele may "empty" a rectocele of contrast material as it slides down the rectovaginal septum, thus giving the false impression of a completely emptying rectum (Figure 6-8).

Current thinking attributes rectocele formation to a defect in the rectovaginal septum, most commonly seen as an avulsion of Denonviellers fascia from its attachment to the perineal body. Other fascial defects described include midline or lateral tears.[25] Retaining rectoceles on defecography typically have a "hockey puck" type appearance (Figure 6-7) that intraoperatively can be confirmed as a detachment of the rectovaginal septum. These may then be repaired simply by suturing the detached fascial edge to the perineal body.

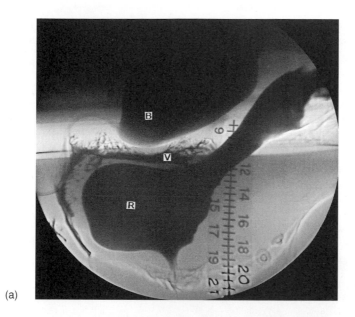

(a)

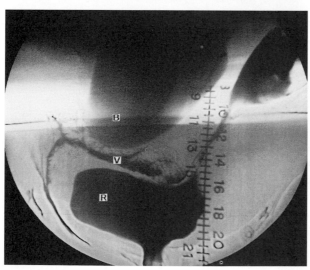

(b)

Figure 6-7. Rectocele; (a) straining; (b) post-evacuation. This rectocele became apparent as the patient emptied her rectum of contrast material. It has a classic "hockey puck" appearance. It retains a significant amount of contrast even after the patient reports that she has completely emptied. *R*, rectocele; *B*, bladder; *V*, vagina.

Rectoceles that form during the course of emptying the rectum of contrast material but do not retain contrast at the conclusion of the study are more difficult to interpret with an eye to surgical correction (Figure 6-9). In the symptomatic patient complaining of incomplete fecal emptying, they should be

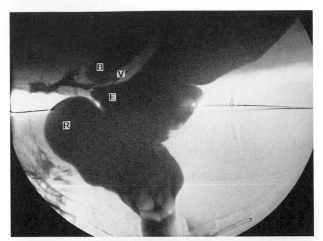

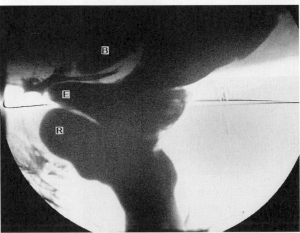

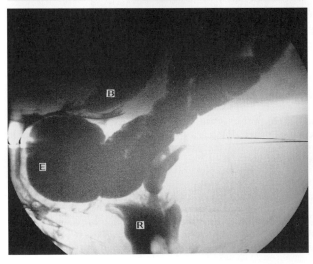

Figure 6-8. Enterocele emptying rectocele. This series of views demonstrates an enterocele that "empties" a large rectocele of contrast material. As the patient strains, the enterocele slides down the rectovaginal septum and compresses the rectum, potentially confusing the diagnosis of a rectocele. *E*, enterocele; *R*, rectocele; *B*, bladder; *V*, vagina.

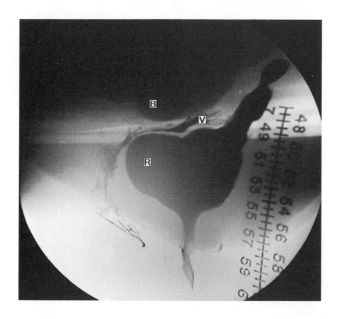

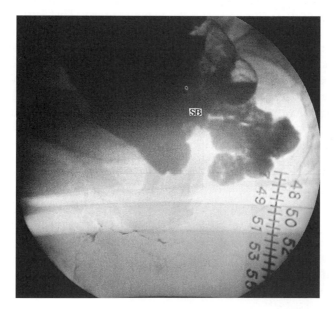

Figure 6-9. Rectocele that does not retain contrast material. This patient has a rectocele that forms during her cystoproctogram. However, by the conclusion of the study it has emptied completely of contrast material. Clinically, this patient presented with a complaint of fecal incontinence and was not noted to have a significant rectocele on physical examination. *R*, rectocele; *B*, bladder; *V*, vagina; *SB*, small bowel.

addressed. In the otherwise asymptomatic patient, they must be taken in context with the remainder of the patient's pelvic floor. A patient with a large cystocele that is "buttressing" the posterior vaginal wall may well return postoperatively with a clinically significant rectocele if this radiographically identified, but initially asymptomatic rectocele is not addressed at the initial operative setting.

Other Findings

Additional findings that may be discovered on a dynamic proctogram include disorders that not uncommonly accompany pelvic organ prolapse due to their similar risk factors for occurrence. These include rectal prolapse, rectal intussesseption, and a nonrelaxing puborectalis muscle in the patient complaining of severe constipation or defecatory disorder.

MAGNETIC RESONANCE IMAGING

Magnetic resonance imaging (MRI) has also been advocated as an adjunct to physical examination and a means of evaluating all pelvic floor hernias with one study.[26,27] Unlike dynamic cystoproctography, it has the advantage of also imaging the muscular and connective tissue supports of the pelvis.[28]

MRI, however, is performed with the patient supine. This is the least optimal position for examining a patient with pelvic organ prolapse. Additionally, the images obtained are static and therefore may not reflect the true extent of a dynamic condition such as incontinence or prolapse. Even "fast" MR imaging requires the patient to hold completely still for at least 6 seconds to avoid artifact in the final image.[26] Many patients are not able to hold a pelvic floor muscle contraction or maximal Valsalva for the length of time required to image their pelvic floor during these maneuvers. These restrictions limit MRI usefulness in the routine management of patients with urinary incontinence and urogenital prolapse.

Nevertheless, MRI does play an important role in continuing to advance our knowledge of both the normal and prolapsed female pelvic floor. Normal muscular and connective tissue support can be readily identified via MRI. This information can then be applied to those patients with prolapse and urinary incontinence to document the anatomic defects that may be leading to their symptoms. As DeLancey[29] has noted, it is important for pelvic surgeons to first understand normal pelvic floor anatomic support before commenting upon the defects that may lead to functional impairment.

ULTRASONOGRAPHY

Ultrasound imaging of the female pelvis is a technique with broad application across the field of obstetrics and gynecology. Multiple studies have now compared its results in the evaluation of urethral mobility in stress urinary incontinent patients to the traditional bead chain cystograms and Q-tip test. Ultrasound is also being used to image bladder-neck funneling. More recently, transurethral ultrasonography has given us additional insight into the anatomy of the urethra and its sphincter.

In the management of incontinent patients, abdominal ultrasound has largely been abandoned as improved technology has permitted clearer visualization of the urethra and bladder base with perineal and vaginal probes. Vaginal probes have been placed either at the level of the introitus just below the external urethral meatus[30] or just within the vagina. This allows for evaluation of UVJ mobility using the pubic symphysis as a fixed bony landmark.[31,32] Disadvantages of these techniques are largely related to the concern for probe impingement upon urethral mobility although many authors report comparable values obtained between measurements derived from cystourethrography and vaginal ultrasound.[31,33] This technique also would not be appropriate in the patient with a large cystocele where the UVJ may proceed beyond the pubic symphysis. An additional concern with vaginal ultrasonography when used concomitantly with urodynamic testing is the potential influence of the probe on urodynamic parameters. Beco and coworkers[34] and Wise and coworkers[35] both demonstrated increased urethral closure pressures with the probe in place.

Perineal ultrasound may be a better choice for sonographic evaluation of patients with urinary incontinence as the probe location does not interfere with UVJ mobility. It may be performed during urodynamic testing for real-time bladder and urethral observation without altering pressure measurements. It is also easier to perform in the upright patient position than introital or vaginal ultrasonography. A 3.5–5 MHz curved array probe is placed sagittally on the vulva.

Multiple authors have compared its use to lateral cystourethrography and found comparable values with respect to measurement of the posterior urethro-vesical angle and urethral mobility.[36–38] However, they suggest that perineal ultrasonography is preferred in that it is not invasion, simple to perform and does not require patient x-ray exposure. One major concern with the use of perineal ultrasound in the diagnosis of urethral hypermobility however, is a lack of standardization among reports as to the reference point for making these measurements.[39] The most common site is the inferior edge of the pubic symphysis with an excursion of 1 cm or more being considered excessive.[40–42]

Perineal ultrasound has also been compared to Q-tip assessment of urethral mobility by Caputo and Benson.[42] They question the validity of the Q-tip test as the Q-tip missed 75% of patients with hypermobility as documented by ultrasound imaging, yet incorrectly diagnosed hypermobility in 22% of patients with stable urethras. In this study, Q-tip testing was performed in the supine position while perineal ultrasound was performed with the patient sitting.

Bladder neck funneling during Valsalva or stress maneuvers may also be evaluated with perineal ultrasonography. Schaer and associates[43] commented that lateral cystourethrography maintained one advantage over perineal ultrasound as the contrast material outlining the UVJ allowed for more reliable diagnosis of urinary incontinence and bladder-neck funneling. Therefore, he added ultrasound contrast material to patients bladders and subsequently performed perineal ultrasonography. With this technique bladder-neck funneling was diagnosed in 38 of 39 stress-incontinent women performing a maximum Valsalva maneuver as compared to only 19 of 39 when perineal ultrasonography was performed without contrast material.

Finally, perineal ultrasound imaging provides a more complete overview of the pelvic floor, allowing for functional assessment of the musculature involved in bladder neck support. Wijma and colleagues[44] used perineal ultrasonography to observe levator ani contractility in continent and stress incontinent women. Both groups were able to elevate the UVJ with active contraction of the pelvic floor musculature. He additionally found no significant difference between UVJ descent with Valsalva maneuver in the two patient groups. However, in the stress incontinent group, fixation of the UVJ with coughing was lost as there was no contraction of the pelvic floor muscles to support it. Peschers and collaborators[45] have also demonstrated impairment of levator ani contractility postpartum via perineal ultrasonography.

Preliminary studies of intraurethral ultrasonography using a 20 MHz intravascular array probe in incontinent patients and controls have now been published.[46,47] Urethral circumference and surface area can be calculated along with

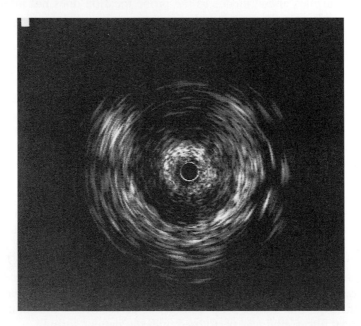

Figure 6-10.   Urethral ultrasound in patient without stress urinary incontinence by urodynamic testing. The hyperechoic band represents the urethral mucosa and submucosa, while the hypoechoic band represents the urethral skeletal muscle sphincter. (Photograph courtesy of Dr. Michael Heit, University of Louisville.)

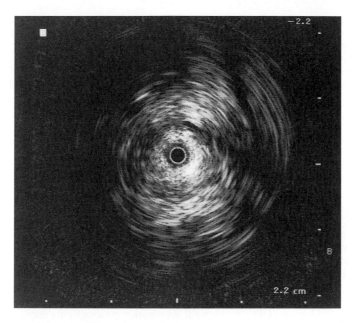

Figure 6-11. Urethral ultrasound imaging in patient with stress urinary incontinence by urodynamic testing. As compared to the previous image, the hypoechoic band representing the urethral sphincter has been significantly attenuated. (Photograph courtesy of Dr. Micheal Heit, University of Louisville.)

direct visualization of the anatomy of the urethral sphincter and its surrounding tissue. It is hoped that this technology may prove particularly useful in the evaluation of those patients with intrinsic sphincteric deficiency (Figures 6-10 and 6-11).

REFERENCES

1. Stevens WE, Smith SP. Roentgenological examination of the female urethra. *J Urol* 1937; **37**: 194–201.
2. Green TH Jr. Development of a plan for the diagnosis and treatment of urinary stress incontinence. *Am J Obstet Gynecol* 1962; **83**: 632–648.
3. Hodgkinson CP. Relationships of the female urethra and bladder in urinary stress incontinence. *Am J Obstet Gynecol* 1953; **65**: 560–573.
4. Jeffcoate TNA, Roberts H. Observation of stress incontinence of urine. *Am J Obstet Gynecol* 1952; **64**: 721–738.
5. Drutz HP, Shapiro BJ, Mandel F. Do static cystograms have a role in the investigation of female incontinence? *Am J Obstet Gynecol* 1978; **130**: 516–520.
6. Kitzmiller JL, Manzer GA, Nebel WA, Lucas WE. Chain cystourethrogram and stress incontinence. *Obstet Gynecol* 1972; **39**: 333–340.
7. Greenwald SW, Thronbury JR, Dunn LJ. Cystourethrography as a diagnostic aid in stress incontinence: An evaluation. *Obstet Gynecol* 1967; **29**: 324–327.

8. Wall LL, Helms M, Peattie AB, Pearce M, Stanton SL. Bladder neck mobility and the outcome of surgery for genuine stress urinary incontinence. *J Reprod Med* 1994; **39**: 429–435.
9. Burhenne HJ. Intestinal evacuation study: A new roentgenologic technique. *Radiol Clin* 1964; **33**: 79–84.
10. Shorvon PJ, McHugh S, Diamant NE, Somers S, Stevenson GW. Defecography in normal volunteers: Results and implications. *Gut* 1989; **30**: 1737–1749.
11. Goei R. Anorectal function in patients with defecation disorders and asymptomatic subjects: Evaluation with defecography. *Radiology* 1990; **174**: 121–123.
12. Goei R, van Engelshoven J, Schouten H, Baeten C, Stassen C. Anorectal function: Defecographic measurement in asymptomatic subjects. *Radiology* 1989; **173**: 137–141.
13. Lash AF, Levin B. Roentgenographic diagnosis of vaginal vault hernia. *Obstet Gynecol* 1962; **20**: 427–433.
14. Bethoux A, Bory S, Huguier M, Sheao SL. Le colpocystogramme. *J Chir (Paris)* 1965; **8**: 809–828.
15. Lazarevski M, Lazarov A, Novak J, Dimcevski D. Colpocystography in cases of genital prolapse and urinary stress incontinence in women. *Am J Obstet Gynecol* 1975; **122**: 704–716.
16. Kelvin FM, Maglinte DDT, Benson JT, Brubaker LP, Smith C. Dynamic cystoproctography: A technique for assessing disorders of the pelvic floor in women. *AJR* 1994; **163**: 368–370.
17. Kelvin FM, Maglinte DDT, Benson JT. Evacuation proctography (defecography): An aid to the investigation of pelvic floor disorders. *Obstet Gynecol* 1994; **83**: 307–314.
18. Brubaker LP, Retzky S, Smith C, Saclarides T. Pelvic floor evaluation with dynamic fluoroscopy. *Obstet Gynecol* 1993; **82**: 863–868.
19. Hinton JM, Lennard-Jones JE, Young AC. A new method for studying gut transit times using radioopaque markers. *Gut* 1969; **10**: 842–847.
20. Mezwa DG, Feczko PJ, Bosanko C. Radiologic evaluation of constipation and anorectal disorders. *Radiol Clin North Am* 1993; **31**: 1375–1393.
21. Jorge JMN, Yang Y, Wexner SD. Incidence and clinical significance of sigmoidoceles as determined by a new classification system. *Dis Colon Rectum* 1994; **37**: 1112–1117.
22. Fenner DE. Diagnosis and assessment of sigmoidoceles. *Am J Obstet Gynecol* 1996; **175**: 1438–1442.
23. Yoshioka K, Matsui Y, Yamada O, Sakaguchi M, et al. Physiologic and anatomic assessment of patients with rectocele. *Dis Colon Rectum* 1991; **34**: 704–708.
24. Kenton K, Brubaker L. Fluoroscopic rectal parameters during defecation: A study of rectocele formation. [Abstract]. *Int. Urogynecol J* 1995; **6**: 308.
25. Richardson AC. The rectovaginal septum revisited: Its relationship to rectocele and its importance in rectocele repair. *Clin Obstet Gynecol* 1993; **36**: 976–983.
26. Yang A, Mostwin JL, Rosenshein NB, Zerhouni EA. Pelvic floor descent in women: Evaluation with fast MRI imaging and cinematic display. *Radiology* 1991; **179**: 25–33.
27. Goodrich MA, Webb MJ, King BF, Bampton AEH, Campeau NG, Riederer SJ. Magnetic resonance imaging of pelvic floor relaxation: Dynamic analysis and evaluation of patients before and after surgical repair. *Obstet Gynecol* 1993; **82**: 883–891.
28. Strohbehn K, Ellis JH, Strohbehn JA, DeLancey JOL. Magnetic resonance imaging of the levator ani with anatomic correlation. *Obstet Gynecol* 1996; **87**: 277–285.
29. DeLancey JOL. Anatomy and biomechanics of genital prolapse. *Clin Obstet Gynecol* 1993; **36**: 897–909.
30. Koelbl H, Bernaschec G. A new method for sonographic urethrography and simultaneous pressure-flow measurements. *Obstet Gynecol* 1989; **74**: 417–422.

31. Mouritsen L, Strandberg C. Vaginal ultrasonography versus colpocystourethrography in the evaluation of female urinary incontinence. *Acta Obstet Gynecol Scand* 1994; **73**: 338–342.

32. Mouritsen L, Strandberg C, Moller MC. Bladder neck anatomy and mobility effect of vaginal probe. *Br J Urol* 1994; **74**: 749–752.

33. Mouritsen L, Rasmussen A. Bladder neck mobility evaluated by vaginal ultrasonography. *Br J Urol* 1993; **71**: 166–171.

34. Beco J, Leonard D, Lambotte R. Study of the artifacts induced by linear array transvaginal ultrasound scanning in urodynamics. *World J Urol* 1994; **12**: 329–332.

35. Wise BG, Burton G, Cutner A, Cardozo LD. Effect of vaginal ultrasound probe on lower urinary tract function. *Br J Urol* 1992; **70**: 12–16.

36. Koelbl H, Bernaschek G, Wolf G. A comparative study of perineal ultrasound scanning and urethrocystography in patients with genuine stress incontinence. *Arch Gynecol Obstet* 1988; **244**: 39–45.

37. Kohorn E, Scioscia AC, Jeanty P, Hobbins JC. Ultrasound cystourethrography by perineal scanning for assessment of female stress urinary incontinence. *Obstet Gynecol* 1986; **68**: 269–274.

38. Gordon D, Pearce M, Norton P, Stanton SL. Comparison of ultrasound and lateral chain urethrocystography in the determination of bladder neck descent. *Am J Obstet Gynecol* 1989; **160**: 182–185.

39. Demirci F, Fine PM. Ultrasonography in stress incontinence. *Int Urogynecol J* 1996; **7**: 125–132.

40. Johnson JD, Lamensdorf H, Hollander IN, Thurman AE. Use of transvaginal endosonography in the evaluation of women with stress urinary incontinence. *J Urol* 1992; **147**: 421–425.

41. Bergman A, Ballard CA, Platt LD. Ultrasonic evaluation of urethrovesical junction in women with stress urinary incontinence. *J Clin Ultrasound* 1988; **16**: 295–300.

42. Caputo RM, Benson JT. The Q tip test and urethrovesical junction mobility. *Obstet Gynecol* 1993; **82**: 892–896.

43. Schaer GN, Koechli OR, Schuessler B, Haller U. Improvement of perineal sonographic bladder neck imaging with ultrasound contrast medium. *Obstet Gynecol* 1995; **86**: 950–954.

44. Wijma J, Tinga DJ, Visser GHA. Perineal ultrasonography in women with stress incontinence and controls: The role of the pelvic floor muscles. *Gynecol Obstet Invest* 1991; **32**: 176–179.

45. Peschers U, Schaer GN, Anthuber C, DeLancey JOL, Schuessler B. Changes in vesical neck mobility following vaginal delivery. *Obstet Gynecol* 1196; **88**: 1001–1006.

46. Klein HM, Hermanns RK, Lagunilla J, Gunther R. Assessment of incontinence with intraurethral ultrasonography: Preliminary results. *Radiology* 1993; **187**: 141–142.

47. Hermanns RK, Klein HM, Muller U, Schafer W, Jakse G. Intraurethral ultrasound in women with stress incontinence. *Br J Urol* 1994; **74**: 315–318.

PART IV

GENUINE STRESS INCONTINENCE

CHAPTER 7

Nonsurgical management of genuine stress incontinence in women

KARL M. LUBER

As the demographics of developed nations change in favor of a more mature population, we see an increasing number of women affected by urinary incontinence. It is now estimated that over 13 million Americans suffer from urinary incontinence and that the cost of caring for this disease is in excess of $15 billion annually.[1] Historically, genuine stress incontinence, which represents over 50% of women with urinary incontinence, has been treated using one of over 200 described surgical techniques with variable success rates. Over the last decade, there has been increasing interest in the nonsurgical management of genuine stress incontinence. This is the result of the simultaneous recognition that surgical failure rates are higher than previously believed, ranging between 16% and 33% for retropubic and transvaginal procedures respectively, and that conservative management of women with genuine stress incontinence can provide symptomatic relief for a large percentage of women.[2–4] The cost of providing surgery, the morbidity associated with the surgery, and the recognition of higher surgical failure rates has challenged us to provide satisfactory alternatives to surgery in an ever-growing and better educated population of women with genuine stress incontinence. Advances in the nonsurgical management of genuine stress incontinence have made this task more complex but more satisfying as well.

Genuine stress incontinence is caused by a combination of poor urethral support, termed an extrinsic defect, and poor urethral function, termed an intrinsic defect. The degree of contribution of these two defects varies greatly within a population of women with genuine stress incontinence; patients with *hypermobility stress incontinence* have primarily a defect of support with lesser contribution from poor urethral function. Patients with *intrinsic sphincter deficiency* have primarily a defect of intrinsic urethral function with or without a defect of urethral support. It is, however, understood that even women with *hypermobility stress incontinence* have some component of poor urethral function. How else to explain the large number of women with urethrovesical junction hypermobility, that is, a support defect, who are entirely continent.[5] Thus, it is important that conservative management of women with genuine stress incontinence consider both extrinsic defects of support and intrinsic defects of function.

The techniques used to treat genuine stress incontinence nonsurgically can be grouped according to their mechanisms of action: those which address the extrinsic support defect and those which address the deficiency of intrinsic urethral function. More recently, a third group of treatments that obstruct the urethra have been introduced. These approaches compliment one another and should be combined to optimize improvement in a patient's symptoms. Women considering conservative management of genuine stress incontinence should also be given realistic expectations, remembering that incontinence is a quality of life issue and that patients may be satisfied without being objectively cured.

EXTRINSIC SUPPORT

The continence mechanism in women depends upon adequate support of the proximal urethra. This is provided by a hammock formed by the anterior vaginal wall and its lateral insertion into the pelvic muscles. Defects in this support mechanism allow descent of the proximal urethra under stress and thus allow urine to continue to move through the patent urethra resulting in the symptom of stress incontinence.[6] Nonsurgical techniques which serve to improve support of the proximal urethra have been shown to be effective means of treating genuine stress incontinence. These include improved pelvic muscle support and tone (through pelvic muscle rehabilitation) and intravaginal devices which help to stabilize the anterior vaginal wall and proximal urethra.

Pelvic Muscle Rehabilitation

In 1948, Dr. Arnold Kegel formalized the concept that exercising the muscles of the pelvis could improve or eliminate the symptoms of genuine stress incontinence in a large portion of women. The concepts he put forth included the need to assess and often teach pelvic muscle exercises, the need for immediate patient feedback during exercises for which he utilized a perineometer and the need for close follow-up and active encouragement. He reported a success rate of 84% with follow-up of 6 months in a large group of women.[7] Since then, many techniques of pelvic muscle rehabilitation have been introduced, including those in which exercises are done independently, those in which a form of resistance is used such as vaginal cones, and those in which biofeedback is used either by direct palpation, using pelvic muscle electrodes, or vaginal pressure devices. More recently, electrical stimulation of the pelvic muscles using a vaginal probe or *functional electrical stimulation*, has also been proposed. Although the methods are varied, the goals of these techniques of pelvic muscle rehabilitation remain the same; to improve the strength and the responsiveness of the muscles of the pelvis and thus provide improved support to the anterior vaginal wall and proximal urethra. The original concepts put forth by Kegel including assessment, teaching, feedback and encouragement remain the foundation of pelvic muscle rehabilitation. The efficacy and cost effectiveness of the different treatment modalities remains an area of lively debate.

Contraction of the muscles of the pelvic floor does not always come naturally. There are several studies which have demonstrated that simple verbal instruction of pelvic muscle contractions provided to patients may, at best, leave a percentage of patients not contracting the pelvic muscles well and at worse, may leave a significant portion of women performing a Valsalva maneuver rather than contracting the pelvic muscles.[8,9] Thus, it is imperative that one takes time to assess the patient's ability to contract the pelvic muscles. There are several subjective scales in use which may be adopted in a clinic or office setting to enhance consistency from patient to patient and visit to visit.[10] In patients who are unable to optimally contract their pelvic muscles, it is important to provide further instruction and enhancement. Without biofeedback, these patients lack an internal measure of pelvic muscle contraction and are unlikely to progress. Biofeedback is available in many forms which range from a single measurement of vaginal pressure or electromyographic (EMG) activity of the pelvic muscles to multimeasurement techniques which monitor pelvic muscle activity, abdominal muscle activity and detrusor muscle activity. There is evidence in the literature that biofeedback enhanced pelvic muscle rehabilitation is superior to nonenhanced pelvic floor contractions.[11] However, optimal technique and protocol have not been standardized.

As early as 1963, electrical stimulation of the pelvic muscles was being considered in the treatment of fecal and urinary incontinence[12] (Figure 7-1). A large body of basic science literature followed which supported the concept

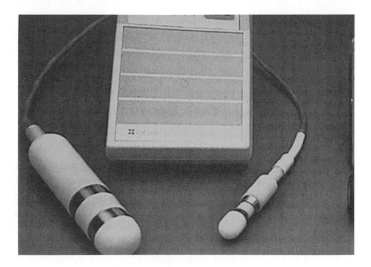

Figure 7-1. Functional electrical stimulation unit with vaginal and anal electrodes. (InCare Medical Products, Libertyville IL.)

and helped explain the presumed mechanism by which electrical stimulation improved continence.[13] Multiple noncontrolled clinical trials followed, many of which showed great promise.[14,15] More recently, several randomized clinical trials have demonstrated mixed results. Sand and colleagues[16] reported on a group of 52 women enrolled in a trial of electrical stimulation for genuine stress incontinence. Based upon improvement in both subjective and objective outcome measures, they concluded that electrical stimulation was effective in treating genuine stress incontinence. However, when cure was considered, there was no difference noted between the treated and control groups. Additionally, the drop out rate in the treated group was four fold that of the control group and this was not considered in the final analysis. More recently, Brubaker and coworkers[17] and Luber and Wolde-Tsadik[18] reported on similar trials with no significant difference in success rate observed between the treatment and control population. Combined, these studies indicate that there is much to learn regarding electrical stimulation. Many practitioners specializing in pelvic muscle rehabilitation feel that electrical stimulation is an excellent tool to facilitate pelvic muscle contraction in patients otherwise unable to contract their pelvic muscles. Few, however, feel that it should be used as a stand alone therapy for genuine stress incontinence. Modifications in stimulation protocol and device parameters may alter the role of electrical stimulation in the future.

The exact mechanism by which pelvic muscle rehabilitation improves genuine stress incontinence symptoms is not completely understood. The striated musculature of the pubococcygeus and puborectalis muscles as well as that of the intrinsic urethral sphincter must be considered. It is important to recall the composition of the pelvic muscles and general rules of muscle rehabilitation when counseling patients and developing a pelvic muscle exercise protocol. The pelvic muscles represent a heterogenous mixture of both long-acting (type I) and short-acting (type II) muscle fibers. Thus, a regimen in which long contractions, ideally for ≥ 10 seconds, followed by a series of short bursts of activity or "quick flicks" should be followed by a rest of ~20 seconds. Like all muscle groups, the pelvic muscles are prone to fatigue when initially exercised. For that reason, patients should be warned that their pelvic muscles may feel uncomfortable afterward and that this may extend to discomfort with coitus.

Along with consideration of muscle type and fatigue, we must consider the duration of therapy and patient compliance. In Bo's excellent review article[11] of pelvic muscle exercises, she found that protocols in which the exercise period was <5 months often reported poor outcomes. She also notes that close patient contact and follow-up are essential. With a well-considered protocol, close follow-up, encouragement, adequate duration of treatment, and biofeedback enhancement when indicated, 60–70% of patients with genuine stress incontinence can expect a good response from pelvic muscle rehabilitation.[4,19,20] As with all muscle groups, consistent exercise of the pelvic muscles is necessary for long-term maintenance of gains.

Vaginal Support Devices

When a woman places a vaginal tampon or support pessary, the anterior vaginal wall is often less mobile thus providing better support to the proximal urethra. Indeed, in some women, this will be associated with less stress incontinence.[21,22] As a result, several pessarylike devices have been developed for the specific purpose of treating genuine stress incontinence by mechanically improving the support of the anterior vaginal wall. Preliminary results with these devices are promising. In an uncontrolled trial using the Introl bladder-neck prosthetic device (Johnson and Johnson, Dallas, TX), an 83% cure rate was observed in a population of 32 women with genuine stress incontinence[23] (Figure 7-2). Urodynamic parameters mimicked those of women having had a colposuspension. Experience with the incontinence ring (Milex, New York, NY) has demonstrated similar results. Not all women can be comfortably fitted with these devices and poor introital support or concomitant pelvic organ prolapse can make it difficult to retain the device. However, in those women able and willing to utilize these devices, a symptomatic improvement rate in excess of 50% can be anticipated. Once an initial in-office fitting of the device has been done, it is important that patients be educated regarding the use of these intravaginal devices. This can be facilitated through well-trained nursing personnel. Likewise, as with any vaginal pessary, vaginal estrogen cream is recommended to enhance the resiliency of the vaginal mucosa and prevent vaginal erosions. Although there is a theoretical risk of voiding difficulties with the vaginal incontinence devices in place, this has not been observed to a significant degree in clinical trials.

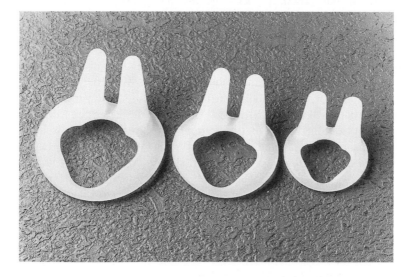

Figure 7-2. Introl bladder neck prosthetic device. (Johnson and Johnson, Dallas, TX.)

INTRINSIC URETHRAL FUNCTION

Although surgical treatment of women with genuine stress incontinence focuses on the correction of the support of the urethra, recent evidence suggests that women with genuine stress incontinence have compromise of their intrinsic urethral function as well. The evidence that so many women in whom hypermobility is appreciated are continent of urine forces us to consider what distinguishes the incontinent woman with hypermobility from a woman with hypermobility but no incontinence.[5] Women with hypermobility stress incontinence have been demonstrated to have an increase in the pudendal motor terminal latency when compared to continent controlled subjects.[24] There is also a subset of women in whom profound stress incontinence occurs despite excellent urethral support, the result of marked compromise of intrinsic urethral function. In light of this evidence, it is impossible to consider hypermobility stress incontinence a defect of external urethral support alone. Treatment of genuine stress incontinence, with or without hypermobility, should consider treatments that improve intrinsic urethral function as complementary to other modalities that address urethral support. Currently available treatments to improve urethral function are primarily pharmacologic and include alpha agonists and estrogen. The role of pelvic muscle exercises in improving intrinsic urethral striated muscle tone is not clear; there is evidence that pelvic muscle exercises benefit intrinsic urethral function as well as the levator ani muscle groups.[20,25]

The urethra is sensitive to both estrogen and progesterone. An absence of estrogen or an excess of progesterone may have a detrimental effect upon urethral function.[26–28] Progesterone should be considered in the evaluation of women with urinary incontinence who are using progestational-based contraceptive methods such as Depo Provera and Norplant. This is particularly important if these patients have initiated a progestational-based contraceptive method immediately postpartum. Treating their incontinence may involve discontinuing progesterone. Likewise, the absence of estrogen should be considered in all postmenopausal and nonmenstruating women.

The theoretical benefit of estrogen is logical given the similar embryologic origin of the distal vagina and urethra.[29] However, evidence regarding the benefit of estrogen in treating women with genuine stress incontinence is inconclusive. While studies by Wilson and colleagues[30] and Walter and colleagues[31] have demonstrated a subjective improvement in stress symptoms in women receiving estrogen therapy, Sansioe and colleagues[32] failed to show any difference between treatment and placebo groups. In 1994, Fantl and associates[33] reviewed 17 uncontrolled trials along with 6 randomized clinical trials. Using standard meta-analytical techniques they concluded that a subjective benefit was realized using estrogen treatment over placebo. More recently, Fantl and associates[34] reported on a randomized clinical trial of 83 postmenopausal women with genuine stress incontinence treated with cyclic hormone replacement therapy in which no improvement in clinical or quality of life parameters was realized for the estrogen treatment group over the control group. In this article, Fantl and colleagues queried the potential contribution of progesterone to the lack of clinical efficacy. The use of estrogen therapy in women with genuine stress incontinence remains a standard treatment until more definitive data is available.

Urethral function is also mediated by alpha adrenergic stimulation of smooth muscle within the proximal urethra.[35,36] This provides the theoretical basis for using alpha adrenergic stimulants to treat genuine stress incontinence. Like estrogen, studies using alpha-adrenergic stimulation to treat women with genuine stress incontinence have demonstrated mixed results. Phenylpropanol-amine represents the prototype alpha agonist and is most commonly used in doses of 25–100 mg b.i.d. There are seven randomized, controlled trials in which phenylpropanolamine was used to treat genuine stress incontinence. These studies demonstrate subjective improvement in between 19% and 60% of patients with three studies reporting cures in a small minority of patients (9–14%).[31,37–42] Given a subjective response rate of between 19% and 60% and the low incidence of side effects, alpha-adrenergic agonists should be considered in treating women with genuine stress incontinence nonsurgically. The recommended dosage of 75 mg of phenylpropanolamine is available in many prescription upper respiratory infection preparations as well as over the counter diet pills. Relative contraindications to alpha adrenergic agonists include hypertension, coronary artery disease, and dysrhythmias. Studies have demonstrated no risk of hypertension in the majority of women using alpha-agonists. However, it appears that a subset of women will respond with an elevated blood pressure and therefore, all women using alpha-agonists should have their blood pressure checked for several weeks following initiation of therapy.

Conversely, women using alpha antagonistic preparations to treat their hypertension may see their symptoms of stress incontinence improve when these agents are discontinued. Both Dwyer and coworkers[43] and Wall and Addison[44] demonstrated this in a small series of women. Thus, women using alpha-antagonistic agents to control hypertension may consider an alternative antihypertensive regimen in the face of genuine stress incontinence.

OBSTRUCTIVE DEVICES

The techniques discussed thus far all have their effect by improving the native continence mechanism through enhancing urethral support and function. It may, however, be possible to offer therapy for incontinence which ignores the native continence mechanism and seeks only to obstruct the urethra between voiding episodes. Such temporary obstruction may be accomplished at either the level of the internal urethral meatus or the external urethral meatus. Several devices are available that attempt to serve this function.

Obstruction at the level of the internal urethral meatus could theoretically be accomplished by placing a Foley catheter-like balloon at the level of the internal meatus and holding it stably in place. The Reliance device (Uromed, Deedham,

MA) is a 14 Fr molded, thermoplastic elastomer catheter with a small balloon at its proximal end and a soft tab at the distal end to stabilize the device upon the external meatus (Figure 7-3). The device is intended to be placed by the patient following a void and removed at the time of the next void using a small string which permits deflation of the balloon. The device is specifically designed for single use and a new device is placed after voiding if so desired. Short-term clinical studies indicate that over a 4-month trial, 37% of patients discontinued device use for a variety of reasons. Objective assessment of those remaining in the study at 4 months demonstrated no loss of urine in 80% of the patients. Urinary tract infections and hematuria occurred frequently in the study population but did not necessitate discontinuation of device use.[45]

Obstruction at the level of the external urethral meatus has been proposed by the developers of several devices. The Mini shield (Uromed, Deedham, MA) is a self-applied adhesive patch which is placed directly over the external urethral meatus between voids. The Fem Assist (Insight Medical, Bolton, MA) is similarly applied but depends upon a negative pressure created by the device to remain in place. Initial trials with the Mini shield were encouraging with 85% of patients reporting good tolerance of the device and 82% of the patients remaining in the trial reporting subjective improvement, with 46% reporting that they were completely dry.[46]

The relative usefulness of obstructive devices to care for urinary incontinence as compared to other nonsurgical techniques is not clear. The long-term risks of such devices on urethral function have not been defined. Additional clinical trials and patient experience will help us better understand the role of such obstructive devices in our armamentarium of nonsurgical techniques.

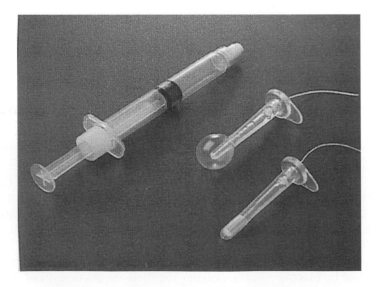

Figure 7-3.   The Reliance device. (Uromed, Deedham, MA.)

CONCLUSIONS

Women with genuine stress incontinence who wish to pursue nonsurgical management have an expanding array of options. These include improved urethral support using pelvic muscle rehabilitation or intravaginal support devices, improved urethral function through the elimination of detrimental medications and the addition of beneficial prescriptions such as estrogen and alpha-agonists, and possibly the use of obstructive devices. The use of nonsurgical techniques to help women with genuine stress incontinence does not preclude surgery. It does, however, select a population of women who may be satisfactorily treated without being exposed to the risks and costs of surgery. Given the large and expanding population of women with genuine stress incontinence and the finite success achieved through surgery, it is appropriate to consider nonsurgical management first in all women with genuine stress incontinence.

REFERENCES

1. Fantl JA, Newman DK, Colling J, et al. *Urinary Incontinence in Adults: Acute and Chronic Management. Clinical Practice Guidelines.* No. 2, 1996 Update. Rockville, MD: U.S. Department of Health and Human Services. Public Health Service. Agency for Health Care Policy and Research. AHCPR Publication No. 96–0682. March 1996.
2. Alcalay M, Ash M, Stanton SL. Burch colposuspension: A 10–20 year follow-up. *Br J Obstet Gynecol* 1995; **102**: 740–745.
3. Leach G, Appell R, Blaivas J, et al. The surgical treatment of female stress urinary incontinence. *Urology* 1997; **158**: 875–880.
4. Dougherty M, Bishop K, Mooney R, Gimotty P, Williams B. Graded pelvic muscle exercise: Effect on stress urinary incontinence. *J Reprod Med* 1993; **39**: 684–691.
5. Walters MD, Diaz K. Q-Tip Test: A study of continent and incontinent women. *Obstet Gynecol* 1987; **70**: 208–211.
6. Delancey JOL. Structural support of the urethra as it relates to stress urinary incontinence: The hammock hypothesis. *Am J Obstet Gynecol* 1994; **170**: 1713–1723.
7. Kegel AH. A progressive resistance exercise in the functional restoration of the perineal muscles. *Am J Obstet Gynecol* 1948; **56**: 238–248.
8. Bump RC, Hertz WG, Fantl A, et al. Assessment of Kegel pelvic exercise after brief verbal instruction. *Am J Obstet Gynecol* 1991; **165**: 322–329.
9. Bo K, Larsen S, Oseid S, et al. Knowledge about and ability to correct pelvic floor muscle exercises in women with urinary stress incontinence. *Neurourol Urodyn* 1988; **73**: 261–262.
10. Wall LL, Norton PA, DeLancey JOL. In: Wall LL, Norton PA, DeLancey JOL (eds) *Conservative Management of Stress Incontinence in Practical Urogynecology.* Baltimore: Williams and Wilkins, 1993.
11. Bo K. Pelvic floor muscle exercise for the treatment of stress urinary incontinence: An exercise physiology perspective. *Int Urogynecol J* 1995; **6**: 282–291.
12. Caldwell K. The electrical control of sphincteric incontinence. *Lancet* 1963; **2**: 174–175.
13. Fall M, Erlandson BE, Carlson CA, et al. The effect of intravaginal electrical stimulation on the feline urethra and urinary bladder: Neuronal mechanisms. *Scand J Urol Nephrol Suppl* 1977; **44**: 19–30.

116 *Genuine stress incontinence*

14. Ericksen BC, Eik-Nes SH. Long term electrical stimulation of the pelvic floor: Primary therapy in female stress incontinence? *Urol Int* 1989; **44**: 90–95.
15. Fall M, Ahlstrom K, Carlsson CA, et al. Contelle: Pelvic floor stimulator for female stress-urge incontinence. *Urology* 1986; **17**: 282–287.
16. Sand PK, Richardson DA, Staskin DR, et al. Pelvic floor electrical stimulation in the treatment of genuine stress incontinence: A multicenter placebo-controlled trial. *Am J Obstet Gynecol* 1995; **173**: 72–79.
17. Brubaker L, Benson JT, Clark A. Transvaginal electrical stimulation is effective for the treatment of detrusor overactivity. *Proceedings of the American Urogynecologic Society, September 1996.*
18. Luber KM, Wolde-Tsadik G. The efficacy of functional electrical stimulation in treating genuine stress incontinence: A randomized clinical trial. *Int Urogynecol J* 1995; **6**: 302.
19. Ferguson K, McKey PL, Bishop KR, et al. Stress urinary incontinence: Effect of pelvic muscle exercise. *Obstet Gynecol* 1990; **73**: 671–675.
20. Benvenuti F, Caputo GM, Bandinelli S, et al. Re-educative treatment of female genuine stress incontinence. *Am J Phys Ther* 1987; **66**: 155–168.
21. Bhatia NN, et al. Urodynamic effects of a vaginal pessary in women with stress urinary incontinence. *Am J Obstet Gynecol* 1983; **147**: 876–884.
22. Nygaard IE, et al. Treatment of exercise incontinence with a vaginal pessary: A preliminary study. *Int Urogynecol J* 1993; **4**: 133–137.
23. Davila GW, Ostermann KV. The bladder neck support prosthesis: A nonsurgical approach to stress incontinence in adult women. *Am J Obstet Gynecol* 1994; **171**: 206–211.
24. Snooks SJ, Swash M, Henry MM, et al. Risk factors in childbirth causing damage to the pelvic floor innervation. *Int J Colorectal Dis* 1986; **1**: 20–24.
25. Bo K, Hagan RM, Kvarstein B, et al. Pelvic floor muscle exercises for the treatment of female Stress urinary incontinence III. Effects of two different degrees of pelvic floor muscle exercises. *Neurourol Urodyn* 1990; **9**: 489–502.
26. Benness C, Abbot D, Cardozo L, et al. Do progestogens exacerbate urinary incontinence in women on HRT? *Neurourol Urodyn* 1991; **10**: 316–317.
27. Ioseph CS, Batraa SC, EK A, et al. Estrogen receptors in the human female lower urinary tract. *Am J Obstet Gynecol Scand* 1981; **141**: 817–820.
28. Ingelman-Sundberg A, Rosen J, Gustafsson SA, et al. Cytosol estrogen receptors in the urogenital tissues in stress incontinent women. *Acta Obstet Gynecol Scand* 1981; **60**: 585–586.
29. Zuckerman S. The histogenesis of tissues sensitive to estrogens. *Biol Rev* 1940; **15**: 231–271.
30. Wilson PD, Faragher B, Butler B, et al. Treatment with oral piperazine and oestrone sulphate for genuine stress incontinence in postmenopausal women. *Br J Obstet Gynaecol* 1987; **94**: 568–574.
31. Walter S, Kjaergaard B, Lose G, et al. Stress urinary incontinence in postmenopausal women treated with oral estrogen (Estriol) in an alpha adrenoceptor stimulating agent (phenylpropanolamine): A randomized double-blind placebo controlled study. *Int Urogynecol J* 1990; **1**; 74–79.
32. Sansioe G, Jansson I, Mellstrom D, et al. Occurrence, nature and treatment of urinary incontinence in a 70-year old female population. *Maturitas* 1985; **7**: 335–342.
33. Fantl JA, Cardozo L, McClish DK. Hormones and urogenital therapy committee.' Estrogen therapy in the management of urinary incontinence in postmenopausal women: A meta analysis: First report of the Hormones in Urogenital Therapy Committee. *Obstet Gynecol* 1994; **83**: 12–18.
34. Fantl JA, Bump RC, Robinson D, et al. Efficacy of estrogen supplementation in the treatment of urinary incontinence. *Obstet Gynecol* 1996; **88**: 745–749.
35. EK A, Alm P, Andersson KE, et al. Adrenergic and cholinergic nerves of the human

urethra and urinary bladder. A histochemical study. *Acta Physiol Scand* 1977; **90**: 345–352.

36. Gosling JA, Dixon J, Lendon RJ. The autonomic innervation of the human male and female bladder neck and proximal urethra. *J Urol* 1977; **118**: 302–305.

37. Colste L, Lindskog M. Phenylpropanolamine in treatment of female stress urinary incontinence: A double blind placebo-controlled study in 24 patients. *Neurourol Urodyn* 1987; **30**: 398–403.

38. EK Á, Andersson KE, Gullberg B, et al. The effects of long term treatment with norephedrine on stress incontinence and urethral closure pressure profile. *Scand J Urol Nephrol* 1978; **12**: 105–110.

39. Fossberg E, Beisland HO, Lundgren RA. Stress incontinence in females: Treatment with phenylpropanolamine: A urodynamic and pharmacologic evaluation. *Urol Int* 1983; **38**: 293–299.

40. Hilton P, Tweddell AL, Mayne C. Oral and intravaginal estrogens alone and in combination with alpha adrenergic stimulation in genuine stress incontinence. *Int Urogynecol J* 1990; **1**: 80–86.

41. Lehtonen T, Rannikko S, Lindel O, et al. The effect of phenylpropanolamine on female stress urinary incontinence. *Ann Chir Gynaecol* 1986; **75**: 236–241.

42. Wells T, Brink C, Diokno A, et al. Pelvic muscle exercise for stress urinary incontinence in elderly women. *J Am Geriatr Soc* 1991; **39**: 785–791.

43. Dwyer PL, Tweele JS. Prazosin: A neglected cause of genuine stress incontinence. *Obstet Gynecol* 1992; **79**: 117–121.

44. Wall LL, Addison WA. Prazosin-induced stress incontinence. *Obstet Gynecol* 1990; **75**: 558–560.

45. Staskin D, Babendam T, Miller J, et al. Effectiveness of a urinary control insert in the management of stress urinary incontinence: Early results of a multicenter study. *Urology* 1996; **47**: 629–636.

46. Harris T, Gleason D, Diokno, et al. External urethral barrier for urinary stress incontinence: A multi-center trial. *Neurourol Urodyn* 1994; **13**: 381–382.

CHAPTER 8

Anterior compartment prolapse, urinary incontinence, and the effects of anterior colporrhaphy and paravaginal repair

SANDRA R. VALAITIS ───────────────────────────────

Genitourinary prolapse and urinary incontinence are common problems, but the etiology of these conditions remains unclear. It is estimated that approximately 400,000 surgical procedures have been described for the treatment of prolapse and it is easy to imagine the cost, both medically and in terms of time off work, that these operations necessitate.[1] Urinary incontinence may occur with or without prolapse and it is estimated that over 15 billion dollars (>2% of total healthcare costs) are spent annually in managing this condition.[2] Because of these estimates, a great deal of research has been undertaken to better understand the causes and ascertain the prevention of these conditions.

Within the anterior compartment of the vagina lies the bladder, urethra, uterus, and supportive connective tissue ligaments and muscles that maintain the correct anatomic position of these structures. This chapter focuses on the anatomic relationships in normal support, and in cases of prolapse and urinary incontinence. It also describes some of the risk factors thought to be related to the development of these conditions. Finally, it describes the means of identifying associated anatomic defects and surgical procedures performed to treat these common clinical problems.

ANATOMY OF PELVIC SUPPORT

Intimate structural relationships of the organs and tissues in the anterior compartment of the vagina help maintain the position of the bladder, urethra, uterus, and vagina. In turn, the anatomic associations between these organs help to preserve the continence mechanism. Prolapse and urinary incontinence result from displacement of the pelvic organs from their original anatomic position through rupture or denervation of connective tissue supports.[3,4] Therefore, before attempts at surgical correction of prolapse or urinary incontinence are made, it is important to identify the structural and physiologic defects that lead to the development of these conditions.

The vagina, cervix, and urethra are held in place by varying connective tissue supports. Proceeding in a proximal to distal direction, there are three different levels of support that attach these organs to adjacent structures (Figure 8-1).[5] The most proximal portion (level I) suspends the vaginal apex and cervix to the pelvic wall. This connective tissue complex consists of the uterosacral and cardinal ligaments which are made up of neurovascular and fibrous connective tissue. Damage to these supports leads to descent of the vaginal apex, uterine and vaginal vault prolapse, and enterocele formation. The second level of support (level II) is found in the midvagina, and is made up of connective tissue attachments of the endopelvic fascia to the arcus tendineus fasciae pelvis and the superior fascia of the levator ani. Damage to these supportive structures anteriorly results in cystocele formation. This can be differentiated into two components: central and lateral or paravaginal defects. Defects in the endopelvic fascia in the central portion of level II result in formation of a distention cystocele (Figure 8-2).[7] This can be repaired with anterior colporrhaphy. Lateral detachments of the endopelvic fascia to the arcus tendineus fasciae result in paravaginal defects, or a displacement cystocele, which can be repaired with a

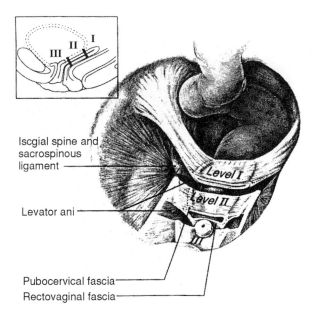

Figure 8-1. Level I (suspension) and level II (attachment). In level I the paracolpium suspends the vagina from the lateral pelvic walls. Fibers of level I extend both vertically and also posteriorly toward the sacrum. In level II, the vagina is attached to the arcus tendineus fasciae pelvis and superior fascia of levator ani. (From DeLancey JOL. Anatomic aspects of vaginal eversion. *Am J Obstet Gynecol* 1993; **166**: 1717, with permission.)

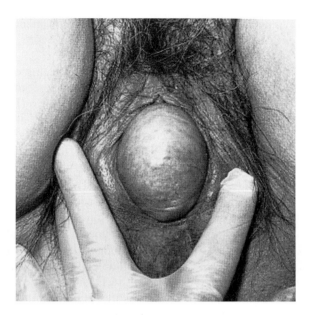

Figure 8-2   Distension cystocele. Note the relative lack of rugal folds. (From reference 8, permission sought.)

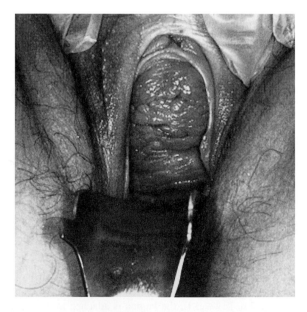

Figure 8-3.   Displacement cystocele. Note obliteration of the urethrovesical crease in the vagina. (From reference 8, permission sought.)

paravaginal repair (Figure 8-3).[9] Distally, the vagina and urethra are held in place by the endopelvic fascia which attaches to the arcus tendineus fasciae pelvis and medial fascia of the levator ani. Defects in this area result in urethrocele formation, bladder neck hypermobility, and genuine stress incontinence.

The levator ani muscles and connective tissue ligaments work together to support the pelvic organs. The levator ani muscles (pubococcygeus, iliococcygeus, and puborectalis) form a supportive diaphragm that elevates these organs. DeLancey[10] describes the phenomenon of a "ship . . . floating on the water attached by ropes on either side to a dock (Figure 8-4)". In this analogy the ship is representative of the pelvic organs, the water, of the levator ani, and the ropes, of the endopelvic fascia and connective tissue supports. If the level of water decreases below the ship's hull, all of the support of the ship would rest on the ropes and eventually the load would cause the ropes to break. Such is the support provided by the levator ani. With weakening of this pelvic diaphragm more tension is placed on the connective tissue supports to hold the pelvic structures in place, and once this load becomes too great, rupture occurs with lengthening or detachment of the ligaments. This is followed by prolapse and possibly urinary incontinence. This phenomenon has been described by Klutke and colleagues[11] who utilized magnetic resonance imaging (MRI) to assess differences in pelvic support in women with and without stress urinary incontinence. They found defects in the musculofascial attachments of the urethra and

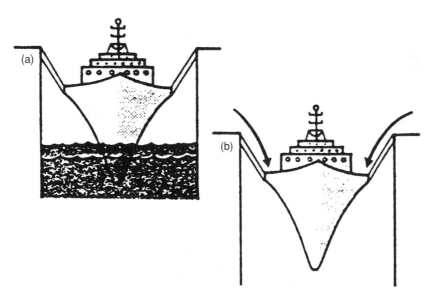

Figure 8-4. "Boat in dry dock." Conception of pelvic floor disorders. This boat is suspended by water (the pelvic floor musculature) and held in place by its mooring (the pelvic ligaments and fascia). (a) If the water is removed, the moorings are suddenly placed under great strain. (b) Likewise, loss of pelvic floor tone may place excessive force on the pelvic ligaments and fascia. (From reference 5, with permission.)

bladder neck in women with stress incontinence when compared to normally supported continent women.

ANTERIOR COMPARTMENT PROLAPSE AND THE CONTINENCE MECHANISM

Although the exact cause of stress urinary incontinence is not completely clear, it is likely that preservation of the continence mechanism greatly depends on the anatomic position and integrity of the structures located within the anterior compartment. However, even with the development of prolapse within the anterior compartment, urinary continence may be maintained. This is related to the degree of structural support of the bladder neck and urethra.

The urethra utilizes several supportive structures to maintain urinary continence. It has been observed in continent patients that with coughing, distal urethral pressure exceeds abdominal pressure to maintain positive urethral closure pressure.[12] DeLancey's cadaveric studies[13] concluded that this augmentation of urethral pressure may occur due to the attachment of the compressor urethrae muscles to the perineal membrane. Therefore, voluntary contraction of the muscles within the perineal membrane help to increase distal urethral pressure in preparation for an increase in intraabdominal pressure. Contraction of the levator ani muscles promotes urinary continence in several ways. The fascia overlying the levator muscles provides a point of attachment for the endopelvic fascia which supports the urethra and anterior vagina. Also, recent MRI studies have shown that portions of the levator ani muscles fuse to the distal vagina.[14] The levator ani muscles are composed of slow-twitch type I and fast-twitch type II fibers. The type I fibers provide continuous tone in the pelvic floor and urethra. The type II fibers are recruited during periods of stress such as with sudden increases in intraabdominal pressure. Voluntary contraction of these muscles results in increasing tension in the suburethral area providing greater urethral support and an increase in urethral closure pressure. This provides the therapeutic basis for utilizing pelvic floor exercises in the treatment of stress incontinence.

STRESS URINARY INCONTINENCE AND ANTERIOR VAGINAL PROLAPSE

The development of stress incontinence in the presence of bladder neck hypermobility is thought to occur due to a loss of suburethral support and an inability to maintain positive urethral pressure. One hypothesis is that with laxity of the suburethral tissues pressure transmission to the urethra decreases, resulting in decreased compression of the urethra and lower urethral closure pressure.[15] However, if there is adequate support and stability of the suburethral tissues, even in the presence of a cystocele, continence is maintained (Figure 8-5).

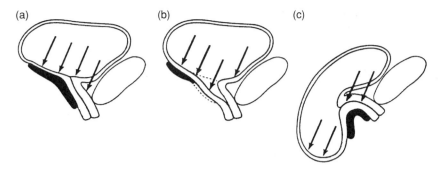

Figure 8-5. Hypothesis concerning affect of abdominal pressure on urethra and pelvic floor depending on stability of the supportive layer. (a) Abdominal pressure (*arrows*) forces urethra against stable supportive layer (*black*) and compresses urethra closed. (b) Unstable supportive layer (*shaded*) is ineffective in providing resistant backstop against which urethra can be compressed. (c) In spite of low, extraabdominal position of urethra and presence of cysto-urethrocele supportive layer is firm and provides adequate backstop against which urethra may be compressed closed. (From DeLancey JOL. Structural support aspects of the urethra as it relates to stress urinary incontinence: The hammock hypothesis. *Am J Obstet Gynecol* 1994; **170**: 1713–1723, with permission.)

OCCULT INCONTINENCE AND PROLAPSE

In some situations urinary continence may be observed even without adequate suburethral support. This has been described in cases of severe genitourinary prolapse. Many of these women will develop postoperative difficulties with stress incontinence despite subjective preoperative continence. In this situation continence occurs due to kinking of the urethra by the prolapse or because of absorption of intraabdominal pressure by the large cystocele.[16] Preoperative urodynamic testing, as described later in this chapter, may help identify patients at risk for postoperative stress incontinence. Many of these women may also have voiding difficulties resulting in retention and recurrent urinary tract infection due to urinary stasis within the displaced large cystocele.

RISK FACTORS ASSOCIATED WITH THE DEVELOPMENT OF PROLAPSE AND URINARY INCONTINENCE

Although the exact causes of prolapse and urinary incontinence continue to elude investigators, it appears that these conditions are progressive and associated with certain physiologic and traumatic events, and may be exacerbated by certain habits.

The vagina, urethra, and bladder all arise from a common embryonic origin: the urogenital sinus. All of these structures, therefore, have similarities in innervation, blood supply, structural support, and hormone receptor status. Estrogen promotes an increase in urethral submucosal vascularity which is also thought to improve urethral tone and support. This is believed to occur due to improvements in mucosal coaptation and pressure transmission during stress.[17] Estrogen also increases the amount of mucosal superficial cells leading to improvements in mucosal atrophy and potentially decreasing symptoms of irritation, frequency and urgency.[18] Although a metanalysis of a 20-year review of the literature on the efficacy of estrogens in treating urinary incontinence confirmed a subjective improvement, randomized controlled trials revealing objective data to support this are lacking.[19] Therefore, it is likely that an estrogen-deficient state alone does not explain the increased frequency of urinary incontinence and prolapse in postmenopausal women.

Childbirth also appears to be linked to the etiology of incontinence and prolapse. Sultan and colleagues[20] found a higher incidence of perineal descent and prolongation of pudendal nerve terminal motor latencies in women who had labored and or delivered vaginally when compared to women who had undergone elective cesarean section, and that these changes were most pronounced in primiparas. This suggests that the first delivery in particular results in stretching of and neurologic trauma to the pelvic floor. Other studies[21,22] have also described histologic changes suggestive of neurologic injury in tissues taken from patients with prolapse and incontinence, and Thind and Lose[23] found decreased resting urethral pressures in women after bilateral pudendal nerve blockade. Cervical ripening and dilatation occur through the activation of various collagenases and elastases that degrade the connective tissue matrix of the cervix and it is possible that a similar process may occur to the connective tissue supports elsewhere in the vagina.[24] Despite these theories and observations, it is still unclear how prolapse can occur in nulliparous women and why 16% of the nulliparous nurses polled in Wolin's study[25] had admitted to experiencing symptoms of incontinence.

Previous surgery and the healing process may be associated with the development of incontinence and prolapse. Prolapse of the vaginal vault is thought to occur in 0.2–1% of women following hysterectomy.[26] This may be due to inadequate attention to supporting structures during the hysterectomy. Surgery for prolapse is associated with a significant degree of failure. Some of this may be due to a lack of recognition of other pelvic floor defects at the time of the first procedure. Others note that certain procedures may predispose to the later development of prolapse in a different area, such as the 7.6% incidence of enterocele formation in patients undergoing a Burch procedure.[27] Wiskind and coworkers[28] also found a higher incidence of postoperative prolapse in patients undergoing a Burch who had a very large cystocele. This may have to do with postoperative changes in pressure transmitted to the vaginal vault. As one area is elevated and supported another area may be left more vulnerable to the pressure exerted over that area, leading to weakening of connective tissue supports and postoperative prolapse. Some surgical treatments for prolapse may also predispose to the later development of incontinence. A 12% incidence of new onset stress incontinence was reported by one review of patients undergoing abdominal sacrocolpopexy for vaginal vault prolapse.[29] Similar results were also described by Nichols[30] in patients undergoing sacrospinous suspension. He attributed this to "straightening of the vesicourethral junction with restoration of vaginal length and depth". Also, wound healing may lead to an alteration in the original composition of the tissues at the operative site. One study showed that after a lacerated muscle heals, very little of the muscle is regenerated and the injured site is replaced by connective tissue.[31] This alteration in histologic composition of tissue may compromise the usual supporting mechanisms promoting continence and preventing prolapse.

Another predisposing factor leading to the development of incontinence and prolapse may be a congenital weakness of connective tissue. Norton and associates[32] found that patients with joint hypermobility had a higher incidence of genitourinary prolapse. A similar relationship was noted by Al-Rawi and Al-Rawi[33] who found joint hypermobility more frequently in women with prolapse than controls without prolapse. Joint hypermobility is frequently seen in patients with connective tissue disorders such as Marfan syndrome and Ehlers-Danlos syndrome. It may be that these patients are at high risk for the development of prolapse although this association is still under investigation.

The anatomic position of the spine may also influence the development of prolapse and incontinence. Patients with thoracic kyphosis have a higher incidence of uterine prolapse; whereas those with lumbar lordosis have a decreased incidence of prolapse.[34,35] This likely has to do with the amount of intraabdominal pressure transmitted to the pelvis. With thoracic kyphosis, the pelvic inlet aligns with the vertical axis and a greater degree of intraabdominal pressure is transmitted to the pelvic floor. The opposite is true for lumbar lordosis, since, in this situation, the sacral promontory protrudes farther anteriorly and the pelvic inlet assumes a more horizontal axis. Therefore, intraabdominal pressure is transmitted to and absorbed by the sacrum and symphysis pubis.

Different habits and conditions associated with chronically increased intraabdominal pressure may also be associated with the later development of prolapse and urinary incontinence. Nurses who do heavy lifting at work are at greater risk of developing genital prolapse than the general female population.[36] This may also be true of patients with other conditions or habits that increase intraabdominal pressure, such as patients who suffer from asthma, chronic obstructive pulmonary disease, chronic cough, or constipation. On the other hand, it has been noted that women who are raised in certain geographic areas where squatting to void is practiced suffer less frequently from urinary incontinence than women who used a commode for toiletting.[37] This may be due to better development of pelvic floor muscle control and tone.

Obviously, many risk factors have been identified, and many of these overlap. Still others leave unanswered questions as to why some patients with none of the previously mentioned risk factors go on to develop prolapse and incontinence, and for this reason the treatment and prevention of these conditions remains a dilemma.

EVALUATION OF ANTERIOR SEGMENT PROLAPSE AND ASSESSMENT OF THE CONTINENCE MECHANISM

Vaginal examination is the best method for assessing various types and degrees of genitourinary prolapse. However, the examiner may have difficulty in determining the cause of prolapse through simple inspection or use of a bivalved speculum. This is because a large rectocele may obscure an underlying cystocele or uterine descensus or vice versa. Use of the Sims speculum allows for separate assessment of each individual compartment of the vagina. Central defects can further be distinguished from lateral defects by reduction of the central portion of the cystocele. If the prolapse is reduced completely then it is more likely caused by a central defect. If bilateral elevation with a ring forceps accomplishes reduction of the prolapse, then its cause can be attributed to a lateral defect. Therefore, by looking at each area separately one can reduce the opposite compartment to better view the area exposed (Figure 8-6).

The position of the patient during vaginal examination greatly affects the examiner's ability to assess the degree of genitourinary prolapse. Nichols recommends that patients be examined in the standing position as depicted in Figure 8-7. By asking the patient to strain, the examiner will then be able to

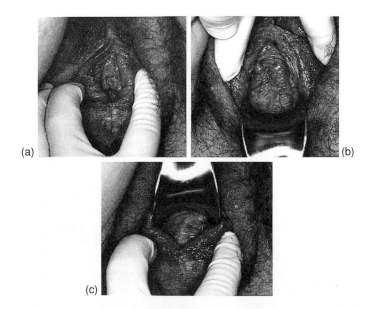

(a)   (b)   (c)

Figure 8-6.   Examination of the individual portions of the vagina. (a) Cursory inspection of the vagina when the patient strains demonstrates minimal prolapse. (b) Examination of the anterior vagina while retracting the posterior vaginal wall reveals a moderate cystocele. (c) Examination of the posterior vagina while retracting the anterior vaginal wall reveals a moderate rectocele. (From reference 7, permission sought.)

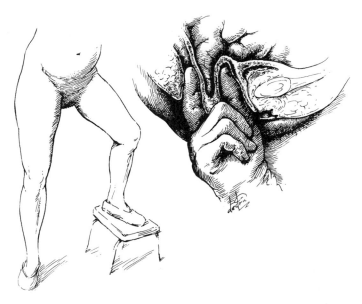

Figure 8-7. Examination of a patient with prolapse. Examination of the patient in a standing position permits the thumb in the vagina to note and replace any descent of the vaginal vault, while the index finger introduced into the rectum permits evaluation of any possible rectocele. When the patient strains, any enterocele present is evidenced by palpation of a bowel-filled sac prolapse dissecting the rectovaginal septum. (From reference 8, permission sought.)

assess the degree of prolapse. However, the degree of bladder neck hypermobility may be more accurately assessed in the supine position. The Q-tip test has been described as an inexpensive method for assessing the degree of bladder neck hypermobility associated with stress incontinence.[39] Handa and co-workers[40] documented greater changes in Q-tip angles from the resting to straining position while the patient was examined in the supine position. This may also explain why supine ultrasonography reveals greater hypermobility than standing lateral bead chain cystography.[41] For these reasons it is important to examine the patient in several positions to more accurately assess the degree of genitourinary prolapse and its effect on the bladder neck.

Multichannel urodynamic testing remains the gold standard for eliciting the presence of genuine stress incontinence. However, other less expensive simpler methods have been described. Wall and colleagues[42] compared the efficacy of detecting urinary incontinence during simple bladder filling and a cough stress test with multichannel subtracted cystometry. They found that simple bladder filling had a sensitivity of 88.1%, a specificity of 77.1%, a negative predictive value of 84.4%, and a positive predictive value of 82% for detecting genuine stress incontinence when compared to multichannel cystometry. They feel that this simpler, less expensive test can be used as a means of testing before low-risk treatment and evaluation for the selection of patients who may "need more extensive evaluation".

Others have promoted use of the Bonney or Marshall Marchetti test to assess if support of the hypermobile bladder neck will prevent stress incontinence. This is not a sensitive test and its effectiveness has been questioned since some argue that manually supporting the bladder neck during a cough may actually result in compression and obstruction of the bladder neck.[43]

Perineal ultrasonography can also demonstrate the degree of mobility of the bladder neck in women with prolapse and stress incontinence. This method is useful in comparing degrees of prolapse before and after surgery and may help elucidate how correction of anterior compartment prolapse postoperatively affects the anatomy of the posterior compartment.[44]

Although it says little about the cause of incontinence, a lateral chain cystometrogram helps to elucidate the anatomic location of the bladder neck and has been used frequently in the past to assess pre- and postoperative differences in bladder-neck position.[45] Cystourethroscopy may also be utilized to assess the degree of voluntary and involuntary urethral sphincter function and may detect the presence of a diverticulum as a cause of incontinence.

The pessary can also be a useful tool to preoperatively assess patients with anterior compartment prolapse. Bergman and collaborators[46] found that using a pessary to reduce prolapse they were able to mimic postoperative changes resulting from bladder neck repair. They felt this was superior to the Bonney test as is was not associated with urethral compression. Others promote the use of pessaries to elevate a very large cystourethrocele to look for occult incontinence, as the prolapse may cause kinking and obstruction of the urethra.[47] Bump and colleagues[48] explain this by observing that with placement of the pessary urethral closure pressures decrease significantly to values associated with genuine stress incontinence. They postulate that larger degrees of prolapse caused a "mechanical obstruction of the less mobile urethra".

TREATMENT OF ANTERIOR SEGMENT PROLAPSE

Given that cystoceles may or may not be accompanied by incontinence depending on the degree of urethral support or obstruction, it is important to fully assess the anatomic causes of the cystocele and to correct the associated defects without neglecting a repair of the continence mechanism in patients with occult or overt stress incontinence associated with prolapse.

Central Defects

Anterior colporrhaphy remains the main operation for correcting a cystocele caused by a central defect. The technique involves vaginal dissection either as a single or as a V-shaped incision (Figure 8-8). The vagina is freed from the underlying pubocervical fascia and bladder with blunt and sharp dissection. Sutures are then placed in the fascia to plicate the urethra and bladder neck. The location

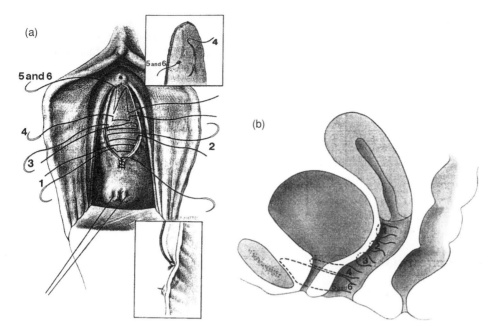

Figure 8-8. (a) Anterior colporrhaphy suture placement. Placement of no. 1 chromic catgut, vertical mattress sutures (*1, 2, and 3*) plicating the fascia under the bladder base with long axis of the needle parallel to the fascial surface (*also bottom insert*). Number 1 polyglycolic suture (*4*) is inserted into fascia at the bladder neck with long axis of the needle at right angles to the fascial surface (*also top insert*). Figure-of-eight no. 1 polyglycolic sutures (*5 and 6*) are inserted into the pubocervical fascia, scratching the back of the symphysis pubis with long axis of the needle held at right angles to the fascial surface (*also top insert*). (b) Anterior repair placement of sutures. Placement of the sutures as in Figure A in sagittal view. When tied, the fascia under the bladder base is plicated. Overcorrection of cystocele is avoided. When sutures *5* and *6*, in fascia under and around the urethra, are tied, the urethra is elevated more than the bladder base (and is tightened). (From reference 49, with permission.)

of this suture placement varies dependent upon the surgeon. Beck and co-workers[49] encourages the use of a delayed absorbable suture such as Dexon, and placing it "under and around the urethra . . . (so that it) scratches the back of the symphysis pubis to ensure that it is of adequate depth". After plication of the fascia is completed, the vaginal mucosa is trimmed and reapproximated.

Although the anterior repair is well tolerated and associated with fewer voiding difficulties, the complications associated with the procedure include bladder and urethral injury, vaginal narrowing, recurrent prolapse, hemorrhage, and incontinence.[50] The ability of this operation to treat genuine stress incontinence is debatable. Beck reports the highest degree of subjective success.[49] Of 194 patients, 165 were considered to be cured at 6 months or more postoperatively. Others report lower rates especially if the patients are objectively studied with postoperative urodynamic testing.[51–53] This may be because the tissues plicated as representatve of pubocervical fascia may vary in content dependent on the area where the stitches are placed. In one study, 14 patients presenting for anterior repair to treat a symptomatic cystocele underwent biopsy of what was felt to be representative of pubocervical fascia on the vaginal and bladder aspects of the dissection. Although there was a trend in increased amounts of collagen in samples taken from the vaginal side, no statistically significant differences were found between samples taken from either side (S.R. Valaitis, V.A. Thomas, and S.L. Stanton, unpublished data). However, these results may represent a type II error due to a small sample size. The varying techniques used to plicate the pubocervical fascia and the quality of tissue plicated may affect the ability of treating prolapse and incontinence with anterior colporrhaphy. The variable success in treating prolapse and incontinence with anterior colporrhaphy is likely a reflection of the differing surgical techniques, suture placement, and tissues chosen for plication and support of the bladder neck.

Lateral Defects

The paravaginal repair is utilized to correct lateral vaginal defects associated with cystocele formation. The technique is traditionally performed through a

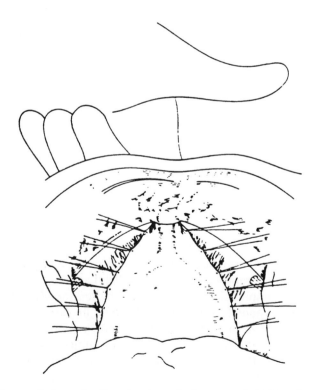

Figure 8-9. Paravaginal repair. Completed repair demonstrating approximation of anterior vaginal wall to white line bilaterally. (From reference 58, with permission.)

retropubic approach. Stitches are first placed in the anterolateral vaginal sulcus after the bladder is reflected medially. The needle is then passed through the arcus tendineus fasciae pelvis (Figure 8-9). Richardson reports subjective cure of stress incontinence in 95% of patients using this approach.[47] Others have reported performing paravaginal repairs through a vaginal approach but the success of this method is still under study.[54]

One complication associated with the paravaginal repair includes a persistent cystocele. This may be due to an unrecognized central defect at the time of the procedure. Other complications include hemorrhage, thrombosis, enterocele formation, detrusor instability, and stress incontinence.[55]

BLADDER NECK SURGERY AT THE TIME OF ANTERIOR PROLAPSE REPAIR

Since variable rates of success have been reported for the treatment of genuine stress incontinence during anterior colporrhaphy and paravaginal repair, if this condition exists some recommend specific bladder neck correction at the time of the repair to prevent potential postoperative stress incontinence. This can be done either by placing several sutures through Cooper's ligament at the time of para-vaginal repair to better elevate the bladder neck or by including a needle suspension procedure into the vaginal repair of a cystocele.[47,55,56] Some have promoted that plication of the posterior pubourethral ligaments at the time of anterior repair may provide greater support of the bladder neck and prevent post-operative stress incontinence. However, a recent study revealed that not only does this add to greater voiding difficulties and prolonged catheterization, but no differences were found in preventing postoperative stress incontinence with this method.[57]

CONCLUSIONS

Genitourinary prolapse and urinary incontinence are common and difficult clinical problems to correct. Approaches for treatment require an adequate understanding of the anatomic relationships and structural supports of the organs in the pelvis, an ability to identify the defects associated with various types of prolapse and urinary incontinence, and a knowledge of several approaches used to surgically correct these anatomic defects. As more answers unfold regarding the causes of these frustrating conditions, clinicians will gain a better understanding not just of how to best treat these problems, but, more importantly, how to prevent them from occurring in the future.

REFERENCES

1. Norton PA. Pelvic floor disorders: The role of fascia and ligaments. *Clin Obstet Gynecol* 1993; **36**: 926–938.
2. Urinary incontinence in adults: acute and chronic management. In: *Clinical Practice Guideline Number 2* (1996 Update) AHCPR Publication No. 96-0682: March, 1996.
3. Richardson AC, Lyon JB, Williams NL. A new look at pelvic relaxation. *Am J Obstet Gynecol* 1976; **126**: 568–573.
4. Smith ARB, Hosker GL, Warrell DW. The role of partial denervation of the pelvic floor in the aetiology of genitourinary prolapse and stress incontinence of urine. A neurophysiologic study. *Br J Obstet Gynecol* 1989; **96**: 24–28.
5. DeLancey JOL. Anatomy and biomechanics of genital prolapse. *Clin Obstet Gynecol* 1993; **36**: 897–909.
6. DeLancey JOL. Anatomic aspects of vaginal eversion. *Am J Obstet Gynecol* 1992; **166**: 1717.
7. In: Nichols DH, Randall CL, eds. *Vaginal Surgery*. Baltimore, MD: Williams and Wilkins; 1989: 239–268.
8. Wall IL, Norton PA, Delancey JOL. *Practical Urogynecology*. Baltimore, MD: Williams and Wilkins, 1993.
9. Richardson AC, Edmonds PB, Williams NL. Treatment of stress urinary incontinence due to paravaginal fascial defect. *Obstet Gynecol* 1981; **57**: 357–362.
10. DeLancey JOL. Anatomy and biomechanics of genital prolapse. *Clin Obstet Gynecol* 1993; **36**: 897–909.
11. Klutke C, Golomb J, Barbaric Z, et al. The anatomy of stress incontinence: Magnetic resonance imaging of the female bladder neck and urethra. *J Urol* 1990; **14**: 563–566.
12. Hilton P, Stanton SL. Urethral pressure measurement by microtransducer: The results in symptom-free women and in those with genuine stress incontinence. *Br J Obstet Gynecol* 1993; **90**: 919–933.
13. DeLancey JOL. Structural aspects of the extrinsic continence mechanism. *Obstet Gynecol* 1988; **72**: 296–301.
14. Strohbehn K, Ellis JH, Strohbehn JA, et al. Magnetic resonance imaging of the levator ani with anatomic correlation. *Obstet Gynecol* 1996; **87**: 277–285.
15. DeLancey JOL. Structural support of the urethra as it relates to stress urinary incontinence: The hammock hypothesis. *Am J Obstet Gynecol* 1994; **170**: 1713–1723.
16. Bergman A, Koonings PP, Ballard CA. Predicting postoperative urinary incontinence development in women undergoing operation for genitourinary prolapse. *Am J Obstet Gynecol* 1988; **158**: 1171–1175.
17. Bhatia NN, Bergman A, Karram MM. Effect of estrogen on urethral function in women with urinary incontinence. *Am J Obstet Gynecol* 1989; **160**: 176–181.
18. Natchigall LE. Emerging delivery systems for estrogen replacement: Aspects of trans-dermal and oral delivery. *Am J Obstet Gynecol* 1995; **173**: 993–997.
19. Fantl JA, Cardozo L, McClish DK and the Hormones and Urogenital Therapy Committee. Estrogen therapy in the management of urinary incontinence in post-menopausal women: A meta-analysis. First report of the Hormones and Urogenital Therapy Committee. *Obstet Gyencol* 1994; **83**: 12–18.
20. Sultan AH, Kamm MA, Hudson CN. Pudendal nerve damage during labor: A prospective study before and after childbirth. *Br J Obstet Gynecol* 1994; **101**: 22–28.
21. Smith ARB, Hoskins GL, Warrell DW. The role of pudendal nerve damage in the aetiology of genuine stress incontinence in women. *Br J Obstet Gynecol* 1989; **96**: 29–32.
22. Snooks SJ, Swash M. Abnormalities of the innervation of the urethral striated sphincter musculature in incontinence. *Br J Obstet Gynecol* 1984; **56**: 401–405.
23. Thind P, Lose G. The effect of bilateral pudendal blockade on the static urethral closure function in healthy females. *Obstet Gynecol* 1992; **80**: 906–911.

24. Norton PA. Pelvic floor disorders: The role of fascia and ligaments. *Clin Obstet Gynecol* 1993; **36**: 926–938.
25. Wolin LH. Stress incontinence in young healthy nulliparous female subjects. *J Urol* 1969; **101**: 545–549.
26. Symmonds RE, Williams TJ, Lee RA, et al. Posthysterectomy enterocele and vaginal vault prolapse. *Am J Obstet Gynecol* 1981; **140**: 852–859.
27. Burch JC. Cooper's ligament urethrovesical suspension for stress incontinence. *Am J Obstet Gynecol* 1968; **100**: 764–774.
28. Wiskind AK, Creighton SM, Stanton SL. The incidence of genital prolapse after the Burch colposuspension. *Am J Obstet Gynecol* 1192; **167**: 399–405.
29. Valaitis SR, Stanton SL. Sacrocolpopexy: A retrospective study of a clinician's experience. *Br J Obstet Gynecol* 1994; **101**: 518–522.
30. Nichols DH. Sacrospinous fixation for massive eversion of the vagina. *Am J Obstet Gynecol* 1982; **142**: 901–904.
31. Garrtett W, Nikolaou P, Ribbeck B, et al. The effects of muscle architecture on the biomechanical failure properties of skeletal muscle under passive extension. *Am J Sports Med* 1988; **16**: 7–12.
32. Norton PA, Baker JE, Charp HC, et al. Genitourinary prlapse and joint hypermobility in women. *Obstet Gynecol* 1995; **85**: 225–228.
33. Al-Rawi ZS, Al-Rawi ZT. Joint hypermobility in women with genital prolapse. *Lancet* 1982; **i**: 1439–1441.
34. Lind LR, Lucente V, Kohn N. Thoracic kyphosis and the prevalence of advanced uterine prolapse. *Obstet Gynecol* 1996; **87**: 605–609.
35. In Nichols DH, Randall CL. *Vaginal Surgery*. Baltimore, MD: Williams and Wilkins; 1989: 64–81.
36. Jorgensen S, Hein HO, Gyntetlberg F. Heavy lifting at work and risk of genital prolapse and herniated lumbar disc in asistant nurses. *Occup Med* 1994; **44**: 47–49.
37. Shershah A, Ansari RL. The frequency of urinary incontinence in Pakistani women. *J Pakistan Med Assoc* 1989; **39**: 16–17.
38. Nichols DH. Repair of enterocele and prolapse of the vaginal vault. In: Barber H (ed). *Goldsmith's Practice of Surgery*. Philadelphia: JB Lippincott, 1981.
39. Crystle CD, Charme LS, Copeland WE. Q-tip test in stress urinary incontinence. *Obstet Gynecol* 1971; **38**: 313–315.
40. Handa VL, Jensen JK, Ostergard DR. The effect of patient position on proximal urethral mobility. *Obstet Gynecol* 1995; **86**: 273–276.
41. Schaer GN, Koechli OR, Schuessler B, et al. Perineal ultrasound for evaluating the bladder neck in urinary stress incontinence. *Obstet Gynecol* 1995; **85**: 220–224.
42. Wall LL, Wiskind AK, Taylor PA. Simple bladder filling with a cough stress test compared with substracted cystometry for the diagnosis of urinary incontinence. *Am J Obstet Gynecol* 1994; **171**: 1472–1479.
43. Bhatia NN, Bergman A. Urodynamic appraisal of the Bonney test in women with stress urinary incontinence. *Obstet Gynecol* 1983; **62**: 696–699.
44. Creighton SM, Pearce JM, Stanton SL. Perineal video-ultrasonography in the assessment of vaginal prolapse: Early observations. *Br J Obstet Gynecol* 1992; **99**: 310–313.
45. Kitzmiller JL, Manzer GA, Nebel WA, et al. Chain cystourethrogram and stress incontinence. *Obstet Gynecol* 1972; **39**: 333–340.
46. Bhatia NN, Bergman A. Pessary test in women with urinary incontinence. *Obstet Gynecol* 1985; **65**: 220–226.
47. Richardson DA, Bent AE, Ostergard DR. The effect of uterovaginal prolapse on urethrovesical pressure dynamics. *Am J Obstet Gynecol* 1983; **146**: 901–905.
48. Bump RC, Fantl JA, Hurt WG. The mechanism of urinary continence in women with severe uterovaginal prolapse: Results of barrier studies. *Obstet Gynecol* 1988; **72**: 291–295.

49. Beck RP, McCormick S, Nordstrom L. A 25-year experience with 519 anterior colporrhaphy procedures. *Obstet Gynecol*. 1991; **78**: 1011–1018.
50. Stanton SL. Stress incontinence: Why and how operations work. *Clin Obstet Gynecol* 1985; **12**: 369–377.
51. Stanton SL, Cardozo L. A comparison of vaginal and suprapubic surgery in the correction of incontinence due to urethral sphincter incompetence. *Br J Urol* 1979; **51**: 497–499.
52. Stanton SL, Hilton P, Norton C, et al. Clinical and urodynamic effects of anterior colporrhaphy and vaginal hysterectomy for prolapse with and without incontinence. *Br J Obstet Gynecol* 1982; **89**: 459–463.
53. Bergman A, Elia G. Three surgical procedures for genuine stress incontinence: Five year follow-up of a prospective randomized study. *Am J Obstet Gynecol* 1995; **173**: 66–71.
54. Shull BL, Benn SL, Kuehl TJ. Surgical management of prolapse of the anterior vaginal segment: An analysis of support defects, operative morbidity, and anatomic outcome. *Am J Obstet Gynecol* 1994; **171**: 1429–1439.
55. Shull BL, Baden WF. A six-year experience with paravaginal defect repair for stress urinary incontinence. *Am J Obstet Gynecol* 1989; **160**: 1432–1440.
56. Raz S, Little NA, Juma S, et al. Repair of severe anterior vaginal wall prolapse (grade IV cystourethrocele). *J Urol* 1991; **146**: 988–992.
57. Columbo M, Maggioni A, Zanetta G, et al. Prevention of postoperative urinary stress incontinence after surgery for genitourinary prolapse. *Obstet Gynecol* 1996; **87**: 266–271.

CHAPTER 9

Retropubic urethropexy

ASH MONGA AND STUART STANTON ────────────────────

The aims of surgery for stress incontinence are:

1. Restoration of the proximal urethra and bladder neck to the zone of intra-abdominal pressure transmission
2. To increase urethral resistance
3. A combination of both

Retropubic urethropexy is the most frequently utilized surgical procedure for the control of stress urinary incontinence caused by urethral sphincter incompetence (genuine stress incontinence [GSI]). The two techniques to be discussed in this chapter are the Marshall-Marchetti-Krantz (MMK) and Burch colposuspension procedures. The MMK procedure[1] has lost popularity over the last decade, largely because of its inherent complications; colposuspension is therefore by far the most frequently performed operation for stress incontinence. Hence, this chapter will concentrate on the Burch colposuspension procedure.

The purpose of the colposuspension and MMK procedures is to elevate the bladder neck, and to place the proximal urethra in a position where it is compressed against the posterosuperior border of the symphysis pubis during increases in intraabdominal pressure.

PREOPERATIVE EVALUATION

History and Examination

Prior to considering continence surgery, the symptom of stress incontinence must be established as a significant problem to the woman. It is our practice to actively encourage women to try physiotherapist-taught conservative measures including pelvic floor exercise, weighted vaginal cone therapy, functional electrical stimulation and use of a variety of occlusive devices. If these have failed, the woman is mentally better prepared to face surgery.

In the urogynecologic history, particular emphasis is placed on symptoms suggesting detrusor instability (DI), voiding difficulty, neurologic disease, fistula or recurrent urinary tract infection as these may complicate or contraindicate surgery. Previous pelvic surgery such as hysterectomy and anterior or posterior colporrhaphy, and prior radiotherapy can produce significant vaginal scarring. The history must take into account any menstrual problems, prolapse and anal incontinence, as additional surgery may then be required. The patient must be asked if her family is completed.

Abdominal examination should exclude any masses and a neurologic examination should focus on deficits in S2–S4 innervation. Pelvic examination should assess urogenital atrophy, residual urine volume, prolapse and uterine and adnexal pathology. A significant cystourethrocele will contraindicate the MMK procedure. Bladder-neck mobility should be assessed. Neither a colposuspension or an MMK procedure will be possible if the bladder neck cannot be elevated. Vaginal capacity and mobility are estimated to see whether the lateral paravaginal fornices can be approximated to the pelvic side walls—a requirement for performing a Burch colposuspension. Signs of stress incontinence must be confirmed clinically or by investigation prior to surgery.

Investigations

Urinary tract infection must be excluded. It is advisable to perform urodynamic investigations prior to continence surgery, particularly when previous continence surgery has failed, as there is poor correlation between symptoms and diagnoses.[2] It is our practice always to perform subtracted cystometry and pressure flow voiding studies to confirm an objective diagnosis of GSI and detect coexistent detrusor instability or voiding dysfunction. Videocystourethrography is reserved for patients with previous failed continence surgery or women with voiding difficulty and incontinence. It is not our practice to perform Valsalva leak point pressure (VLPP) measurements to exclude intrinsic sphincter deficiency, although this is used more routinely in the United States. To date there appears to be no standardization of VLPP with investigators using different patient position, bladder volumes and catheter size. Urethral pressure profilometry is performed on all women who have had previous failed continence surgery. Ambulatory monitoring and pad testing may be required when conventional investigations objectively fail to demonstrate stress incontinence.

INDICATIONS AND CONTRAINDICATIONS

The decision to undergo surgery should be made by the patient after informed discussion of all the options, their success rates and complications. The main indication for a retropubic urethropexy is the objective urodynamic diagnosis of GSI and a bladder neck which needs elevation. The Burch colposuspension will correct concurrent cysturethrocele whilst the MMK procedure will not. Retropubic urethropexy may also be indicated at the time of surgery for vaginal vault prolapse.

The main contraindication is the presence of a foreshortened, scarred and immobile vagina where elevation of the bladder neck or lateral vaginal fornices is unlikely.[3] Failure rates of 55%[4] are reported after colposuspension in women with these pelvic examination characteristics.

It has been demonstrated that preoperative DI has an adverse affect on the outcome of continence surgery;[5,6] this appears to be accentuated in patients with systolic detrusor instability compared with low compliant detrusor instability,[7] and the height of systolic contraction has an inverse relationship with success.[8] It is therefore important to treat coexistent DI prior to surgery. Colombo and colleagues (1996)[9] compared the success rates of colposuspension in 44 women with stress incontinence and stable bladders with 44 women matched for age, parity, by mass index (BMI), previous surgery and urethral pressure profilometry, with stress incontinence and detrusor overactivity. At 2-year follow-up the cure rates were 95% and 75% respectively. If stress incontinence remains a substantial complaint, then a retropubic urethropexy can be performed as long as the patient is aware of lower success rates[9] and the likely reappearance of symptoms of DI.[10]

Voiding difficulty may be a relative contraindication and must be assessed by pressure flow studies and measurement of residual urine. Bhatia and Bergman (1984)[11] reported that patients with low preoperative voiding pressure of less than 15 cmH_2O had increased postoperative voiding difficulty. The delay in resumption of normal voiding was greater in those women with low maximum flow rate. The predictive value of low voiding pressure has been confirmed by Lose and colleagues (1987).[12]

A low maximum urethral closure pressure (MUCP) and functional urethral length (FUL) have been shown to predispose to an adverse outcome in women with GSI undergoing colposuspension[13] and Marshall-Marchetti-Krantz[14] procedures.

McGuire (1981)[15] reported a 41% failure rate for colposuspension if the MUCP was less than 20 cmH_2O. Sand and coworkers (1987)[16] noted that in 86 women undergoing colposuspension, a preoperative MUCP less than 20 cmH_2O was three times more likely to give an unsatisfactory outcome. Bowen and colleagues (1989)[17] performed a case-controlled study with 21 patients in each group. Of the successfully treated patients, 81% had a MUCP >20 cmH_2O compared with 23% of failures. These findings were confirmed by Wolf and colleagues (1989).[18] In the latter study, success rates fell from 91% to 75% if the MUCP was <20 cmH_2O prior to colposuspension. In a prospective study of 79 women, Monga and Stanton (1997)[19] found that an MUCP of <20 cmH_2O was only associated with adverse outcome if the women had undergone previous bladder-neck surgery, but not primary colposuspension.

The role of electrophysiological measurements in patient selection remains controversial, with studies demonstrating conflicting results.[19,20]

As with any continence procedure, the patient should have completed her family beforehand, as pregnancy and vaginal delivery may weaken the bladder-neck supports and lead to recurrence of incontinence. This may be overcome by an elective cesarean section which must be discussed with the patient prior to surgery.

If the women is physically and mentally fit, age is not a bar to colpo-suspension. Cure rates of 89% are reported in selected women over the age of 65 years,[21] however it is a major operation and other alternatives need to be considered for less fit women. Timing of surgery should be optimized to patient fitness, for example patients with chronic obstructive pulmonary disease should avoid surgery during the winter months.

THE PROCEDURES

Preoperative preparation

Subcutaneous low molecular weight heparin is administered pre- and post-operatively until the patient is fully mobile, and patients are instructed to wear thromboembolic deterrent stockings. 500 mg of cephradine and 1 g metronidazole are administered at induction of anesthetic. This is supported by a comparative study showing a reduction in febrile morbidity and hospital stay in women receiving prophylactic antibiotics.[22] The procedure may be performed under regional or general anesthesia. The patient is positioned in the horizontal lithotomy position with the legs supported in Lloyd-Davies or similar stirrups. The abdominal, vaginal and perineal regions are prepared in a sterile manner. A transurethral resection drape is used to cover the perineum, allowing access to the vagina during the operation by means of a sterile condom. A 14 Fr, Foley urethral catheter is inserted, to allow continous drainage throughout the operation, delineate the bladder neck and facilitate filling of the bladder prior to placement of the suprapubic catheter when the procedure is completed. In some centers where postoperative bladder drainage is achieved by clean intermittent self-catheterization, patients need to be fully competent with the technique preoperatively.

MARSHALL-MARCHETTI-KRANTZ PROCEDURE

Since the first description in 1949,[1] this procedure has risen and subsequently fallen in popularity. As long as the clinical and urodynamic findings are appropriate the MMK procedure may be used for primary or secondary surgery. However, we no longer utilize this technique. In the original account, three No. 1 chromic catgut sutures were placed in the paraurethral tissues, taking a double bite to ensure a secure hold. A fourth suture was placed at the level of the bladder neck. The sutures were inserted into the periosteum of the pubis and also the symphiseal cartilage where feasible. When tied, the urethra and bladder neck were apposed to the symphysis and posterior aspect of the rectus muscles. Additional sutures were placed in the anterior wall of the bladder and posterior aspect of the rectus muscle. Krantz (1980)[23] suggested a much simpler version using just two Mersilene sutures, one either side of the bladder neck and attached to the pubic periosteum.

BURCH COLPOSUSPENSION PROCEDURE

In the original description Burch (1961)[24] approximated the paravaginal fascia to the ipsilateral white line; later he utilized the ileopectineal ligament.

A low Pfannenstiel or Cherney incision is made approximately 1-finger breadth above the symphysis pubis to allow access to the retropubic space. A Denis Browne 4-blade self-retaining retractor is used to enhance exposure and the bladder is carefully dissected from the symphysis using blunt dissection. Sharp dissection is preferred when previous retropubic surgery has been performed.

With the space of Retzius exposed, the operator places a forefinger into the vagina and elevates a lateral fornix. Beginning laterally the bladder is dissected medially, off the paravaginal fascia using a swab on a holder in the abdominal hand. Scissor dissection may be required if previous continence surgery or an anterior repair has been performed. Large paravesical veins should be diathermied or ligated. The paravaginal fascia is recognized as white tissue and is exposed from the bladder neck to the apex of the vagina. Two or three No. 1 nonabsorbable Polybutylate-coated polyester sutures are then inserted into the paravaginal fascia. The most distal (caudal) suture is placed at the level of the bladder neck. The sutures are tied to secure hemostasis and to prevent them from sliding through the tissue. The lateral vaginal fornix is elevated each time by the operator's finger towards the ipsilateral ileopectineal ligament as the corresponding suture is being placed through the ligament to ensure accurate positioning. This ensures approximation of the paravaginal tissue with minimal "bow string" effect. This procedure is repeated on the opposite side. The most caudal sutures elevate the bladder neck and produce continence: the more cephalad sutures will correct the cystocele.

Once all the sutures are in position, the most caudal are tied first. The remaining sutures are tied on alternating sides to provide a balanced approximation to each ileopectineal ligament. If bladder integrity is in doubt, instillation of milk or methylene blue will locate the leak. A suction drain is left in the space of Retzius. A suprapubic Bonnano catheter is inserted under direct vision before wound closure to prevent damage to surrounding structures. The urethral catheter is removed.

Additional Surgery

Abdominal hysterectomy for coexistent pathology (e.g. menorrhagia or prolapse), or coaptation of the uterosacral ligaments when there is a large cystocele (to prevent a future enterocele)[25] are performed prior to the colposuspension. If a posterior repair is necessary it is usually deferred for 3–6 months, as simultaneous posterior repair is associated with a high recurrence of rectocele.[26]

Postoperative Management

Postoperative care is usually straightforward. Accurate fluid balance is recorded. Early mobilization is encouraged and the suction drain removed after 24 hours. On the morning of the second postoperative day, the suprapubic catheter is clamped for 6–8 hours or until the patient has discomfort. At the end of this time the patient voids once more and the catheter is unclamped for 30 minutes and the residual urine measured. Once the patient is able to void volumes >200 ml with residual volumes <200 ml, the catheter is clamped overnight. The patient is awakened by the nursing staff to void once or twice during the night; if the voided volume is >200 ml and the morning residual is <200 ml, then the catheter is removed. Early clamping results in 65% of patients voiding by the third day.[27] Patients unable to void satisfactorily are taught the clamping regimen or clean intermittent self-catheterization before being allowed home. Daily contact is maintained.

The patient is discharged on day 4 or 5, and returns for clinical and uro-dynamic assessment after 2–3 months. Heavy lifting and sexual intercourse are avoided for 3 months.

COMPLICATIONS

Marshall-Marchetti-Krantz Procedure

Mainprize and Drutz (1988)[35] reviewed 56 articles examining the results of 2712 MMK procedures. The overall complication rate was 21.1%. Osteitis pubis was reported in 2.5%, prolonged retention in 3.6%, urinary tract injury in 1.6% and fistulae in 0.3%. In a metanalysis of 213 articles. Jarvis (1994)[36] reported post-operative detrusor instability in 11% and voiding difficulty in 11–12%.

Burch Colposuspension

Intraoperative complications are infrequent and include venous hemorrhage, injury to the bladder and urethral and ureteric obstruction. Venous hemorrhage is controlled by diathermy and usually ceases when elevation of the paravaginal fascia is completed. Transfusion is required in 0.7–2.3% of cases.[10] Injury to bladder or urethra is repaired with one or two layers using a 3.0 polyglycolic acid suture and the bladder drained for 7 days. Ureteric ligation is rare: ureteric kinking due to acute elevation of the anterior vaginal wall is a more likely cause of obstruction. Postoperative lumbar pain and pyrexia should alert the clinician; an ultrasound will confirm the diagnosis. Renal obstruction may be relieved with percutaneous nephrostomy or retrograde ureteric stent insertion. Cystoscopy may reveal a suture that can be retrieved.

Urinary tract infection is uncommon, especially when using a suprapubic catheter, but may be exacerbated by residual urine.

The cure of stress incontinence is usually accompanied by a decreased flow rate and raised maximum voiding pressure: voiding difficulties are well-documented with reported incidences of up to 25%.[10] There does not seem to be a relationship between delayed spontaneous voiding after colposuspension and long-term voiding problems, or between voiding difficulty and cure of stress incontinence. The adjunctive use of cholinergic or alpha-blocking agents does not confer any benefit. Early reports using prostaglandins are encouraging.[28] Increasing age and postmenopausal status have been found to reduce resumption of spontaneous voiding,[29,30] but concomitant hysterectomy and vaginal repair appear to have no effect.[31]

Another well-recognized complication is the development of postoperative DI in up to 25% of patients.[32] This appears to be more common in women who have undergone previous bladder-neck surgery. Over 50% can be improved with anti-cholinergic therapy and in most symptoms improve at 10-year follow-up.[33] In women with mixed incontinence, if urgency and urge-incontinence symptoms were antecedent to the symptom of stress incontinence, DI is more likely to persist postoperatively.[34]

The development of postoperative rectocele, enterocele or uterine prolapse requires surgical correction in up to 27% of cases.[10] The etiology may be due to mechanical disruption of the middle and posterior compartments of the pelvic floor due to the anterior wall elevation, or to an intrinsic weakness in the pelvic floor of these women.

Occasionally persistent groin pain occurs, and this may be relieved by suture removal.

RESULTS

Comparison of results is hampered by variable follow-up, and many studies still report only subjective results. The results of the Marshall-Marchetti-Krantz procedure and Burch colposuspension are shown in Tables 9-1 and 9-2

Table 9-1   Results of MMK

	n	*FU (months)*	*Cure (%)*
Kujansuu (1983)[37]	7	15	57
Milani et al. (1985)[38]	42	22–73	71
Krantz (1986)[23]	3861	0–372	96
Riggs (1986)[39]	411	6–204	85
Spencer et al. (1987)[40]	54	21–118	57
Park and Miller (1988)[41]	227	60–120	72
Mainprize and Drutz (1988)[35]*	2712	–	86
Jarvis (1994)[36]*			89

* Metanalysis.

Table 9-2   Results of Burch colposuspension

	n	FU (months)	Cure (%)
Burch (1961)[24]	143	12	93
Stanton and Cardozo (1979)[42]	88	12	88
Walter (1982)[43]	38	14	84
Mundy (1983)[44]	26	12	73
Gillon (1984)[21]	35	36–60	89
Bhatia (1985)[45]	32	12	98
Lose (1987)[46]	80	26	75
Galloway (1987)[47]	50	54	84
Pigne (1988)[48]	370	12	95
Hilton (1988)[49]	150	40	92
Bergman (1989)[50]	101	12	87
Eriksen et al. (1990)[51]	86	60	71
Kiilholma et al. (1993)[52]	186	24	91
Herbertsson and Iosif (1993)[53]	72	96–144	90
Feyereisl et al. (1994)[54]	87	60–120	82
Alcalay et al. (1995)[33]	109	120–240	69
Kjolhede and Ryden (1995)[55]	232	72	63
Kinn (1995)[56]	153	60	78
Langer et al. (1998)[57]	109	120–180	94

respectively. Colombo and colleagues (1994)[58] randomized 80 women to either MMK procedure or Burch colposuspension. Although the success rates of both procedures was similar, there was a greater incidence of retropubic hematoma, voiding difficulty and detrusor instability associated with the MMK operation. In the review by Jarvis (1994),[36] success and complication rates for both procedures were similar.

The colposuspension procedure is the most widely used operation for primary and secondary surgery worldwide[59] and appears to give the most consistent subjective and objective outcomes. However, there is a lack of randomized prospective studies that have sufficient evidence to substantiate this statement based on rigorous scientific analysis. Studies suffer from lack of standardization on definition, severity and diagnosis of stress incontinence. Information on detrusor instability, prior surgery, quality of life measurements, surgical technique, length of follow-up and external validity are often not available. A systematic review of the effectiveness of surgery for stress incontinence in women (Black and Downs, 1996)[60] identified 11 randomized control trials, 20 nonrandomized trials/prospective cohort studies and 45 retrospective cohort studies of sufficient quality to be analysed from 943 citations.

Four randomized control trials and 11 nonrandomized prospective studies suggest that colposuspension appears to be more effective in curing and improving stress incontinence compared with anterior colporrhaphy at 1 year (85% vs 50–70%). The benefits of colposuspension are sustained for at least 5 years, whilst those of anterior colporrhaphy diminish rapidly. Two randomized and two nonrandomized studies reported a higher success rate for colposuspension (85% vs 50–70%). There is no convincing evidence that the effectiveness of colposuspension and slings differ. However, less than 150 patients have ever been included in prospective studies.

REFERENCES

1. Marshall V. Marchetti A, Krantz K. The correction of stress incontinence by simple vesico-urethral suspension. *Surg Gynecol Obstet* 1949; **44**: 509–518.
2. Cardozo LD, Stanton SL. Genuine stress incontinence and detrusor instability: A review of 200 cases. *Br J Obstet Gynaecol* 1980; **87**: 184–190.
3. Stanton SL. Colposuspension. In: Stanton SL (ed). *Surgery of Female Incontinence*. New York: Springer-Verlag: 1986: 95.
4. Bergman A, Koonings PP, Ballard CA. Negative Q-tip test as a risk factor for failed incontinence surgery in women. *J Reprod Med* 1989; **34**: 193.
5. Stanton SL, Cardozo L, Williams J, Ritchic D, Allan V. Clinical and urodynamic features of failed incontinence surgery in the female. *Obstet Gynecol* 1978; **51**: 515–520.
6. Pow-Sang J, Lockhart J, Suarez A, Lansman H, Politano V. Female urinary incontinence: Preoperative selection, surgical complications and results. *J Urol* 1986; **136**: 831–833.
7. Wilkie D, Barzilai M, Stanton SL. Combined urethral sphincter incompetence and detrusor instability: Does colposuspension help? *Proceedings of the 16th Annual Meeting of the International Continence Society*, Boston, 1986; 618–620.
8. Lockhart J, Vorstman B, Politano V. Anti incontinence surgery in females with detrusor instability. *Neurourol Urodynam* 1984; **3**: 201–207.
9. Colombo M, Zanetta G, Vitobello D, Milani R. The Burch colposuspension for women with and without detrusor activity. *Br J Obstet Gynaecol* 1996; **103**: 255–260.
10. Wiskind AK, Stanton SL. The Burch colposuspension for genuine stress incontinence. In: Thompson JD, Rock JA (eds). *TeLinde's Operative Gynecology Updates*. Philadelphia: JB Lippincott, 1993; **1**: 1–13.
11. Bhatia NN, Bergman A. Use of preoperative uroflowmetry and simultaneous urethrocystometry for predicting risk of prolonged postoperative bladder drainage. *Urology* 1986; **28**: 440–445.
12. Lose G, Jorgensen L, Mortenson SO, Molsted-Pedersen L, Kristensen JK. Voiding difficulties after colposuspension. *Obstet Gynecol* 1987; **69**: 33–38.
13. Hilton P, Stanton SL. A clinical and urodynamic assessment of the Burch colposuspension for genuine stress incontinence. *Br J Obstet Gynaecol* 1983; **90**: 934–939.
14. Behr J, Winkler L, Schwiersch U. Urodynamic observations on the Marshall-Marchetti-Krantz operation. *Geburtshilfe Frauenheilkunde* 1986; **46**: 649–653.
15. McGuire EJ. Urodynamic findings in patients after failure of stress incontinence operations. *Prog Clin Biol Res* 1981; **78**: 351–360.
16. Sand PK, Bowen LW, Panganiban R, Ostergard DR. The low pressure urethra as a factor in failed retropubic urethropexy. *Obstet Gynecol* 1987; **69**: 399–402
17. Bowen LW, Sand PK, Ostergard DR, Franti CE. Unsuccessful Burch retropubic urethropexy. A case controlled urodynamic study. *Am J Obstet Gynecol* 1989; **160**: 452–458.
18. Wolf H, Coburg P, Maass H. Recidivrate nach Intontinenzoperationen bei Patrentinnen mit Hypotoner Urethra. *Geburtshilfe und Frauenheilkunde* 1989; **49**: 865–871.

19. Monga AK, Stanton SL. Predicting outcome of colposuspension—a prospective evaluation. *Neurourol Urodynam* 1997; **16**: 354–355.
20. Kjolhede P, Lindehammar H. Pelvic floor neuropathy in relation to the outcome of Burch colposuspension. *Int Urogynecol J Pelvic Floor Dysfunct* 1997; **8**: 61–65.
21. Gillon G, Stanton SL. Long-term follow up of surgery for urinary incontinence in elderly women. *Br J Urol* 1984; **56**: 478–481.
22. Bhatia NN. Role of antibiotic prophylaxis in retropubic surgery for stress urinary incontinence. *Obstet Gynecol* 1989; **74**: 637–639.
23. Krantz KK. Marshall-Marchetti-Krantz procedure. In: Stanton SL, Tanagho EA (eds). *Surgery of Female Incontinence*. Heidelberg: Springer-Verlag; 1986.
24. Burch J. Urethrovaginal fixation to Cooper's ligament for correction of stress incontinence, cystocele and prolapse. *Am J Obstet Gynecol* 1961; **81**: 281–290.
25. Wiskind AK, Creighton SM, Stanton SI. The incidence of genital prolapse after the Burch colposuspension. *Am J Obstet Gynecol* 1992; **167**: 399–404.
26. Alacalay et al. 1997; (unpublished work).
27. Montz F, Stanton SL. Suprapubic bladder catheterisation: Use and management in the gynecologic patient. *Contemp Obstet Gynecol* 1987; **25**: 31–34.
28. Koonings PP, Bergman A, Ballard CA. Prostaglandins for enhancing detrusor function after surgery for stress incontinence in women. *J Reprod Med* 1990; **35**: 1.
29. Kremer CC, Freeman RM. Which patients are at risk of voiding difficulty immediately after colposuspension. *Int Urogynecol J* 1995; **6**: 257–261.
30. Heit M, Vogt V, Brubaker L. An alternative statistical approach for predicting prolonged catheterisation after Burch colposuspension during reconstructive pelvic surgery. 1997; **8**: 203–208.
31. Sze EHM, Miklos JR, Karram MM. Voiding after colposuspension and effects of concomitant pelvic surgery: Correlation with preoperative voiding mechanism. *Obstet Gynecol* 1996; **88**: 564–567.
32. Vierhout ME, Mulder AFP. De novo detrusor instability after Burch colposuspension. *Acta Obstet Gynecol Scand* 1992; **72**: 414–416.
33. Alcalay M, Monga AK, Stanton SL. Burch colposuspension: A 10–20 year follow up. *Br J Obstet Gynaecol* 1995; **102**: 740–745.
34. Scotti RJ, Angell G, Flora R, Greston WM. Burch colposuspension for detrusor instability: Predictive value of preoperative history. *Neurourol Urodynam* 1996; **15**: 286.
35. Mainprize TC, Drutz HP. The Marshall Marchetti Krantz procedure: A critical review. *Obstet Gynecol Surv* 1988; **43**: 724–729.
36. Jarvis GJ. Surgery for genuine stress incontinence. *Br J Obstet Gynaecol* 1994; **101**: 371–374.
37. Kujansuu E. Urodynamic analysis of successful and failed incontinence surgery. *Int J Gynaecol Obstet* 1983; **21**: 355–360.
38. Milani R, Scalambrino S, Quadri G, et al. Marshall-Marchetti-Krantz procedure and Burch colposuspension in the surgical management of female urinary incontinence. *Br J Obstet Gynaecol* 1985; **92**: 1050–1053.
39. Riggs J. Retropubic cystourethropexy: A review of two operative procedures with long term follow up. *Obstet Gynecol* 1986; **68**: 98–105.
40. Spencer J, O'Connell V, Schaeffer A. The comparison of endoscopic suspension of the vesicle neck with suprapubic vesicourethropexy for the treatment of stress urinary incontinence. *J Urol* 1987; **137**: 411–415.
41. Park G, Miller E. Surgical treatment of stress urinary incontinence in comparison with kelly plication, Marshall-Marchetti-Krantz and Pereyra procedures. *Obstet Gynecol* 1986; **71**: 575–579.
42. Stanton SL, Cardozo L. Results of the colposuspension for incontinence and prolapse. *Br J Obstet Gynaecol* 1979; **86**: 693–697.
43. Walter S, Olesen KP, Hald T, Jensen HK, Pedersen PH. Urodynamic evaluation after vaginal repair and colposuspenion. *Br J Urol* 1982; **54**: 377–380.

44. Mundy AR. A trial comparing the stamey bladder neck suspension with colposuspension for the treatment of stress incontinence. *Br J Urol* 1983; **55**: 687–690.
45. Bhatia NN, Bergman A. Modified Burch versus Pereyra retropubic urethropexy for stress urinary incontinence. *Obstet Gynecol* 1985; **66**: 255–261.
46. Lose G, Jorgensen L, Mortensen SO, Molsted-Pedersen L, Kristensen JK. Voiding difficulties after colposuspension. *Obstet Cynecol* 1987; **69**: 33–38.
47. Galloway NT, Davies N, Stephenson TP. The complications of colposuspension. *Br J Urol* 1987; **60**: 122–124.
48. Pigne A, Keskes J, Maghioracos P, Boyer F, Marpeau L, Barrat J. Clinical and urodynamic results of Burch colposuspension operation in the treatment of female stress incontinence. A study apropos of 370 cases. *J Gynecol Obstet Biol Reprod Paris* 1988; **17**: 22–30.
49. Hilton P, Stanton SL. A clinical and urodynamic assessment of the Burch colposuspension for genuine stress incontinence. *Br J Obstet Gynaecol* 1983; **90**: 934–939.
50. Bergman A, Koonings PP, Ballard CA. Primary stress urinary incontinence and pelvic relaxation: prospective randomised comparison of three different operations. *Am J Obstet Gynecol* 1989; **161**: 97–101.
51. Eriksen BC, Hagen B, Eik-Nes SH, Molne K, Mjolnerod OK, Romslo I. Long term effectiveness of the Burch colposuspension in female urinary stress incontinence. *Acta Obstet Gynecol Scand* 1990; **69**: 45–50.
52. Kiilholma P, Makinen J, Chancellor MB, Pitkanen Y, Hirvonen T. Modified Burch colposuspension for stress urinary incontinence in females. *Surg Gynecol Obstet* 1993; **176**: 111–115.
53. Herbertsson G, Iosif CS. Surgical results and urodynamic studies 10 years after retropubic colpourethrocystopexy. *Acta Obstet Gynecol Scand* 1993; **72**: 298–301.
54. Feyereisl J, Dreher E, Haenggi W, Zikmund J, Schneider H. Long term results after Burch colposuspension. *Am J Obstet Gynecol* 1994; **171**: 647–652.
55. Kjolhede P, Ryden G. Prognostic factors and long term results of the Burch colposuspension. A retrospective study. *Acta Obstet Gynecol Scand* 1994; **73**: 642–647.
56. Kinn AC. Burch colposuspension for stress urinary incontinence. 5 year results in 153 women. *Scand J Urol Nephrol* 1995; **29**: 449–455.
57. Langer R, Halperin R, Schneider D, Bukovsky I. Burch colposuspension a 10–15 year follow up. *Neurourol Urodynam* 1998; **17**: 458–459.
58. Colombo M, Scalambrino S, Maggioni A, Milani R. Burch colposuspension versus modified Marshall-Marchetti-Krantz urethropexy for primary genuine stress incontinence: A prospective randomised clinical trial. *Am J Obstet Gynecol* 1994; **171**: 1573–1579.
59. Greunwald I, Monga AK, Stanton SL. Surgery for stress incontinence: A global perspective. *Neurourol Urodynam* 1996; **15**: 400–401.
60. Black NA, Downs SH. The effectiveness of surgery for stress incontinence in women: A systematic review. *Br J Urol* 1996; **78**: 497–510.

CHAPTER 10

Transvaginal needle suspension procedures

NEERAJ KOHLI AND MICKEY M. KARRAM

The optimal operation for the correction of genuine stress incontinence is still controversial, as more than 150 different procedures have been described. Procedures aimed at stabilizing the urethrovesical junction can be broadly classified as retropubic suspensions, transvaginal needle suspension procedures, and vaginal suburethral plication.

Transvaginal needle suspension procedures were first described in 1959 by Pereyra.[1] In an attempt to improve cure rates and minimize complications, over 15 modifications of the original Pereyra technique have been described.[2] Although current literature seems to suggest that the transvaginal needle suspension procedures have lower long-term cure rates compared to the retropubic approach,[3] they are still commonly performed procedures. Claimed advantages when compared to the retropubic procedures include the ability to readily perform concurrent vaginal repairs, decreased perioperative and post-operative morbidity, and shorter hospitalization and recovery.[4] The following chapter will review the history, surgical anatomy, indications, techniques, results, and complications of transvaginal needle suspension procedures.

HISTORY

Armand J. Pereyra became chief medical officer at the California Institution for Women after retiring from a 26-year career as an obstetrician-gynecologist in the United States Navy. While treating prison inmates with recurrent urinary incontinence following previous Marshall-Marchetti-Krantz procedures, Pereyra began to develop a surgical technique which could be performed transvaginally without splitting of the anterior abdominal fascia or extensive retropubic dissection.[5] His original technique, published in the 1959 edition of *Western Journal of Surgery, Obstetrics, and Gynecology*, utilized a special needle carrier passed through an abdominal stab incision penetrating the undissected vaginal wall. Extension of a stylet would result in a Y-shaped double unilateral vaginal perforation. Suture material, originally No. 30 steel wire, was passed through the needle, transferred to the abdominal site, and tied over the rectus sheath, resulting in vaginal wall elevation. Unfortunately, this original technique, reported on 31 patients followed for 14 months, had a high rate of recurrent anatomic defects because the vaginal loops eventually pulled through the vagina.[6]

Based on the collaborative efforts of Pereyra with Dr. Thomas Lebherz, the second modification of the original Pereyra technique was reported in 1967. This report summarized their experience by using No. 1 chromic suture with a technique of suprapubic angulation and suspension in conjunction with vesical neck plication to create a suburethral shelf that would help reduce strain on the suspensory sutures and minimize the pull-through effect. Although the article reported an initial success rate of 94% in 210 patients, long-term follow-up by Pereyra[7-9] found the failure rate to increase to 16% due to suture failure. Nonabsorbable suture would be shown to pull through the tissue, while absorbable sutures would subsequently weaken and break.[10]

Over the next decade, Pereyra and Lebherz experimented with various suture materials and operative techniques. In 1979, they described a subsequent modification which is recognized today as the modified Pereyra procedure. This modification included vaginal entrance into the retropubic space followed by release of the anterolateral attachments of the periurethral tissue from the pubic rami. A helical nonabsorbable suture was passed through the detached endopelvic fascia and posterior pubourethral ligaments. Traction on the sutures resulted in ruffling and thickening of the periurethral tissues, thus preventing suture pull-through. The suspensory sutures were then transferred to the abdominal site by using a newly developed needle carrier and anchored to the anterior rectus fascia. Pereyra and Lebherz[8,11] reported this modification to be associated with success rates ranging from 84–95% with variable long-term follow-up.

In 1965, Harer and Gunther[12] reported the first modification of the original Pereyra technique, which used a vaginal incision to cover the suspending sutures, continuous chromic catgut suture instead of wire to suspend the paraurethral tissue, and simultaneous performance of a vaginal urethroplasty to correct funneling. Their initial experience resulted in a cure rate of 83% with variable short-term follow-up. In 1973, Stamey[13] first described his technique, which was performed under cystoscopic guidance to visualize the urethrovesical junction and incorporated a Dacron buffer in the periurethral suture to prevent tissue pull-through. In his series of 203 patients, Stamey[14] reported a short-term cure rate of 91%. In 1975, Mason and Soderstorm[15] advocated the use of an infant cystoscope suprapubically to ensure proper passage of the needle from the vagina to the suprapubic area. No postoperative results were reported. Using a specially designed double-pronged needle in their 1978 modification, Cobb and Radge[16] used No. 2 nylon with a centrally tied barrel knot to suspend the urethra bilaterally to the anterior rectus sheath through two transverse suprapubic skin incisions. Their results reported 56 of 62 women to be continent with a mean follow-up of 11 months.[16]

The Raz[17] modification, introduced in 1981, altered the modified Pereyra approach in that the suspension sutures incorporated full-thickness vaginal wall (excluding the epithelium) in addition to the endopelvic fascia. Among 100

consecutive patients undergoing the Raz procedure, 96 were noted to subjectively have "excellent control" of their stress incontinence. In 1982, Muzsnai
and colleagues[18] described a transvaginal needle colposuspension, stabilizing the
urethra by suspending full-thickness vagina (excluding epithelium) to the
anterior rectus sheath using a Pereyra needle. Ninety-eight patients were
monitored for up to 6 months with a 95% cure rate. In an effort to make the
needle suspension procedure minimally invasive, Gittes and Loughlin[19]
described a no-incision pubovaginal suspension procedure in 1987. In their
initial study of 38 patients, they reported an 87% overall cure rate, noting six
failures early in the series. In 1988, Leach[20] described a bone fixation technique
stabilizing the paraurethral fascia to the pubic tubercle by using a helical permanent suture. This series reported a cure rate of 95% in 115 consecutive cases with
few postoperative complications. Further modifications of the bone anchoring
procedure led to a percutaneous technique described by Benderev[21] who reported
on 150 women undergoing this procedure.

Additional modifications using a variety of sutures, different anchoring
tissues, and laparoscopic guidance have also been described, but these results are
limited by insufficient sample size and a lack of long-term follow-up data.

SURGICAL ANATOMY

The anatomy of the anterior pelvic compartment is complex and the exact
mechanism of urinary continence is poorly understood. Current concepts empha-
size the role of urethral hypermobility and ineffective abdominal pressure transmission to the proximal urethra in the pathophysiology of genuine stress
incontinence. Lack of a clear understanding as well as inconsistency in
terminology describing the anatomic supports of the urethra and bladder has led
to much confusion regarding the many modifications of the needle suspension
procedures.

Traditionally, the urethra and bladder have been described to rest on a sheet of
endopelvic fascia that envelops the vagina and attaches laterally to the arcus
tendineus fasciae pelvis and the levator ani muscles. The anterior portion of the
arcus in the area of the pubis is a thin tendinous band that widens out posteriorly
as it approaches the ischial spine.[22] Urethral support is provided by the anterior
and posterior pubourethral ligaments. Contrary to their description, these fascial
attachments do not actually insert directly onto the pubic bone.[23] Recent studies
have revealed these ligaments to be a dense band of connective tissue that
supports the urethra and is composed of a muscular component that attaches the
connective tissue of the vagina to the levator ani muscles and a fascial
component that connects the endopelvic fascia between the urethra and vagina
laterally to the arcus tendineus fasciae pelvis.[24]

Recent data have challenged our traditional understanding of the "vaginal
fascia". Based on histologic and anatomic studies, Weber and Walters[25] have
noted that the layer previously referred to as the "pubocervical fascia" is in fact

the adventitial layer of the vagina, which lies above the muscularis. The vagina is separated from the bladder anteriorly by the continuation of loose areolar tissue that merges with the vagina adventitia. At the level of the urethra, the adventitia is less distinct, and the muscular layers of the vagina and urethra are fused. The lateral aspects of the vagina are attached on each side by fibrous connections to the parietal fascia overlying the the levator ani muscles. This fibrous connection forms the arcus tendineus fasciae pelvis and results in support of the vagina and the overlaying bladder. The urethral supports are composed of the anterior vagina and the perineal membrane with its muscular components, the urethrovaginal sphincter and compressor urethrae.

The surgical anatomy of the needle bladder neck suspension has recently been described by Fitzpatrick and colleagues.[22] Based on cadaver studies, the point of entry into the retropubic space lies between the levator ani and its superior fascia, lateral to the arcus tendineus fascia pelvis, the paraurethral vascular plexus, and bladder neck. Suspension sutures placed during the needle urethropexy incorporate the portion of the endopelvic fascia that lies between the vagina and the urethra and, usually, the arcus tendineus fasciae pelvis, stabilizing the bladder neck by providing an alternate point of lateral fixation. As these procedures are often performed blindly through the retropubic space, knowledge regarding the surgical anatomy of the needle bladder neck suspension is very important for obtaining the appropriate tissue as well as avoiding complications such as hemorrhage and urinary tract injury.

INDICATIONS

Transvaginal needle suspension procedures are indicated for the correction of genuine stress incontinence, which is felt to be due to urethral hypermobility. These procedures achieve continence through support and stabilization of the proximal urethra and bladder neck, resulting in restoration of positive pressure transmission to the proximal urethra. Although some investigators have advocated the use of needle suspension procedures in the surgical management of intrinsic sphincter deficiency (type III incontinence), alternative treatment options such as suburethral slings, periurethral collagen injections, and artificial sphincters probably yield better results. Urodynamic studies are recommended before surgical correction to document bladder compliance and rule out intrinsic sphincter deficiency.

TECHNIQUES

The following section will provide a brief review of the commonly performed modifications of the needle suspension procedures with pertinent aspects of the surgical techniques. Comparison of the various modifications is illustrated in Figure 10-1. Table 10-1 notes the difference among the procedures.

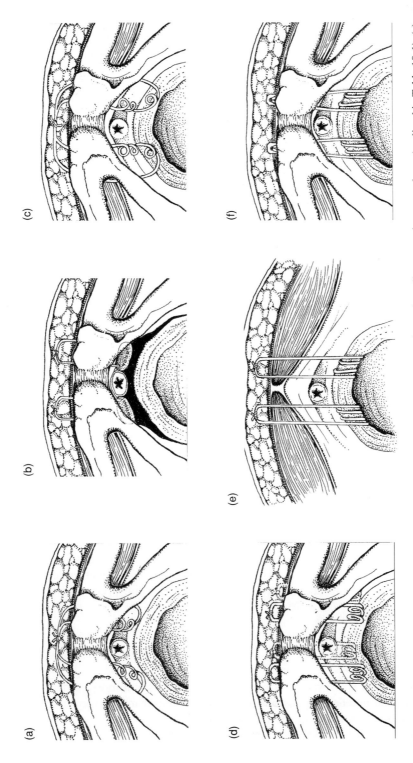

Figure 10-1. Cross-sectional view of anchoring tissue used in the commonly performed needle suspension procedures (outlined in Table 10-1). (a) Modified Pereyra procedure: helical stitch through pubourethral ligament and detached endopelvic fascia. (b) Stamey procedure: Dacron buttresses placed on each side of the bladder neck. (c) Raz procedure: helical stitch through detached endopelvic fascia and anchored in vaginal wall excluding epithelium. (d) Muzsnai: two stitches on each side of the bladder neck through vaginal wall excluding epithelium. (e) Gittes procedure: stitches through full-thickness vaginal wall. (f) Percutaneous bone fixation: stitches through full-thickness vaginal wall attached to bone anchors.

Table 10.1. Differences among various needle suspension procedures

Procedure	Vaginal incision	Needle passage	Anchoring tissue	Use of cystoscopy
Modified Pereyra	Midline	Direct finger guidance	Pubourethral ligament and endopelvic fascia	Rule out injury
Stamey	T-shaped	Blindly	Pubocervical fascia	Confirm suture placement
Raz	Inverted U	Direct finger guidance	Endopelvic fascia and vaginal wall	Rule out injury
Muzsnai	Midline	Direct finger guidance	Vaginal wall (excluding epithelium)	Rule out injury
Gittes	None	Blindly	Full thickness of vaginal wall	Confirm suture placement
Percutaneous bone fixation	None	Blindly	Full thickness of vaginal wall	Rule out injury

These procedures can be performed under general, spinal, or epidural anesthesia with the patient in the dorsolithotomy position. DVT prophylaxis and preoperative antibiotics are recommended for all patients. The lower abdomen and perineum are cleansed and draped in a sterile fashion, and a Foley catheter is inserted into the bladder to facilitate bladder drainage and identify the anatomic location of the urethrovesical junction.

Modified Pereyra Procedure

A midline anterior vaginal wall incision is made through the epithelium beginning 2 cm superior to the external urethral meatus and extending down to just beyond the urethrovesical junction. Using Metzenbaum scissors, the epithelium is mobilized laterally on each side to reveal the underlying endopelvic fascia. At the level of the bladder neck, the dissection is extended laterally to the inferior pubic ramus. The anterolateral attachments of the periurethral tissue are released using a fingertip directed against the inferior posterolateral pubic ramus. This detachment of the endopelvic fascia can be performed either sharply (Figure 10-2) or bluntly (Figure 10-3). The surgeon's fingertip is then flexed medially to hook the edge of the detached fascia, which is then grasped and brought down into the vaginal field (Figure 10-4). A No. 0 polypropylene suture is passed in a

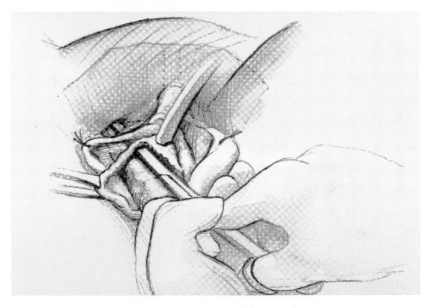

Figure 10-2.   Technique of sharp entrance into the retropubic space. The endopelvic fascia is perforated at the inferior margin of the pubic ramus by using Metzenbaum scissors guided by the surgeon's finger. After perforation of the endopelvic fascia, the blades of the scissors are separated slightly to allow insertion of a finger into the retropublic space. (From reference 71, with permission.)

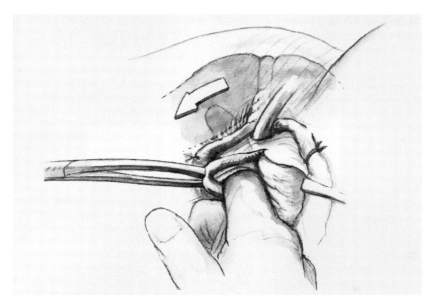

Figure 10-3. Technique of blunt dissection into the retropubic space. With the tip of the index finger flexed anteriorly against the posterior surface of the pubic ramus, the paraurethral attachment of the endopelvic fascia to the pubic bone is perforated downward and lateral, allowing easy insertion of a finger into the retropubic space. (From reference 71, with permission.)

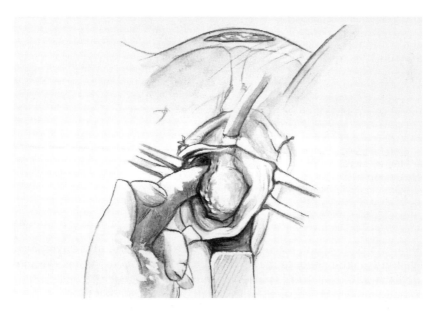

Figure 10-4. Identification of endopelvic fascia. Once the retropubic space has been entered, the surgeon's finger is flexed medially behind the detached endopelvic fascia, mobilizing it into the vaginal field to facilitate placement of the anchoring suture in a helical fashion. (From reference 71, with permission.)

helical fashion several times through this detached fascia. Traction of this suture confirms correct placement in strong supportive tissue (Figure 10-5).

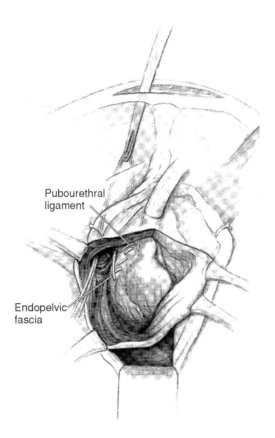

Figure 10-5.   Modified Pereyra procedure. Permanent suture is anchored to the detached endopelvic fascia in a helical fashion. (From reference 71, with permission.)

A small transverse skin incision is made 2 cm above the pubic symphysis and the incision is taken down to the level of the anterior rectus fascia. The Pereyra ligature carrier (Figure 10-6) is introduced through the lateral aspect of this skin incision and advanced retropubically into the vaginal wound under direct finger guidance. (Figure 10-7) Each suspension suture is transferred from the vagina to the suprapubic incision, and cystoscopy is performed to ensure no bladder injury or stitch penetration has occurred. The sutures are then tied over the anterior rectus fascia.

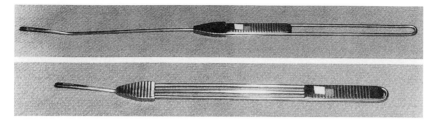

Figure 10-6. Pereyra ligature carrier. Shown in the open (*top*) and closed (*bottom*) position. (Courtesy of EI Ney Industries, Inc. Upland, CA.) (From reference 71, with permission.)

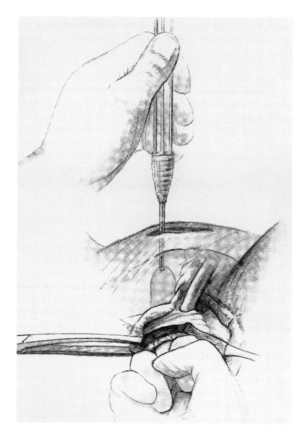

Figure 10-7. Suprapubic transfer of the suspension sutures. A small suprapubic incision is made, and the rectus fascia is perforated with the needle which is passed through the retropubic space to the vaginal area under direct finger guidance. Care should be taken to guide the needle laterally along the posterior surface of the pubic symphysis to prevent injury to the bladder. (From reference 71, with permission.)

Stamey Procedure

Two small transverse suprapubic incisions are made 3 fingerbreadths above the pubic symphysis on each side of the midline and taken down till the anterior rectus fascia is exposed. Next, a T-shaped incision is made on the anterior vaginal mucosa and the vaginal wall is dissected off the underlying urethra and bladder, exposing the bladder neck. One of three special needles (Figure 10-8), each angled at different degrees, is passed blindly through the retropubic space alongside the vesical neck, which is identified by gentle traction on the Foley balloon. A 70-degree cystoscope is then inserted to ensure lateral motion of the needle produces indentation or movement of the vesical wall at the bladder neck. Once proper placement is confirmed, the tip of the needle is advanced into the vagina, threaded with No. 2 monofilament nylon suture, and withdrawn suprapubically. The needle is again passed through the same incision 1 to 2 cm lateral to the original entry to exit in the vagina ~1 cm distal to the previous needle exit site. The vaginal end of the nylon suture is passed through a 1-cm tube of 5-mm knitted Dacron arterial graft to buttress the vaginal tissue, threaded through the the eye of the needle, and pulled out suprapubically. This procedure is repeated on the opposite side (Figure 10-9).

The vaginal incision is irrigated with antibiotic solution and closed, burying the Dacron buttresses below the suture line. Gentle traction is placed on the suspension sutures, which are then tied loosely on each side.

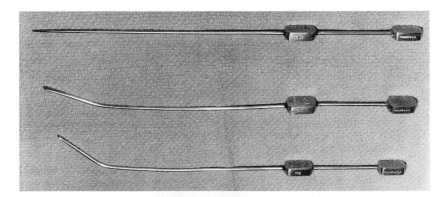

Figure 10-8. Series of Stamey needles. Straight needle (*top*), 15-degree angled needle (*middle*), and 30-degree angled needle (*bottom*). (Courtesy of Pilling Co. Fort Washington, PA) (From reference 71, with permission.)

Raz Procedure

The Raz modification differs from the 1978 modification of the Pereyra procedure in its use of vaginal wall in addition to endopelvic fascia as anchoring tissue in stabilizing the bladder neck. The technique begins with an inverted U-shaped incision of the anterior vaginal wall and vaginal dissection lateral to

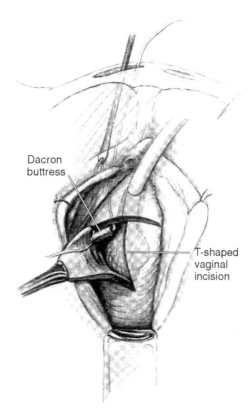

Figure 10-9.   Stamey procedure. The endopelvic fascia is used to anchor surgical polyester fiber (Dacron) loops on each side of the bladder neck. These loops are suspended to the anterior rectus fascia by using nylon sutures. (From reference 71, with permission.)

the urethra and bladder neck. The retropubic space in entered and dissected as previously described, allowing adequate mobility of the vaginal wall, bladder, and urethra. Monofilament suture, typically No. 1 polypropylene, is then placed in a helical fashion through the detached endopelvic fascia and anchored in the full-thickness of the vaginal wall excluding epithelium (Figure 10-10).

Next, a small transverse suprapubic incision is made. The suspension sutures are then transferred suprapubically under direct finger guidance by using a needle ligature carrier, and cystoscopy is performed to assess bladder integrity and ureteral patency. After the vaginal incision is closed, the sutures are tied above the fascia.

Muzsnai Procedure

Muzsnai and colleagues[18] described this modification after observing that the integrity and strength of the detached endopelvic fascia was unpredictable. With

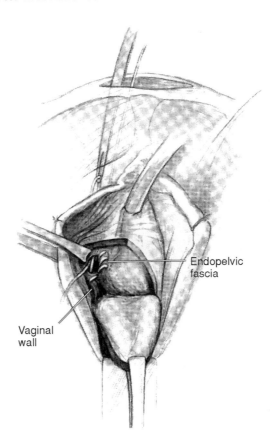

Figure 10-10. Raz procedure. The suspension sutures are incorporated into the detached endopelvic fascia in a helical fashion and anchored into the full-thickness vaginal wall excluding epithelium. (From reference 71, with permission.)

hopes of duplicating the results of the Burch colposuspension, they described a vaginal colposuspension. Using a Foley balloon to identify the urethrovesical junction before opening the anterior vaginal wall, the bladder neck is marked on both sides. The bladder and urethra are dissected off the vaginal wall through a midline vaginal incision. The retropubic space is entered and dissected as previously described. Two nonabsorbable sutures, one at the level of the midurethra and the other at the level of the bladder neck, are then placed in a helical fashion through the inner surface of the vaginal wall excluding epithelium ~2 cm lateral to the edge of the vaginal flap. This procedure is repeated on the opposite side (Figure 10-11).

The sutures are then transferred suprapubically through a midline incision under direct finger guidance. A bridge of rectus fascia between each set of sutures should be maintained during withdrawal. Cystoscopy is performed, and

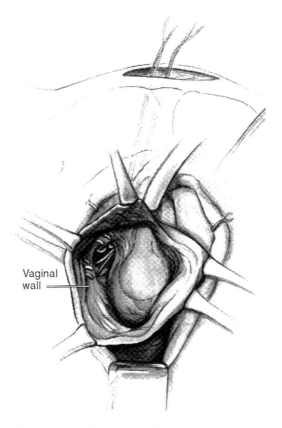

Figure 10-11. Muzsnai procedure. After vaginal dissection, two sets of permanent suture are placed on each side of the bladder neck, incorporating full thickness of the vaginal wall excluding epithelium. (From reference 71, with permission.)

the vagina is closed. With a hand elevating the anterior vaginal wall, the sutures are tied, creating a dimple in the lateral area of the vaginal fornix on each side similar to an abdominal colposuspension.

Gittes Procedure

The Gittes procedure, a no-incision pubovaginal suspension, is similar to the original needle suspension procedure initially described by Pereyra in 1959.[1] No vaginal incision is made in this procedure. A small puncture is made in the suprapubic skin and subcutaneous tissue, 2 cm superior to the pubic bone and 5 cm lateral to the midline on each side. A 30-degree Stamey needle is introduced into this incision, passed through the rectus fascia, and carefully advanced along the posterior aspect of the pubic bone. With the surgeon's other hand elevating the anterior vaginal wall lateral to the bladder neck, identified by palpation of the Foley balloon, the tip of the needle is popped through the unopened vagina. A No. 2 nylon suture is threaded through the eye of the needle which is then withdrawn. A second pass is made through a different site on the rectus facia with the vaginal exit point of the needle to be selected tactilely and visually to be ~2 cm cephalad to the original vaginal penetration. Using a free needle, the suture is anchored to the vaginal wall between the first and second penetration in a helical fashion and then transferred to the suprapubic region (Figure 10-12). Cystourethroscopy is performed during passage of the sutures to assure no inadvertent bladder injury or suture penetration has occurred. The sutures are tied tightly into the stab incision, resulting in elevation of the anterior vaginal wall and bladder neck. The tied sutures are pulled upward and trimmed just above the knot, which then retracts below the skin.

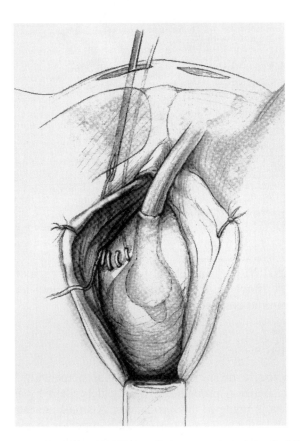

Figure 10-12.   Gittes procedure. Permanent stitches are taken through full thickness of the vaginal wall and transferred suprapubically. No vaginal incision is made. (From reference 71, with permission.)

Bone Fixation Procedure

In an effort to reduce postoperative discomfort and the "pulling sensation" caused by anchoring the sutures to the rectus fascia and to provide a stable anchor point nondependent on patient position or fascial rigidity, Leach[20] described the bone fixation technique for transvaginal needle suspension in 1988. This technique was essentially a modified Pereyra procedure with the exception that the pubic tubercle instead of the anterior rectus fascia was used as a fixation point for the suspension sutures which incorporated the full thickness anterior vaginal wall excluding epithelium.[20]

A current modification of this technique, described by Benderev,[21] employs special instrumentation and bone anchors to perform it as a minimally invasive percutaneous procedure. A 3- to 4-cm midline suprapubic incision is made and the periosteum of the pubic tubercle is exposed. Using a bone locator to establish the correct symmetrical position over the pubic tubercle, a titanium bone anchor with its attached No. 1 permanent monofilament suture is drilled into the cortex of the symphysis bilaterally. Next, one end of the suspension suture is threaded through the eye of a special needle suture passer, which is used to perforate four sites on the unopened anterior vaginal wall ~1 cm lateral to the bladder neck on both sides. The suture passer, operated with a thumb lever and three-position toggle, is guided through the abdominal wall musculature and retropubic space directly behind the pubic bone to perforate the vaginal wall. Cystoscopy is performed to exclude bladder injury by the passer. The passer is then withdrawn into the retropubic space above the endopelvic fascia and then passed again, passing slightly cephalad to its first vaginal exit point. This series of steps is repeated resulting in a Z-shaped suture configuration. Cystoscopy is again performed to assess bladder and urethral integrity. This procedure is repeated on the opposite side. After both sides are completed, traction is placed on the nonanchored end of the suture to confirm adequate strength and location at the level of the bladder neck. The sutures are then tied to the bone anchors using a suture spacer which prevents excessive tension on the suspension sutures. The incision is then irrigated and closed.

RESULTS

Surgical success rates of the various antiincontinence procedures are difficult to evaluate due to limitations of published studies. Success rates are dependent on the extent of preoperative evaluation, the criteria used to determine success, and the time of follow-up. Many previous studies have reported success rates based on subjective evaluation of patient complaints rather than objective urodynamic evaluation. Additionally, length of follow-up is often highly variable and inconsistent even within individual studies. Although few long-term studies exist, longer length of follow-up is generally associated with decreased efficacy rates and may be subject to more recall bias.[26] Second, many studies do not have strict exclusion criteria and compare heterogeneous groups which include variations in age, weight, history of prior surgery, associated medical conditions, associated pelvic prolapse, and coexisting detrusor instability or intrinsic sphincter deficiency. Third, the various modifications in materials and techniques used by individual surgeons make direct comparison of results difficult. Finally, very few studies report postoperative complications such as voiding dysfunction, urge incontinence, or pelvic prolapse. One should keep these limitations in mind when analyzing the published data regarding the surgical efficacy of antiincontinence procedures.

Published results of transvaginal needle suspension procedures report cure rates varying from 40% to 100%, depending on method of postoperative assessment and duration of follow-up[27–37] (Table 10-2). The generally accepted success rate is 85% with variable follow-up based on a review of published results of more than 2000 patients[2,38] (Table 10-3). However, most of these reports are observational studies with limited sample size and nonstandardized follow-up, and few define the severity of incontinence or use objective measures of cure. Furthermore, some modifications have little to no objective long-term data available regarding success rates.

Several studies have investigated the surgical efficacy of the needle suspension procedures in the elderly patient who may benefit from the less invasive transvaginal procedure. In a retrospective analysis of 92 women over the age of 65 with genuine stress incontinence, Nitti and coworkers[39] reported a subjective cure or improvement rate of 68%. Golomb and associates[40] reported a subjective cure rate of 90% in 21 patients studied. The overall follow-up time for both series was 17 months. Unfortunately, studies with objective outcomes analysis and longer follow-up have reported significantly lower cure rates. Peattie and Stanton[41] noted only a 53% subjective cure rate and a 43% objective cure rate at 2 years after a Stamey procedure. Mundy[27] confirmed these findings, reporting a 40% success rate in 51 patients treated with a Stamey procedure who were objectively evaluated at 1 year. Using the modified Pereyra procedure, Stanton and coworkers[42] reported a subjective cure rate of 57% and an objective cure rate of 46% in 35 women with 2-year follow-up.

In a prospective randomized study of 289 patients with primary stress incontinence and coexisting pelvic relaxation treated with either anterior colporrhaphy, modified Pereyra procedure, or retropubic urethropexy, Bergman and associates[33] reported significantly better results with the retropubic approach. Patients were randomized with respect to procedure and surgeon and underwent objective urodynamic evaluation before surgery and at 3 months and 12 months postoperatively. Although objective cure rates were comparable on short-term follow-up, 1-year follow-up revealed the cure rates were significantly higher for the Burch colposuspension compared to the Pereyra needle suspension or the anterior colporrhaphy (87%, 70%, and 69%, respectively).[33] A separate study analyzing 109 patients with isolated genuine stress incontinence randomized in a similar fashion confirmed these results.[31] Bergman and Elia[37] recently published a 5-year objective follow-up of this original study group which noted the Burch

Table 10-2. Published studies comparing needle suspension procedures to other antiincontinence procedures

Investigator(s) (ref).	No. of patients	Outcomes analysis	Cure rate by procedure (%)				Length of follow-up
			Needle suspension	Anterior colporrhaphy	Retropubic urethropexy	Suburethral sling	
Mundy (27)	51	Subjective	76 (S)		89 (BC)		12 m
		Objective	40 (S)		73 (BC)		
Riggs (28)	204	Mixed	77 (P)		86 (MMK)		5–10 y
Spencer et al. (29)	95	Subjective	61 (S)		57 (MMK)		2–10 y
English and Fowler (30)	45	Objective	58 (S)				6 m
Bergman et al. (31)	107	Objective	72 (P)	65	91 (BC)		12 m
Hilton (32)	21	Objective	80 (S)			90	6 m
Bergman et al. (33)	289	Objective	70 (P)	69	87 (BC)		12 m
Karram et al. (34)	93	Subjective	82 (P)				12 m
		Objective	63 (P)				
Trockman et al. (35)	125	Subjective	20 (P)				5–13 y
Korman et al. (36)	106	Subjective	47 (S)				9–45 m
Bergman and Elia (37)	93	Objective	43 (P)	37	82 (BC)		5 y

S, Stamey; P, Pereyra; BC, Burch colposuspension; MMK, Marshall-Marchetti-Krantz, m, months; y, years.

Table 10-3.   Success rates following transvaginal needle bladder neck suspension

Investigator (ref.)	No. of patients	No. of cures	Cure rate (%)	Follow-up (months)
Pereyra, 1959 (1)	31	28	90	14
Harer and Gunther, 1965 (12)	30	25	83	2–36
Pereyra and Lebherz, 1967 (7)	210	198	94	12
Crist et al., 1969	56	30	54	23
Backer and Probst 1971	80	68	85	6–12
Kursh et al., 1972	25	16	64	0–36
Stamey, 1973 (13)	16	11	69	0–36
Portnuff and Ballon, 1973	186	170	91	24–60
Litvak and McRoberts, 1974	35	31	89	36–60
Stamey et al., 1975	44	41	93	10–29
Winter, 1976	9	7	78	1–7
Backer and Probst, 1976	199	163	82	6–108
Cobb and Radge, 1978 (16)	62	56	90	6–18
Pereyra and Lebherz, 1978 (8)	49	49	100	12
Pereyra, 1978 (11)	29	27	93	24–36
Vordermark et al., 1979	20	18	90	3–24
Stamey, 1980 (14)	203	184	91	6+
Raz, 1981 (17)	100	96	96	
Quigley and King, 1981	50	41	82	12–24
Faysal et al., 1981	20	18	90	1
Pereyra et al., 1982 (9)	82	70	85	48–60
Mundy, 1983 (27)	25	10	40	12
Leach and Raz 1984	54	50	94	24
Fleischer et al., 1984	48	38	79	4–41
Diaz et al., 1984	31	28	90	6
Gaum et al., 1984 (64)	60	55	90	6
Ashken et al., 1984	60	46	77	12–24
Richardson et al., 1984	163	150	92	36
Huland and Bucher, 1984	66	47	71	48
Bhatia and Bergman, 1985	20	17	85	12
Leach et al., 1987	20	18	90	14
Spencer et al., 1987 (29)	41	25	61	21
Vamer, 1990 (4)	20	16	80	12–39
Ramon et al., 1990 (39)	62	56	84	10–46
Benderev, 1994 (21)	53	49	92	15
Total	*2096*	*1802*	*85*	

Adapted from reference 2.

colposuspension to maintain its durability over time while the results with anterior colporrhaphy and needle suspension continued to deteriorate, 82% vs 43% vs 37%, respectively.

Based on a hand search of all relevant articles published since 1970, Jarvis[3] recently reported a meta-analysis of 213 studies comparing previously published outcomes data of the different procedures utilized in the surgical treatment of genuine stress incontinence. The cure rate for the transvaginal needle suspension procedures, with or without endoscopic guidance, was consistently lower than retropubic approaches (Marshall-Marchetti-Krantz urethropexy or Burch colposuspension) on both objective and subjective assessment. Further breakdown of studies with objective results confirmed the retropubic approach to have better cure rates than the transvaginal needle suspension procedures for primary incontinence but not necessarily in the treatment of recurrent incontinence (Table 10-4). Based on these data and analysis of associated complications, the author concluded that "this review demonstrates the poor comparative nature of reported studies in the world" and "there is no single genuine stress incontinence operation which should be offered to all women in all situations as a first choice".[3]

Table 10-4. Meta analysis results comparing efficacy of antiincontinence procedures

Procedure	% Objective cure rate		
	All patients	Primary incontinence	Recurrent incontinence
Kelly plication	72.0	67.8	—
MMK procedure	89.2	89.5	—
Burch colposuspension	71.4	89.8	82.5
Nonendoscopic BNS	71.4	70.2	75.0
Endoscopic BNS	70.0	86.7	86.4
Suburethral sling	85.3	93.9	86.1

MMK, Marshall-Marchetti-Krantz; BNS, bladder needle suspension.
Adapted from reference 3.

COMPLICATIONS

Complications of needle suspension procedures can be broadly classified into those mutual for all incontinence procedures and those associated specifically with the transvaginal needle suspension procedures and their modifications.

RECURRENT OR PERSISTENT POSTOPERATIVE INCONTINENCE

Postoperative incontinence may be due to surgical failure, development of *de novo* or worsening of coexisting detrusor instability, intrinsic sphincter deficiency, overflow incontinence, or fistula formation. The most common cause of recurrent incontinence is weakness of the anchoring tissues and inaccurate placement of the suspension sutures that fail to provide adequate urethral support. Suture erosion occurs in 0% to 12% of cases and suture breakage has been reported in up to 6% of suspension procedures.[29,43] Coexisting medical conditions such as chronic abdominal straining or coughing and chronic obstructive pulmonary disease may increase the likelihood of suture erosion or breakage.

Coexisting detrusor instability or intrinsic sphincter deficiency may also lead to recurrent incontinence. Both the Webster[44] and Lockhart[45] groups have reported that more than 50% of women with persistent urinary leakage following antiincontinence surgery have evidence of detrusor instability and urge incontinence. Patients with irritative bladder symptoms should undergo preoperative urodynamics and may require pharmacotherapy postoperatively. Several authors have reported an increased incidence of recurrent or persistent incontinence after antiincontinence surgery in patients with low urethral pressures preoperatively.[46,47] Although genuine stress incontinence associated with coexisting urethral hypermobility and intrinsic sphincter deficiency may improve or resolve in the short-term postoperative period following bladder neck stabilization, long-term results are suboptimal. These patients may benefit more from a suburethral sling procedure, which creates increased resistance at the bladder neck in addition to providing stability to the urethrovesical junction.

Overflow incontinence, an uncommon cause of postoperative urinary leakage, occurs with overdistention of the bladder and can be a manifestation of iatrogenic retention or neurologic disease. This condition can be managed with a combination of fluid restriction and self-catheterization. Fistula formation should be considered in the differential diagnosis of immediate postoperative incontinence, which is persistent.

VOIDING DYSFUNCTION

Voiding dysfunction is a potential complication of any antiincontinence procedure. Although the incidence of immediate postoperative voiding dysfunction varies widely between the different surgical approaches, we believe that the needle suspension procedures are associated with increased postoperative voiding dysfunction and irritative bladder symptoms compared to the retropubic procedures. Various studies have reported the incidence of urinary retention to range from 2% to 50% and chronic incomplete emptying can be seen in up to 20% of patients.[42]

Patients with increased preoperative postvoid residuals, coexisting severe anterior vaginal wall prolapse, or underactive or areflexic detrusor muscles are at increased risk and should be counseled preoperatively. Fortunately, this condition is usually transient and self-limited. The incidence of prolonged voiding dysfunction has been reported to be 2% to 7%.

Postoperative voiding dysfunction can be initially managed with intermittent self-catheterization until a normal voiding pattern returns. The management of persistent urinary retention is controversial, and options should be discussed with the patient on an individual basis. Long-term self-catheterization or placement of a suprapubic tube is the mainstay of therapy. Medical management using prostaglandins, tranquilizers, and alpha-blockers has also been reported. Occasionally, surgical revision with takedown of the suspension sutures may be indicated. Readjustment of the loop tension without excision of the sutures has also been reported.[50]

PELVIC PROLAPSE

Recent studies have noted the rate of recurrent prolapse to be increased when needle suspension procedures are performed in conjunction with other recon- structive vaginal procedures. In a prospective study of 88 women undergoing reconstructive pelvic surgery for advanced pelvic prolapse randomized to the abdominal or vaginal route, Benson and coworkers[51] found that patients under- going abdominal repair had significantly better surgical outcomes and required less reoperation for recurrent incontinence or prolapse. Surgical effectiveness was optimal in 29% of the vaginal group in which needle suspension procedures were the primary antiincontinence procedure and 58% of the abdominal group in which retropubic repair was the primary anticontinence procedure. The re- operation rate was 33% in the vaginal group and 16% in the abdominal group.[51] Kohli and coworkers[52] reported the incidence of recurrent cystocele following transvaginal needle suspension with concurrent anterior colporrhaphy to be as high as 33% on 1-year follow-up compared to 7% when anterior colporrhaphy alone was performed. Sze and associates[53] noted a similarly increased rate of recurrent prolapse to or beyond the hymen in 75 women undergoing sacro- spinous ligament fixation with or without concurrent needle suspension with a mean follow-up of 24 months. Bump and colleagues[54] have also reported that the combination of needle bladder neck suspension with other vaginal operations for advanced prolapse predisposes to early development of anterior vaginal segment support defects and inadequate bladder neck support. Although the etiology of these findings is uncertain, possible theories include pelvic neuropathy produced by vaginal dissection, iatrogenic paravaginal defects created during retropubic mobilization, and significant alteration in the vaginal axis.

INFECTION

Infection can occur after any surgical procedure but is probably more common in needle suspension procedures utilizing nonabsorbable suture, buttresses, and grafts, and in those procedures in which permanent suture penetrate the vaginal lumen. Since most surgeons use permanent suture when performing these procedures, stitch abscesses and wound infections have been reported in 2% to 12% of cases and may present either vaginally or suprapubically.[29,42,55,56] Abscesses rarely occur in the postoperative period, but may present months and even years postoperatively. If an abscess occurs, the wound should be opened to drain and antibiotics begun. If initial management fails, reexploration with removal of sutures or buttresses may be required.[57]

Osteitis pubis has been reported in up to 10% of Marshall-Marchetti-Krantz procedures,[42] and is certainly a concern when performing the bone fixation needle procedure. To date, there are limited data regarding the safety and efficacy of this procedure.

The incidence of postoperative urinary tract infection following needle suspension procedures is highly variable, varying from 1% to 32%.[40,58] Urosepsis has also been reported.[29] This rate is dependent on many factors, including coexisting cystocele, incomplete bladder emptying, type of catheter drainage system used, and length of drainage required postoperatively. Suprapubic catheter drainage systems have been associated with less postoperative bacteriuria compared with transurethral systems.[59] Patients should be treated with appropriate antibiotic treatment and suppression therapy if indicated. Patients with persistent postoperative bacteriuria should undergo cystoscopic evaluation to exclude an anatomic abnormality (i.e., diverticulum) or foreign body (i.e., suture).[60]

Proper precautions, including a sterile preoperative urine, an antibacterial vaginal/abdominal preparation, broad-spectrum intravenous intraoperative antibiotics, and postoperative oral antibiotics while catheters are in place, may minimize the frequency of postoperative infections.[61]

HEMORRHAGE

Bleeding complications, including excessive intraoperative blood loss, need for transfusion, and hematoma formation, are more common after modifications the require vaginal entry into the retropubic space. Excessive intraoperative bleeding may occur during mobilization of the perivesical venous plexus and may be controlled with suture ligature, elevation of the bladder neck resulting in tamponade, or vaginal packing. An alternative technique, described by Kartske and Raz,[62] is the placement of a sponge-wrapped Foley catheter with a 30-ml balloon into the bleeding space to achieve transvaginal tamponade. Excessive electrocautery in the area of the urethra should be avoided, as thermal injury may result in fistula formation. Postoperative transfusion complicating needle suspension procedures has been reported in 1% to 7% of cases.[34,54,63] Reoperation for bleeding is rare, and the rate of hematoma formation has been reported to be 1% to 5% based on several large series.[4,5,10,11,64,65]

Fitzpatrick and associates[22] have identified two groups of vessels vulnerable to injury during retropubic dissection: the branches of the the inferior vesical and vaginal arteries that form the paraurethral vascular plexus, which lie lateral to the urethra just above the paraurethral sulcus, and the branches of the dorsal clitoral vessels, which lie in the perineal membrane. These same vessels can be injured during modifications that require blind insertion of the needle ligature carrier. Since subsequent bleeding may not be identified intraoperatively, a postoperative hematocrit is recommended on all patients. Meticulous surgical technique and knowledge of the surgical anatomy are essential in the prevention and management of vascular injuries during needle suspension procedures.

DETRUSOR INSTABILITY

Detrusor instability is a common cause of postoperative incontinence. Its presence should be evaluated preoperatively as it has been shown to coexist in up to 30% of women with genuine stress incontinence.[66,67] The postoperative course of detrusor instability is highly variable and unpredictable, and patients should be counseled before surgery. From 35% to 75% of patients will experience resolution of their urge-related symptoms following surgery, while 2% to 24% will develop de novo detrusor instability with or without incontinence.[42] This condition is often self-limited and shows improvement over time with observation and reassurance. Urinary culture should be performed to exclude infection as an etiologic agent, and cystoscopy and urodynamic evaluation should be considered in cases with persistent symptomology. Patients with protracted symptoms should be managed with bladder training and anticholinergic pharmacotherapy.

LOWER URINARY TRACT INJURY

Needle suspension-related injury to the bladder can occur during vaginal dissection, needle insertion, or suprapubic transfer of the suspension sutures. Inadvertent stitch penetration into the bladder lumen may be more common in modifications, such as the Stamey or Gittes, which advocate passage of the needle ligature carrier blindly through the retropubic space. Previous pelvic surgery with resulting scarring of the urethra and bladder may be an additional risk factor. Intraoperative cystoscopy should identify bladder injury or inadvertent stitch penetration. If an intravesical suture is noted, it should be removed and passed again under finger guidance. If such an injury is left unrecognized, persistence of a nonabsorbable suture within the bladder lumen may result in postoperative detrusor instability, persistent urinary tract infection, or formation of a bladder calculus.[66] Injury to the urethra or ureters following transvaginal needle procedures is rare.

NERVE DAMAGE

Needle suspension procedures are performed with the patient in the dorsal lithotomy position which, if not correctly done, can put the patient at risk for nerve damage due to compression or stretch injuries. The most frequent nerve involved is the common peroneal nerve, but injury to the obturator, sciatic, tibial, femoral, or saphenous nerves can also occur[69] (Table 10-5). These injuries are

Table 10-5. Nerves susceptible to injury during needle suspension procedures

Nerve	Location of injury	Mechanism of injury	Clinical presentation
Common peroneal	Fibular neck	Compression against brace	Footdrop
Sciatic	Sciatic notch	Compression or stretching during hip flexion	Weakness during knee flexion, or loss of common peroneal or tibial nerve function
Obturator	Pubic ramus	Compression	Weakness of ipsilateral thigh on adduction
Femoral	Inguinal ligament	Compression during hyperflexion of hips	Quadriceps weakness, gait impairment, decreased sensation over anterior thigh and medial calf
Saphenous	Medial aspect of knee	Stretching during hyperflexion of hips	Burning or aching pain in medial calf
Ilioinguinal	Lateral to pubic tubercle	Nerve entrapment by suspension sutures	Pain in medial groin, labia, or inner thigh

Adapted from reference 69.

often self-limited and resolve spontaneously over time. Early recognition and appropriate neurologic and physical medicine consultations are recommended.[60] Careful attention to positioning, abduction and flexion of the thigh, and adequate padding of the legs should minimize risk of position-related injuries.

Surgical injury to the ilioinguinal nerve can occur during placement and tying of the suspension sutures in transvaginal needle procedures. Miyazaki and Shooks[70] reported seven cases of ilioinguinal entrapment in their series of 402 needle suspension procedures. Timing and severity of symptoms is variable, but most patients present with characteristic complaints of pain localized to the medial groin and inner thigh. Three patients were treated with suture removal, while the remaining four had spontaneous resolution of their symptoms. As the nerve is most vulnerable to injury near its exit from the superficial inguinal ring, sutures should be placed medial to the pubic tubercle or body of the symphysis pubis to prevent nerve entrapment.[70]

CONCLUSION

Long-term follow-up of transvaginal needle suspension procedures for stress urinary incontinence has resulted in less than optimal cure rates. Prospective randomized studies have noted retropubic operations to be associated with superior outcomes. Additionally, postoperative complications such as voiding dysfunction and recurrent or iatrogenic prolapse have been seen in a significant percentage of patients after needle suspension procedures.

Vaginal operations for stress urinary incontinence continue to evolve and many procedural details remain controversial. Many currently accepted concepts and practices are advocated empirically with little supporting data. We hope that, with greater understanding of the relevant anatomy, underlying pathophysiology, and techniques of surgery, our understanding of the etiology and management of female incontinence will improve and lead to better long-term surgical outcomes.

REFERENCES

1. Pereyra AJ. A simplified surgical procedure for the correction of stress urinary incontinence in women. *West J Surg* 1959; **67**: 223–226.
2. Karram MM, Bhatia NN. Transvaginal needle bladder neck suspension procedures for stress urinary incontinence: A comprehensive review. *Obstet Gynecol* 1989; **73**: 906–914.
3. Jarvis GJ. Surgery for genuine stress incontinence. *Br J Obstet Gynaecol* 1994; **101**: 371–374.
4. Varner RE. Retropubic long-needle suspension procedures for stress urinary incontinence. *Am J Obstet Gynecol* 1990; **163**: 551–557.
5. Cornella JL, Ostergard DR. Needle suspension procedures for urinary stress incontinence: A review and historical perspective. *Obstet Gynecol Survey* 1990; **45**: 805–816.

6. Pereyra AJ. A simplified surgical procedure for the correction of stress urinary incontinence in women. *West J Surg* 1959; **67**: 223–226.
7. Pereyra AJ, Lebherz TB. Combined urethrovesical suspension and vaginourethroplasty for correction of urinary stress incontinence. *Obstet Gynecol* 1967; **30**: 537–546.
8. Pereyra AJ, Lebherz TB. The revised Pereyra procedure. In: Buschbaum H, Schmidt JD (eds). *Gynecologic and Obstetric Urology*. 1st ed. Philadelphia: WB Saunders, 1978: 208–222.
9. Pereyra AJ, Lebherz TB, Growdon WA, Powers JA. Pubourethral supports in perspective: Modified Pereyra procedure for urinary incontinence. *Obstet Gynecol* 1982; **59**: 643–648.
10. Cornella JL, Pereyra AJ. Historical vignette of Armand J. Pereyra and the modified Pereyra procedure: The needle suspension for stress incontinence in the female. *Int J Urogynecol* 1990; **1**: 25–29.
11. Pereyra AJ. Revised Pereyra procedure using colligated pubourethral supports. In: Slate WG (ed). *Disorders of the Female Urethra and Urinary Incontinence*. Baltimore: William and Wllkins, 1978: 143–159.
12. Harer WB, Gunther RE. Simplified urethral vesical suspension and urethroplasty. *Am J Obstet Gynecol* 1965; **91**: 1017–1021.
13. Stamey TA. Endoscopic suspension of vesical neck for urinary incontinence. *Surg Gynecol Obstet* 1973; **136**: 547–554.
14. Stamey TA. Endoscopic suspension of the vesical neck for urinary incontinence in females. *Ann Surg* 1980; **192**: 465–471.
15. Mason JT, Soderstrom RM. Suprapubic endoscopic evaluation of vesical suspension procedures. *Urology* 1975; **6**: 233–234.
16. Cobb OE, Radge H. Correction of female stress incontinence. *J Urol* 1978; **120**: 418–420.
17. Raz S. Modified bladder neck suspension for female stress incontinence. *Urology* 1981; **17**: 82–84.
18. Muzsnai D, Carrillo E, Dubin C, Silverman I. Retropubic vaginopexy for correction of urinary stress incontinence. *Obstet Gynecol* 1982; **59**: 113–117.
19. Gittes RF, Loughlin KR. No-incision pubovaginal suspension for stress incontinence. *J Urol* 1987; **138**: 568–570.
20. Leach GE. Bone fixation technique for transvaginal needle suspension. *Urology* 1988; **31**: 388–390.
21. Benderev TV. A modified percutaneous outpatient bladder neck suspension system. *J Urol* 1994; **153**: 2316–2320.
22. Fitzpatrick CC, Elkins TE, DeLancey JOL. The surgical anatomy of needle bladder neck suspension. *Obstet Gynecol* 1996; **87**: 44–49.
23. DeLancey JOL. Pubovesical ligament: A seperate structure from the urethral supports ("pubo-urethral ligaments"). *Neurourol Urodyn* 1989; **53**: 53–61.
24. DeLancey JOL. The structural support of the urethra as it relates to stress urinary incontinence: The "hammock hypothesis". *Am J Obstet Gynecol* 1994; **170**: 1713–1720.
25. Weber AM, Walters MD. Anterior vaginal prolapse: Review of anatomy and techniques of surgical repair. *Obstet Gynecol* 1997; **89**: 311–318.
26. Diokno AC, Brown MB, Brock BM, Herzog AR, Normolle DP. Prevalence and outcome of surgery for female incontinence. *Urology* 1989; **33**: 285–290.
27. Mundy AR. A trial comparing the Stamey bladder neck suspension procedure with colposuspension for the treatment of stress incontinence. *Br J Urol* 1983; **55**: 687–690.
28. Riggs JA. Retropubic cystourethrpexy: A review of two operative procedures with long-term follow-up. *Obstet Gynecol* 1986; **68**: 98–105.
29. Spencer JR, O'Conor VJ, Schaeffer AJ. A comparison of endoscopic suspension of the vesical neck with suprapubic vesicourethropexy for treatment of stress urinary incontinence. *J Urol* 1987; **137**: 411–415.

30. English PJ, Fowler JW. Videourodynamics assessment of the Stamey procedure for stress incontinence. *Br J Urol* 1988; **62**: 550–552.
31. Bergman A, Kooning PP, Ballard CA. Comparison of three different surgical procedures for genuine stress incontinonce: Prospective randomized study. *Am J Obstet Gynecol* 1989; **160**: 1102–1106.
32. Hilton P. A clinical and urodynamic study comparing the Stamey bladder neck suspension and sunurethral sling procedures in the treatment of genuine stress incontinence. *Br J Obstet Gynecol* 1989; **96**: 213–220.
33. Bergman A, Kooning PP, Ballard CA. Primary stress urinary incontinence and pelvic relaxation: Prospective randomized comparison of three different operations. *Am J Obstet Gynecol* 1989; **161**: 91–101.
34. Karram MM, Angel O, Koonings P, Tabor B, Bergman A, Bhatia N. The modified Pereyra procedure: A clinical and urodynamic review. *Br J Obstet Gynaecol* 1992; **99**: 655–658.
35. Trockman BA, Leach GE, Hamilton J, Sakamoto M, Santiago L, Zimmern PE. Modified Pereyra bladder neck suspension: 10 year mean followup using outcomes analysis in 125 patients. *J Urol* 1995; **154**: 1841–1847.
36. Korman HJ, Siris LT, Kirkemo AK. Success rate of modified Pereyra bladder neck suspension determined by outcomes analysis. *J Urol* 1994; **152**: 1453–1457.
37. Bergman A, Elia G. Three surgical procedures for genuine stress incontinence: Five-year followup of a prospective randomized study. *Am J Obstet Gynecol* 1995; **173**: 66–71.
38. Ramon J, Mekras JA, Webster GD. The outcome of transvaginal cystourethropexy in patients with anatomical stress urinary incontinence and outlet weakness. *J Urol* 1990; **144**: 106–109.
39. Nitti VM, Bregg KJ, Sussman EM, Raz, S. The Raz bladder neck suspension in patients 65 years old and older. *J Urol* 1993; **149**: 802–807.
40. Golumb J, Goldwasser B, Mashiach S. Raz bladder neck suspension in women younger than 65 years old compared with elderly women: Three years' experience. *Urology* 1994; **43**: 40–43.
41. Peattie AB, Stanton SL. The Stamey operation for the correction of genuine stress incontinence in the elderly woman. *Br J Obstet Gynaecol* 1989; **96**: 983–986.
42. Stanton SL, Reynolds SF, Creighton SM. The modified Pereyra (Raz) procedure for genuine stress incontinence – A useful option in the elderly or frail patient? *Int Urogynecol J* 1995; **6**: 22–25.
43. Spencer JR, O'Connor VJ. Comparison of procedures for stress urinary incontinence. *AUA Update Ser* 1987; **6**: 1–7.
44. Webster GD, Sihelnik SA, Stone AR. Female urinary incontinence: The incidence, identification, and characterization of detrusor instability. *Neurourol Urodyn* 1984; **3**: 235–242.
45. Lockhart JL, Tirado A, Morillo G, Politano VA. Vesicourethral dysfunction following cystourethropexy. *J Urol* 1982; **128**: 943–945.
46. Koonings PP, Bergman A, Ballard CA. Low urethral pressure and stress urinary incontinence in women: Risk factor for failed retropubic surgical procedure. *Urology* 1990; **36**: 245–248.
47. Sand PK, Bowen LW, Panganivan R, Ostergard DR. The low pressure urethra as a factor in failed retropubic urethropexy. *Obstet Gynecol* 1987; **69**: 399–402.
48. Zimmen PE, Hadley HR, Leach GE, Raz S. Female urethral obstruction after Marshall-Marchetti-Krantz operation. *J Urol* 1987; **138**: 517–520.
49. Nygaard IE, Kreder KJ. Complications of incontinence surgery. *Int Urogynecol J* 1994; **5**: 353–360.
50. Araki T, Takamoto H, Fujimoto H, Koga M, Hara T. Readjusting the loop tension for resolving postoperative urination difficulties and recurrent stress incontinence after Stamey suspension of the vesical neck. *Int Urogynecol J* 1992; **3**: 104–109.

51. Benson JT, Lucente V, McClellan E. Vaginal versus abdominal reconstructive surgery for the treatment of pelvic support defects: A prospective randomized study with long-term outcome evaluation. *Am J Obstet Gynecol* 1996; **175**: 1418–1422.
52. Kohli N, Sze EHM, Roat TW, Karram MM. Incidence of recurrent cystocele after anterior colporrhaphy with and without concomitant transvaginal needle suspension. *Am J Obstet Gynecol* 1996; **175**: 1476–1482.
53. Sze EHM, Miklos JR, Partoll L, Roat TW, Karram MM. Sacrospinous ligament fixation with transvaginal needle suspension for advanced pelvic organ prolapse and stress incontinence. *Obstet Gynecol* 1997; **89**: 94–96.
54. Bump RC, Hurt WG, Theofrastous JP, et al. Randomized prospective comparison of needle colposuspension versus endopelvic fascia plication for potential stress incontinence prophlaxis in women undergoing vaginal reconstruction for stage III or IV pelvic organ prolapse. *Am J Obstet Gynecol* 1996; **175**: 325–326.
55. Loughlin KR, Whitmore WF, Gittes RF, Richie JP. Review of an eight-year experience with modifications of endoscopic suspension of the bladder neck for female stress incontinence. *J Urol* 1990; **143**: 44–45.
56. Griffith-Jones MD, Abrams PH. The Stamey endoscopic bladder neck suspension in the elderly. *Br J Urol* 1990; **65**: 170–172.
57. Staskin DR. Complications of female anti-incontinence surgery. In: Smith RB, Erlich RM (eds). *Complications of Urologic Surgery*. Philadelphia: WB Saunders, 1990; 499–517.
58. Kursh ED, Angell AH, Resnick MI. Evolution of endoscopic urethropexy: Seven-year experience with various technique. *J Urol* 1991; **337**: 428–431.
59. Bergman A, Matthews L, Ballard C, Roy S. Suprapubic versus transurethral bladder drainage after surgery for stress urinary incontinence. *Obstet Gynecol* 1987; **69**: 546–549.
60. Phillips TH, Zeidman EJ, Thompson IM, St. Clair SR. Complications following needle bladder-neck suspension. *Int Urogynecol J* 1992; **3**: 38–42.
61. Kelly MJ, Zimmer PE, Leach GE. Complications of bladder neck suspension procedures. *Urol Clin North Am* 1991; **18**: 339–348.
62. Katske FA, Raz S. Use of Foley catheter to obtain ransvaginal tamponade. *Urol Urotechmol* May 1987; 8.
63. Dunton CJ. Epiurethral suprapubic vaginal suspension: A report on 52 cases. *Obstet Gynecol* 1988; **71**: 945–948.
64. Guam I, Riccioti NA, Fair WR. Endoscopic bladder neck suspension for stress urinary incontinence. *J Urol* 1984; **132**: 1119–1121.
65. Muzsnai D, Carrillo E, Dubin C, Silverman I. Retropubic vaginopexy for correction of urinary stress incontinence. *Obstet Gynecol* 1992; **59**: 113–118.
66. Karram MM, Bhatia NN. Management of coexistent stress and urge urinary incontinence. *Obstet Gynecol* 1989; **73**: 4–7.
67. McGuire EJ, Savastano JA. Stress incontinence and detrusor instability/urge incontinence. *Neurourol Urodyn* 1985; **4**: 313–316.
68. Zederic SA, Burros HM, Hanno PM. Bladder calculi in women after urethrovesical suspension. *J Urol* 1988; **139**: 1047–1048.
69. Karram MM. Transvaginal needle suspension. In: Hurt GW (ed). *Urogynecologic Surgery*. Gaithersburg MD, Aspen Publishers, 1992; 61–72.
70. Miyazaki F, Shook G. Ilioinguinal nerve entrapment during needle suspension for stress incontinence. *Obstet Gynecol* 1992; **80**: 246–248.
71. Hurt WG. *Urogynecologic Surgery*. New York: Lippincott-Raven, 1992.

CHAPTER 11

Suburethral sling procedures

ANITA CHEN AND NICOLETTE S. HORBACH

PUBOVAGINAL SLINGS

History

The pubovaginal sling procedure for the treatment of urinary incontinence has a long history. Von Giordano[1] in 1907 pioneered a sling technique using a pedicle graft of gracilis muscle that was passed around the urethra. In 1910, Goebell used a pedicle of pyramidalis muscle that was passed through the retropubic space on either side of the bladder neck and sutured in the midline below the urethra. Frangenheim modified this procedure by incorporating adjacent rectus fascia to the pyramidalis muscle in order to provide sufficient length and less tension. In 1917, Stoeckel further modified the procedure by plicating the vesical neck and raising bilateral rectangular flaps of rectus fascia and pyramidalis muscle that were passed through the retropubic space, around the plicated urethra and sutured in the midline. Further modifications of these techniques became known as the Goebell-Stoeckel-Frangenheim operation.[1,2,3,4] These early procedures were soon abandoned due to the difficulty in maintaining the muscle's blood supply and because of the bulkiness of the suburethral tissue. Other complications included a high rate of urinary infection, hemorrhage and obstruction.

Miller[5] in 1931 described a technique of passing a pedicle graft of pyramidalis or rectus muscle superficial to the pubis and around the urethra. This decreased the need for extensive dissection of the vesical neck and thereby lessened the likelihood of bleeding and injury. In 1942, Aldridge[6] modified this technique using bilateral rectus fascial strips that were detached laterally, passed through the rectus muscle, and sutured beneath the urethra in the midline. Further modification was performed by Studdiford[7] by using a single continuous strip of rectus fascia attached at one lateral margin, passed under the urethra and reattaching the free end to the fascia on the contralateral side. Again, the procedure fell into disfavor because of complications. In 1933, Price[8] first reported a successful free graft of fascia lata as a sling.

The modern era of pubovaginal fascia sling procedures was popularized by McGuire. In 1976, McGuire[9] used a combined abdominal and vaginal approach to obtain a strip of rectus fascia and external oblique muscle with a lateral attachment 2 cm from the midline. The bladder neck was then exposed through the retropubic space and a midline anterior vaginal mucosal incision was made to create a tunnel on either side of the urethrovesical junction. The free end of the sling was then passed through the rectus muscle, around the vesicle neck, back through the rectus muscle and sutured to the contralateral side. Blaivas[10] in 1984 modified the technique using a free graft of rectus fascia. The operative approach is transvaginal with the sling passed around the vesical neck without open dissection through the retropubic space. The sling is then sutured to the rectus fascia on either side.

Over the years, many sling materials have been used (Table 11-1). Organic autologous materials include round ligament, strips of rectus fascia or fascia lata, and palmaris longus tendon. Raz has modified the sling procedure by using a patch of rectus fascia and more recently, a vaginal wall patch.[11,12] Concern exists over the advisability of using rectus fascia for sling material, especially in patients who have undergone multiple previous abdominal or retropubic operations. Thus, fascia lata has been substituted as the graft material. Alternatively, allogenic dural slings using a strip of dura mater cerebri cleansed of its antigenic properties have also been used. These strips are available in lengths of 2×25 cm or 2×30 cm.

Table 11-1.   Sling material

Organic materials	*Synthetic materials*
Autologous	Nylon
Rectus fascia	Marlex mesh
Fascia lata	Mersilene mesh
Vaginal wall patch	Silastic
Gracilis muscle	Gore-Tex
Rectus muscle	
Pyramidalis muscle	
Round ligament	
Palmaris longus tendon	
Heterologous	
Lyophilized ox dura mater	
Porcine dermis	
Cadaveric fascia lata	

A number of surgeons have used synthetic material instead of autologous grafts. The search for a perfectly strong and inert material has progressed from Nylon and Mersilene tape, to gauze hammocks of Mersilene or Marlex, to Dacron and Vicryl mesh, and recently to Silastic bands and polytetrafluorethylene (Gore-Tex).[13–22] The Nylon and Mersilene tapes were quickly abandoned because the 0.5 cm strips under tension would form a narrow cord which could result in urethral obstruction and even potential urethral transection. Moir and the Nichols substituted a 2.5-cm diameter Mersilene mesh in the shape of a hammock 2.5–3.0 cm wide at the central belly.[23,24] This hammock distributes tension more widely and evenly over the entire proximal urethra and distal bladder. Marlex and Mersilene mesh have limited acceptance because of the severe scar formation due to fibroblastic infiltration through the large interspaces of the mesh. Surgeons have recently been using Silastic and polytetrafluorethylene which have less tendency toward fibroblast infiltration, and because they remain freer from surrounding tissue, they are more easily approached for adjusting tension or in removal.[14,24–26]

Indications

The indications for performing a suburethral sling procedure have not been well-defined. Traditionally this procedure has been used for treating complicated cases of recurrent stress urinary incontinence, especially in women with decreased mobility of the urethra secondary to postoperative scarring.[27,28] Many authors believe that a sling procedure, because of its partially obstructive nature, offers better results than a repeat retropubic procedure in those women with fixed, nonfunctioning urethras.[29,30]

The current challenge is to establish criteria to define a poorly functioning urethra. Type III incontinence, low urethral pressure and intrinsic sphincter deficiency have been used interchangeably to refer to a poorly functioning urethra, although these terms may describe different physiologic and clinical states. Regardless of which term is used, a suburethral sling procedure should be considered in those patients with a poor intrinsic urethra in which a simple elevation and stabilization of the urethrovesical junction will not produce continence.

Numerous investigators have attempted to identify risk factors associated with failure of standard retropubic incontinence procedures for genuine stress urinary incontinence.[31–33] In 1976, McGuire[9] and colleagues introduced the concept of two generic types of stress incontinence: urethral hypermobility and intrinsic sphincter deficiency. McGuire added a new category of classification for stress incontinence by defining type III stress incontinence as an absence of urethral hypermobility, a low proximal urethral pressure, and an open vesical neck at rest.[1] In 1978, McGuire and coworkers[34] reported on a group of postsurgical patients who had persistent stress incontinence despite adequate anatomical correction of the position of the urethra. They found that most of the patients in this group had low urethral closure pressures. In this group of patients, a success rate of 80% was obtained after placement of a sling. In subsequent series, McGuire documented success rates of up to 82% in patients who had failed multiple surgical procedures for stress urinary incontinence, with evidence of intrinsic sphincter deficiency as indicated by low (<20 cmH$_2$O) urethral closure pressure both with and without loss of anatomic support.[1]

Several other investigators have examined the surgical outcome of women with intrinsic urethral deficiency as defined by low urethral closure pressures following a variety of surgical procedures.[1,30] These studies have all confirmed

McGuire's initial report that women with low urethral pressure are at high risk for failing standard surgery for incontinence. However, Bergman and colleagues[35] reported a 5-fold increased risk of failing a Burch retropubic urethropexy or Pereyra needle suspension in women with a negative Q-tip test, regardless of their preoperative urethral closure pressures. Summit[26] reported a 20% success rate in women with low urethral pressures and well-supported urethrovesical junctions, compared with a 93% cure rate in the same group of women with urethrovesical junction hypermobility. This would indicate that women with intrinsic sphincter deficiency in the presence of a well-supported urethra are not good candidates for a sling and would be better treated with peri-urethral injections of bulking agents. Otherwise, consideration should be given to intraoperative urethrolysis to remobilize the urethra at the time of a sling procedure. The optimal candidate for a sling procedure is a woman with intrinsic sphincter deficiency and hypermobility of the urethrovesical junction.

In addition to the underlying physiologic factors of urethral closure pressure, urethral mobility, and collagen composition of tissues, preoperative psychosocial factors need to be considered. These include the patient's activity level, use of exogenous corticosteroids, previous radiation therapy to the pelvis, future desire for pregnancy, and underlying medical problems. Medical problems such as bronchitis, asthma and obesity place a woman at high risk for failure of standard antiincontinence procedures, and may make these patients better candidates for a sling. A primary suburethral sling procedure may also be indicated for an active woman whose career or lifestyle is dependent on heavy lifting or strenuous physical exertion. Patients with chronic pulmonary conditions, especially those patients requiring long-term corticosteroid use, are at risk for surgical failure. In addition to patients with chronic cough, obese patients are at risk of increased failure because of sutures pulling out of tissue after a standard retropubic urethropexy operation.

As investigators attempt to identify women who are at risk for surgical failure of standard incontinence procedures, some authors have also advocated the use of the suburethral sling procedure as a primary antiincontinence surgery in high risk patients or in women with severe intrinsic sphincter dysfunction and urethrovesical junction hypermobility.[36-39] Horbach and colleagues[22] found an 85% success rate in primary sling patients with the aforementioned preoperative findings.

PREOPERATIVE EVALUATION

All surgical patients should have a thorough preoperative evaluation. This should include a complete history, general physical and neurologic examination, and urodynamic and endoscopic evaluation to assure proper diagnosis and to exclude any contraindications to a sling procedure. It is imperative that the diagnosis of genuine stress incontinence is confirmed as there are many other causes of urinary leakage that may not be amenable to surgical intervention.

These would include significant detrusor instability, overflow incontinence secondary to atonic bladder, a urethral or bladder fistula, or uninhibited urethral relaxation.

The physical examination should include an assessment of postvoid residual, urine culture, and assessment of urethrovesical junction hypermobility via a Q-tip test or radiologic procedures. The Q-tip test is performed by inserting a sterile lubricated (2% lidocaine gel) cotton-tipped applicator transurethrally into the bladder. The applicator is then slowly withdrawn until resistance is felt, indicating that the cotton tip is at the bladder neck. This is most readily done with the patient in the dorsal lithotomy position at the time of the pelvic examination. The resting angle of the applicator stick to the horizontal is measured with a goniometer. The patient is then asked to perform a Valsalva maneuver and cough so that the maximum straining angle from the horizontal is measured. A straining angle of more than 30 degrees indicates hypermobility.

Cystourethroscopy and multichannel urethrocystometry with urethral pressure profilometry and leak point pressure measurements should be performed. In addition, preoperative voiding patterns need to be determined to screen for patients who may be at risk for postoperative urinary retention. Patients who void with a Valsalva maneuver and have minimal or no bladder contractions need to realize that spontaneous voiding may either be delayed or never resume. These patients may require prolonged postoperative drainage or intermittent self-catheterization either on a temporary or permanent basis. Due to the procedure's obstructive nature, all patients should be taught intermittent self-catheterization preoperatively. Patients with urodynamic evidence of mixed incontinence should be aggressively treated preoperatively and need to understand that the detrusor instability may worsen after the procedure.[29]

OPERATIVE TECHNIQUE

Most of the techniques described for suburethral sling procedure consist of taking either fascial, muscular, or alloplastic sling and inserting this graft around the vesical neck at the base of the urethra. The choice of material is based on accessibility and adequate tensile strength. It should also carry minimal risk of infection, graft rejection, or excessive scarring. In contrast to autologous slings, synthetic material is far more accessible but may be associated with increased risk of graft rejection.[22,40]

Most surgeons perform sling procedures using a combined abdominal-vaginal approach. The procedure can also be performed entirely through an abdominal incision with tunneling under the urethra and bladder, but a separate vaginal incision reduces the likelihood of urethral trauma. The use of preoperative prophylactic antibiotics has prevented any increase in infectious morbidity with a vaginal incision. Finally, most reports on sling procedures describe fixing the sling to the anterior rectus fascia. Other structures can also be used, including the iliopectineal ligament.

ALDRIDGE SLING

The Aldridge sling technique used rectus fascia harvested through a transverse abdominal incision.[4] A strip of fascia is raised on either side, but left attached in the midline anterior to the pubic symphysis (Figure 11-1). The anterior vagina is opened and the bladder neck exposed. The ends of the rectus fascia are passed down through the retropubic space and crossed beneath the bladder neck. Permanent suture is used to sew the vaginal ends of the fascia to the endopelvic fascia. The two fascial ends are then sewn to each other and the vaginal incision closed. The integrity of this technique depends on the secure attachment of the two ends of the rectus fascia. Tension may be harder to determine, because there are two strips of fascia to adjust and each end of the two strips is fixed. Care must also be taken to close the abdominal incision to prevent hernia formation.

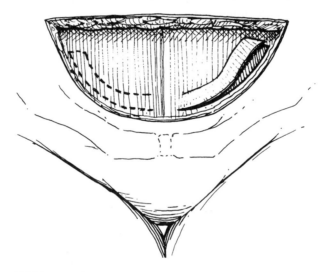

Figure 11-1.   Aldridge modification of the sling procedure. Two strips of rectus fascia are developed, one on each side of the abdomen. The end of each strip of fascia is left attached in the midline just behind the pubic symphysis. (From: Wall LL. Urinary stress incontinence. In: Rock JA, Thompson JD (eds). *TeLinde's Operative Gynecology*. Philadelphia: Lipincott-Raven; 1997: 1125. With permission.)

McGUIRE SLING

The McGuire pubovaginal sling procedure using rectus fascia can be performed in the following way.[41] The patient is placed in Allen Universal stirrups (Edgewater Medical Systems, Cleveland, OH) in a dorsal lithotomy position. The vaginal and lower abdominal area are appropriately prepared and draped.

A 16–18 French Foley catheter is inserted to drain the bladder and delineate the urethra and urethrovesical junction. Injectable saline or a dilute vasopressin (1 : 10 dilution) solution is used to inject beneath the epithelium of the anterior vaginal wall. The anterior vaginal mucosa is incised in the midline from above the vaginal apex to ~1.5 cm proximal to the external urethral meatus. The vaginal epithelium is then dissected off the underlying periurethral and pubocervical fascia. The dissection is carried laterally to the descending pubic ramus.

Transvaginal perforation of the endopelvic fascia is performed by blunt dissection with the surgeon's finger along the posterior surface of the inferior pubic ramus (Figure 11-2). Occasionally entry into the retropubic space is gained by sharp dissection with scissors if scarring is present. To avoid bladder injury, the position of the urethra should be confirmed by palpation of the catheter. Also prior to perforation of the endopelvic fascia, it is essential that no tissue be present between the surgeon's finger and the posterior pubic ramus. Keep in mind that excess medial dissection may result in injury to the urethra, while excess dissection lateral to the pubic tubercle increases risk of injury to the

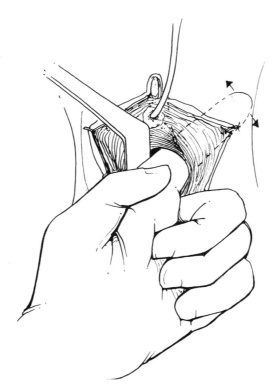

Figure 11-2.   Perforation of the endopelvic fascia into the space of Retzius. (From: Wall LL. Urinary stress incontinence. In: Rock JA, Thompson JD (eds). *Telinde's Operative Gynecology*. Philadelphia: Lipincott-Raven; 1997: 1117. With permission.)

ilioinguinal nerve. Delayed absorbable suture is then used to plicate the sub-urethral tissue in two layers. Correction of any cystocele is then accomplished in the usual manner. The vaginal field is then packed while the rectus fascia is harvested abdominally.

A transverse incision is made just above the symphysis pubis and carried down to the rectus fascia which is exposed and opened. A 10 to 15-cm strip of rectus fascia is mobilized from the lower aspect of the rectus incision. Fascial closure is easier when the sling is cut from the lower leaf rather than the upper leaf. The fascial strip should measure ~0.5 cm wide at the ends and 1–1.5 cm wide in the middle (Figure 11-3). The wider portion is placed under the urethro-vesical junction and proximal urethra to distribute the upward force of the sling over a wider area. This wider portion of the sling also decreases the risk of urethral transection that may occur if a narrower sling is used. Once the graft is harvested, nonabsorbable sutures are sewn into each end of the sling perpen-dicular to the length of the graft, so that the sutures will not tear out of the fascia. The fascial defect is then closed.

The tunnel for the sling is made by placing a vaginal finger upward into the retropubic space while a uterine packing forceps is advanced from the abdominal field. The abdominal side of the sling tunnel is located by retracting the lateal aspect of the rectus muscle medially near its insertion into the pubic bone and dissecting the overlying tissue in this area to gain access to the lateral retropubic space. The vaginal finger then guides the packing forceps from the abdominal incision through the retropubic space into the vaginal field. The sutures at the

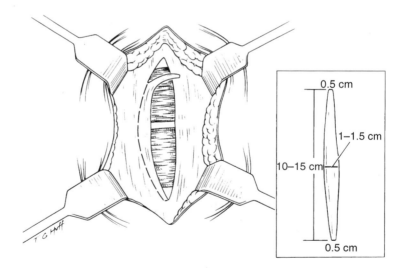

Figure 11-3. Rectus fascia harvest. The sling is harvested from the lower leaf of the fascial incision. The fascial incision runs to the lateral border of the recti muscles. (From: McGuire EJ, Wan J. Pubovaginal slings. In: Hurt WG (ed). *Urogynecologic Surgery*. New York: Raven Press; 1992: 101. With permission.)

ends of the graft are grasped with the forceps and elevated through the retropubic space into the abdominal field. The suture ends are then passed through a small pledget of fascia or synthetic material (Figure 11-4).

Cystoscopy should now be performed to rule out bladder or urethral injury and to ensure that the sling is not in the bladder. Only partial closure of the urethrovesical junction with elevation of the sling should be documented during urethroscopy. Complete closure of the urethrovesical junction results in increased risk of postoperative voiding dysfunction. At this point the sling is then sutured to the periurethral fascia which was previously reinforced. Securing the sling suburethrally holds the sling in place so that the central widest portion stays in contact with the urethra, preventing rolling up or migration of the sling. The vaginal incision is then closed. Sutures at the end of the sling are tied down to a predetermined tension. One may use a Q-tip placed into the urethra to assist with determining the tension applied, so that the urethral axis is horizontal to positive 10 degrees. Some surgeons advocate tying the sling under direct endo-scopic visualization with tension sufficient to partially coapt the urethrovesical junction. Excess tension should be avoided. ("If you think it's too loose, it's probably just right.") A suprapubic catheter is placed and a vaginal pack is placed for 24 hours. Prophylactic antibiotics are administered and voiding trials are started on postoperative day 2–3. The suprapubic catheter is removed once

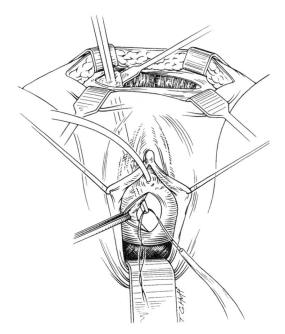

Figure 11-4.   Grasping the sling sutures prior to passing them up into the abdomen. (From: McGuire EJ, Wan J. Pubovaginal slings. In: Hurt WG (ed). *Urogynecologic Surgery*. New York: Raven Press; 1992: 103. With permission.)

the postvoid residuals are below 100 ml or do not exceed 20% of the volume spontaneously voided for 12–24 hours.

In women who have undergone numerous abdominal procedures, other organic or synthetic material may be used as the sling material. Fascia lata may be harvested using a Masson or Wilson fascial stripper (Figure 11-5). Cadaveric fascia lata may also be obtained. Alternatively, 2 to 3-cm wide strips of 1-mm thick Marlex, Silastic or polytetrafluorethylene may be used.

Variations on the sling procedure have been developed over the years. Karram and Bhatia[42] in 1990 described a technique in which a patch of fascia lata is placed suburethrally. The patch should cover an area from the midurethra to ~1 cm beyond the bladder neck. The patch is secured to the suburethral tissue and bladder base using delayed absorbable suture. Helical stitches of No. 1 prolene suture are taken through the long axis of the patch and these ends are then brought up through the retropubic space into a previously made abdominal incision in the usual manner. Raz and colleagues[12] in 1989 described a technique using a patch of *in situ* vaginal skin as sling material. An "A" shaped incision is made in the anterior vaginal mucosa from just below the urethral meatus to 2 cm beyond the bladder neck. The island of tissue represented by the upper portion of the "A" becomes the sling. The vaginal skin lateral to the sling is dissected from its underlying periurethral fascia and the endopelvic fascia is penetrated and opened from the pubic bone to the ischial tuberosity. The flap of tissue in the lower part of the incision is undermined to allow for later advancement over the sling segment. A spiral No. 1 polypropylene suture is placed in each corner of

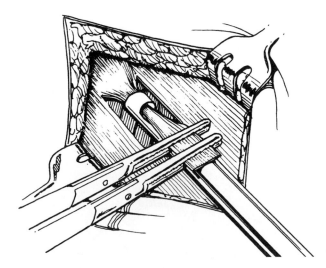

Figure 11-5. Fascia lata harvest. The end of the fascial strip is passed through the Masson fascial stripper and grasped with two Kocher clamps. (From: Wall LL. Urinary stress incontinence. In: Rock JA, Thompson JD (eds). *TeLinde's Operative Gynecology*. Philadelphia: Lipincott-Raven; 1997: 1121. With permission.)

the sling island, incorporating the periurethral fascia. A suprapubic abdominal incision is made and carried down to the fascia and a needle suture carrier, guided by a finger inserted through the vaginal incision, is passed through the rectus sheath into the retropubic space. The needle pulls the ends of the suture through the retropubic tunnel onto the rectus fascia. Each suture is tied to itself and the ipsilateral suture. The suprapubic incision is closed, and the vaginal incision is closed with the mobilized flap advanced over the island sling and sewn to the vaginal skin.

RESULTS

It is difficult to assess sling procedure outcomes because the definition of cure is inconsistent. Most authors report subjective cure rates. Specific guidelines defining surgical cure rates have not been established; therefore, it has been difficult to compare the many different sling procedures and materials. In general, sling procedures appear to be successful in curing patients with stress incontinence.[24,27,43–45] Surgical cure rates are reported in the range of 70–100%. Low[43] and Parker[44] reported 95% and 84% objective cure rates respectively with fascia lata. There does not seem to be any significant difference in cure rate between sling procedures performed with autologous tissue vs synthetic tissue. Subjective cure rates range from 59 to 95%, with objective cure rates ranging from 70–90% for inorganic grafts.[16,22,23,26,39]

The variation in reported surgical cure rates is influenced by many factors. There are multiple modifications described in the literature and it is difficult to compare the results of one investigator's experience with another's. Few studies control for preoperative variables such as preexisting detrusor instability, and also most authors include patients with both primary and recurrent incontinence. The length of follow-up in most series is also variable, ranging from months to years.

Several investigators have examined the effect of surgery on objective urodynamic parameters in an attempt to elucidate the mechanism of surgical care.[11,22,34,37,46–49] The two postoperative changes that occur are an improvement in pressure transmission ratios and a reduction in the peak flow rate during voiding. Surgical success was not consistently predicted based on changes in measurements of functional urethral length of maximum urethral closure pressure.

COMPLICATIONS

Sling procedures are usually associated with a higher incidence of both intraoperative and postoperative complications compared with standard incontinence procedures (Table 11-2).[30] Intraoperative complications include bleeding, intraoperative cystotomy and urethral injuries. Intraoperative cystotomy, especially in patients with increased scarring from previous surgery, may be avoided by using

Table 11-2.   Complications of sling procedures

Complication	Therapy
Intraoperative	
Bladder perforation	Intraoperative cystoscopy
	Closure of cystotomy as indicated
Severe hemorrhage	Tamponade with gauze pack. Look for bladder trauma
Postoperative	
Urinary retention	Intermittent self-catheterization
	Abdominal adjustment of sling tension
	Removal of sling
Recurrent urinary tract infections	Check postvoid residuals, intermittent self-catheterization as needed
Detrusor instability	Bladder retraining
	Anticholinergic medications
Pain in region of sutures	Percutaneous blockage with local anesthesia
	Pledget removal
Fistula tract	Removal of sling material

sharp dissection to enter the retropubic space. Urethral injuries may be avoided by careful vaginal dissection with the urethral catheter in place. Endoscopy is crucial at the conclusion of the procedure, but prior to closure of the incision to detect injuries or the presence of the sling in the bladder.

Since sling procedures significantly increase urethral outlet resistance, most postoperative complications are related to various forms of voiding difficulty and urinary retention. This is especially true in patients who are unable to generate a detrusor contraction during voiding. In extreme cases, complete urinary retention may occur. Traditional treatment modalities include continued intermittent self-catheterization or sling removal or revision. Brubaker[50] described a method for loosening the tension of suburethral sling in order to lessen obstruction in patients with severe voiding dysfunction persisting 6 weeks postoperation. Using an abdominal approach, the abdominal incision is opened and access to the extraperitoneal sites of the sling fixation to the rectus fascia is obtained. The previously placed sling fixation sutures are grasped and elevated. Two new strands of permanent suture material are passed under the knot of the original suture. While the new sutures are elevated, the previous fixation site is circumscribed with a No. 15 scalpel blade. The newly placed sutures which are under the loop of the old suture form an additional length between the sling and the rectus fascia. This fascial plug is then repositioned by tension placed posteriorly on the sling through a universal dilator in the urethra. The fascial plug retracts into the retropubic space and the new sutures are put through the fascia to both secure the sling to the fascia and to close the fascial defect. The abdominal incision is then closed. Alternatively, a vaginal incision may be made and the sling transected in the midline while the two ends are grasped. A small addition of sling material may be inserted suburethrally and sewn to the previously cut sling ends—in essence inserting a suburethral patch of material.

Sudden urgency or frequency symptoms may also occur in the absence of voiding dysfunction.[14,51] These irritative symptoms may occur because many patients did not have normal bladder capacity preoperatively secondary to loss of bladder compliance after long-term severe incontinence. Recurrent urinary tract infections may also be exacerbated by elevated postvoid residuals. Detrusor instability can develop, persist, or worsen in a small group of patients, especially those with an overactive detrusor prior to surgery.

Pain in the area in which sutures are tied may be exacerbated by movement and is also common in the initial postoperative period.[41] Occasionally unilateral pain persists. Percutaneous injection of a local anesthetic in the central area of the sutures usually provides significant relief. If the pain is not alleviated, suture and pledget removal 10 weeks postoperation under local anesthesia may be necessary. It is uncertain whether over time the sling will maintain tension without the suspending sutures.[41] Pain may also occur related to nerve injury.

A number of complications are associated specifically with the use of synthetic rather than autologous graft (Table 11-3). Early reports of sling procedures found up to a 20% incidence of erosion of the graft through the urethra or formation of an abdominal sinus tract have been found.[41] This necessitates the need for sling removal. Since the synthetic grafts are inert, poor healing of the vaginal mucosa over the graft has been reported, especially with polytetrafluorethylene.[1,14,25,40] To decrease the incidence of this complication, a

Table 11-3. Comparison between organic and inorganic slings

	Organic	*Inorganic*
Cured	90.3%	78.9%
Improved	4.27%	6.38%
Failed	5.7%	14.54%
Urinary retention	7.8%	8.11%
Detrusor instability		
De novo	3.38%	14.57%
Persistent	8.63%	8.8%
Urgency/frequency	6.57%	20.7%
Wound infection	2.65%	7.67%
Urinary tract infection	8.6%	11.86%
Urethral/bladder injury	4.25%	6.5%
Sling erosion	0.5%	9.43%
Sling revision	3.29%	24.2%
Sling removal	0	6.62%
Fistula/sinus	1.5%	3.69%

Modified from Ghoniem GM, Shaaban A. Sub-urethral slings for treatment of stress urinary incontinence. *Int Urogynecol J* 1994; **5**: 228–239.

layer of submucosal vaginal tissue can be brought over the sling to interpose tissue between the sling and vaginal mucosa.

CONCLUSION

The pubovaginal sling procedure is indicated in patients with recurrent genuine stress incontinence, intrinsic sphincter deficiency, preferably with urethrovesical junction hypermobility, or in high-risk patients with primary incontinence. The choice of graft material and operative approach should be based on the advantages and disadvantages of the choice for each individual patient. Sling procedures have found a permanent place among the operative procedures to correct incontinence, and surgical outcome is often better than that obtained by standard retropubic procedures. Complications can be minimized by meticulous preoperative evaluation and careful attention to surgical technique.

REFERENCES

1. Blaivas JG. Pubovaginal sling. In: Kursh ED, McGuire EJ (eds). *Female Urology.* Philadelphia: J.B. Lippincott Company; 1994: 239–249.
2. Wheeless CR, Wharton LR, Dorsey JH, TeLinde RW. The Goebell-Stoeckel operation for universal cases of urinary incontinence. *Am J Obstet Gynecol* 1977; **128**: 546–549.
3. Ridley JH. Appraisal of the Goebell-Frangenheim-Stoeckel sling procedure. *Am J Obstet Gynec* 1966; **95**: 714–721.
4. Wall LL: Urinary stress incontinence. In: Rock JA, Thompson JD (eds). *TeLinde's Operative Gynecology.* Philadelphia: Lippincott-Raven Publishers; 1997: 1097–1134.
5. Miller NF. Surgical treatment of urinary incontinence in the female. *JAMA* 1932; **98**: 628.
6. Aldridge AH. Transplantation of fascia for relief of urinary stress incontinence. *Am J Obstet Gynecol* 1942; **44**: 398.
7. Studdiford WE. Transplantation of abdominal fascia for relief of urinary stress incontinence. *Am J Obstet Gynecol* 1944; **47**: 764–775.
8. Price PB. Plastic operations for incontinence of urine and of feces. *Arch Surg* 1933; **26**: 1043.
9. McGuire EJ, Lytton B, Kohorn EL. Stress urinary incontinence. *Obstet Gynecol* 1976; **47**: 255–264.
10. Blaivas JG, Salinas J. Type III stress urinary incontinence: The importance of proper diagnosis and treatment. *Surg Forum* 1984; **35**: 472.
11. Bauer SB. Vesical neck reconstruction. In: Glenn JF (ed). *Urologic Surgery.* Philadelphia: J.B. Lippincott Company; 1991: 509–522.
12. Raz S, Siegel AL, Short JL, et al. Vaginal wall sling. *J Urol* 1989; **141**: 43–46.
13. Hohenfellner R, Petri E. Sling procedures. In: Stanton SL, Tanagho EA (eds) *Surgery of Female Incontinence.* New York: Springer-Verlag; 1986: 105–113.
14. Young SB. Suburethral sling rejection. In: Nichols DH, Delaney JOL (eds). *Clinical Problems, Injuries and Complications of Gynecologic and Obstetric Surgery.* Philadelphia: Williams and Wilkins; 1995: 315–317.
15. Williams TJ, TeLinde RW. The sling operation for urinary incontinence using Mersilene ribbon. *Obstet Gynecol* 1962; **19**: 241–245.

16. Morgan JE. A sling operation using Marlex propropylene mesh for treatment of recurrent stress incontinence. *Am J Obstet Gynecol* 1970; **106**: 369–377.
17. Frutz IIP, Buckspan M, Flax S, et al. Clinical and urodynamic reevaluation of combined abdominovaginal Marlex sling operations for recurrent stress urinary incontinence. *Int Urogynecol J* 1990; **1**: 70–73.
18. Fiano S, Soderberg G. Absorbable polyglactin mesh for retropubic sling operations in female urinary stress incontinence. *Gynecol Obstet Invest* 1983; **16**: 1–6.
19. Spencer TS, Jequier AM, Kersey HJG. The gauze-hammock operation in the treatment of persistent stress incontinence. *J Obstet Gynaecol Br Common* 1972; **79**: 666–669.
20. Kersey J, Martin MR, Mishra P. A further assessment of the gauze hammock sling operation in the treatment of stress incontinence. *Br J Obstet Gynaecol* 1988; **95**: 382–385.
21. Korda A, Peat B, Hunter P. Silastic slings for female incontinence. *Int Urogynecol J* 1990; **1**: 66–69.
22. Horbach NS, Blanco JS, Ostegard DR. A suburethral sling procedure with polytetrafluorethylene for the treatment of genuine stress incontinence in patients with low urethral closure pressure. *Obstet Gynecol* 1988; **71**: 648–652.
23. Moir JC. The gauze-hammock operation: A modified Aldridge sling procedure. *J Obstet Gynaecol Br Common* 1968; 75: 1–13.
24. Nichols DII. The Mersilene mesh gauze-hammock for severe urinary stress incontinence. *Obstet Gynecol* 1973; **42**: 88–92.
25. Chin YK, Stanton SL. A follow-up of silastic sling for genuine stress incontinence. *Br J Obstet Gynaecol* 1995; **102**: 143–147.
26. Summitt RL, Bent AE, Ostergard DR, Harris TA. Suburethral sling procedure for genuine stress incontinence and low urethral closure pressure. A continued experience. *Int Urogynecol J* 1992; **3**: 18–21.
27. Beck RP, McCormick RN, Nordstrom L. The fascia lata sling procedure for treating recurrent genuine stress incontinence of urine. *Obstet Gynecol* 1988; **72**: 699–703.
28. Morgan JE, Farrow GA, Stewart FE. The Marlex sling operation for the treatment of recurrent stress urinary incontinence. A 16 year review. *Am J Obstet Gynecol* 1985; **151**: 224–226.
29. McGuire EJ. Abdominal procedures for stress incontinence. *Urol Clin North Am* 1985; **151**: 224–226.
30. Horbach NS. Suburethral sling procedures. In: Ostergard DR, Bent AE (eds). *Urogynecology and Urodynamics*. Baltimore: Williams and Wilkins; 1991: 449–458.
31. McGuire EJ. Urodynamic findings in patients after failure of stress incontinence operations. *Prog Clin Biol Res* 1981; **78**: 351–360.
32. McGuire EJ, Lytton B. Pubovaginal sling procedures for stress incontinence. *Obstet Gynecol* 1976; **47**: 255–614.
33. Sand PK, Bowen LW, Panganiban R., Ostergard DR. The low pressure urethra as a factor in failed retropubic urethropexy. *Obstet Gynecol* 1987; **69**: 399–402.
34. McGuire EM, Lytton B. The pubovaginal sling in stress urinary incontinence. *J Urol* 1978; **119**: 82.
35. Bergman A, Koonings PP, Ballard CA. Negative Q-tip test as a risk factor for failed incontinence surgery in women. *J Reprod Med* 1989; **34**: 193–197.
36. Spence-Jones C, DeMarco E, Lemieux MC, et al. Modified urethral sling for the treatment of genuine stress incontinence and latent incontinence. *Int Urogynecol J* 1994; **5**: 69–75.
37. Rottenberg RD, Weil A, Brioschi PA, et al. Urodynamic and clinical assessment of the Lyodura sling operation for urinary stress incontinence. *Br J Obstet Gynecol* 1985; **92**: 829–834.
38. McLaren HC. Late result from sling operations. *J Obstet Gynecol Br Common* 1968; **75**: 10–13.

39. Kersey J. The gauze hammock sling operation in the treatment of stress incontinence. *Br J Obstet Gynaecol* 1983; **90**: 945–949.
40. Bent AE, Ostegard DR, Zwick-Zaffuto M. Tissue reaction to expanded polytetra-fluorethylene suburethral sling for urinary incontinence: Clinical and histologic study. *Am J Obstet Gynecol* 1993; **169**: 1198–1204.
41. McGuire EJ, Wan J. Pubovaginal slings. In: Hurt WG (ed). *Urogynecologic surgery*. Maryland: Aspen Publishers: 1992: 97–105.
42. Karram MM, Bhatia NN. Patch procedure: Modified transvaginal fascia lata sling for recurrent or severe stress urinary incontinence. *Obstet Gynecol* 1990; **75**: 461–463.
43. Low JA. Management of severe anatomic deficiencies of urethral sphincter function by a combined procedure with a fascia lata sling. *Am J Obstet Gynecol* 1969; **105(2)**: 149–155.
44. Parker RT, Addison WA, Wilson CJ. Fascia lata urethrovesical suspension for recurrent stress urinary incontinence. *Am J Obstet Gynecol* 1979; **135**: 843–852.
45. Ghoniem GM, Shaaban A. Suburethral slings for treatment of stress urinary incontinence. *Int Urogynecol J* 1994; **5**: 228–239.
46. Henriksson L, Ulsen U. A urodynamic evaluation of the effects of abdominal urethro-cystopexy in women with stress incontinence. *Am J Obstet Gynecol* 1978; **113**: 78–82.
47. Obrink A, Bunne G. The margin of incontinence after three types of operations for stress incontinence. *Scand J Urol Nephrol* 1978; **12**: 209–214.
48. Hilton P, Stanton SL. Clinical and urodynamic evaluation of the polypropylene (Marlex) sling for genuine stress incontinence. *Neurourol Urodyn* 1983; **2**: 145–153.
49. Hilton P. A clinical and urodynamic study comparing stamey bladder neck suspension and suburethral sling procedures in the treatment of genuine stress incontinence. *Br J Obstet Gynecol* 1989; **96**: 213–220.
50. Brubaker L. Suburethral sling release. *Obstet Gynecol* 1995; **86(4)**: 686–688.
51. Karram MM. Surgical correction of genuine stress incontinence secondary to intrinsic urethral sphincter dysfunction. In: Walters MD, Karram MM (eds). *Clinical Urogynecology*. Missouri: Mosby; 1993: 210–216.

CHAPTER 12

Laparoscopic incontinence procedures

STEPHANIE POWELL AND INGRID NYGAARD

Over 100 procedures for stress urinary incontinence have been described in the literature. In reality, the number is much larger, since each surgeon adds modifications from suture types to ancillary procedures. One of the more recent surgical techniques to join this large armamentarium is the laparoscopic approach to the retropubic colposuspension (i.e., Burch procedure). Most gynecologic surgeons at this time recognize that the long-term efficacy of the retropubic colposuspension is higher than that of either the anterior vaginal repair or of the needle suspension procedure.[1–3] However, retropubic colposuspension is also more invasive and associated with a longer hospitalization and recovery time than less invasive procedures. Thus it is not surprising that laparoscopic surgeons began to use their newly acquired laparoscopic techniques in the arena of urinary incontinence.

Proported benefits of the laparoscopic approach to incontinence include avoiding a large incision, shorter hospitalization and convalescence, less need for pain medications, faster return to bowel function, and less time off from work. Disadvantages of the laparoscopic approach include a long operating time in most hands, a steep and prolonged learning curve, and an absence of long-term follow-up data. In addition, it remains to be seen whether laparoscopic retropubic colposuspensions can be easily accomplished by most gynecologic surgeons. Pioneers in this field are among the most skilled laparoscopists in the country and it is unclear whether their success rates are applicable to average laparoscopic surgeons.

The procedures and various modifications of the laparoscopic Burch colposuspension are many (see Table 12-1). Modifications of the procedure include an intraperitoneal or extraperitoneal approach, changes in suture material and numbers or sutures placed, number of ports placed, instruments used for dissection, and methods used to check the integrity of the bladder and suture placement.

Patient selection in most of the series reviewed was similar to that for the abdominal procedure. After confirmation of the presence of genuine stress incontinence by history, a voiding diary, physical examination, cough stress test, or urodynamic evaluation was performed. The presence or absence of prolapse was sometimes documented (but not always mentioned in the final results) as was the history of a prior procedure for incontinence, or need for concomitant procedures.

The trans or intraperitoneal approach to the space of Retzius by laparoscopy usually uses three suprapubic trocars plus the infraumbilical trocar. An anterior peritoneal incision is made 2–3.5 cm between the two obliterated folds of bladder above the pubic symphysis. A variety of instruments, including bipolar or unipolar cautery, the harmonic scalpel, or scissors were used and the operative ports are inserted through this incision for dissection of the retropubic space. Generally, either the operator or the assistant used a vaginal hand to elevate the urethrovesical junction, although both retractors and sutures are also described to perform this function. Several operators described a vaginal illuminator as being extremely helpful in identifying anatomy. Different knot tying mechanisms were reported, with a slip knot pusher and laparoscopic knot tier the most common. One or two sutures were placed bilaterally. Several authors recommended using the Lapra-Ty suture crimper (Ethicon, Cincinnati, Ohio) rather than directly tying the sutures as this often is laborious. In addition, as can be seen from Table 12-1, other modifications such as using bone anchors or mesh were also reported. Both Harewood[4] and Knapp[5] reported doing a Stamey needle suspension under laparoscopic guidance. Advantages given included being able to do the surgery with a single port, deleting the vaginal incisions, eliminating the laborious laparoscopic knot tying, and having improved visualization of exact placement of the sutures. Many investigators used instilled indigo carmine to reveal inadvertent cystotomy during the procedure or performed cystoscopy or cystotomy to confirm ureteral patency.

When an extraperitoneal technique was used, a 2 cm horizontal incision was generally made midway between the umbilicus and the symphysis pubis. Blunt dissection was used to open the retropubic space beneath the rectus laterally to Cooper's ligaments. The dissection was done by balloon filling into this space to a volume of 1000–1500 ml, or by blunt finger dissection. Bilateral 5-mm ports were inserted. Occasionally, a suprapubic port was placed for retraction. Pneumoretzius is created after suturing the rectus sheath around a 10-mm port, using low pressure (8–12 mmHg).

Methods to decrease procedure duration described by experienced laparoscopists include a combination of needle techniques, surgical mesh and staples to elevate the urethrovesical junction. One study described using motorized retractors in place of the gas distension method.[6] Another used the Visiport for direct preperitoneal dissection.[7]

At the time of this writing, only one randomized prospective trial has been presented comparing the laparoscopic and traditional laparotomy approaches to the Burch retropubic urethropexy. Burton[8] randomized 60 women with urodynamically proven moderate or severe genuine stress incontinence to either laparoscopic or open colposuspension. Before embarking on this study he did 10 laparoscopic colposuspensions to familiarize and standardize his techniques. Two 1/0 polyglycolic sutures were used bilaterally. Women were evaluated both

Table 12-1. Surgical techniques of laparoscopic retropubic colposuspension

Author (Ref.)	Approach*	Suspension material	No. sutures per side	Operating time†
Vancaille and Schuessler, 1991 (21)	I	2–0 Ethibond	2	123 (35–175)
Albala et al., 1992 (22)	I	Ethibond	1	MMK: 65 (35–175)
				Burch: 105 (40–160)
Ou et al., 1993 (23)		Prolene mesh, Titanium staples		
Liu, 1993 (24)	I	Gore-Tex	2	73 (50–120)
Seman and O'Shea 1994 (25)	E	N.S.	N.S.	187 (120–300)
McDougall et al., 1995 (14)	I and E	O polyglactin	1	124 (70–175)
Polasciki et al., 1995 (15)	E	2–0 Ticron	2	185 (110–240)
Langebrekke et al., 1995 (26)	I and E	Absorbable	2	75–120
Wallwiener et al., 1995 (27)	I	Gore-Tex and Ethicon mesh	N.S.	45–105
Carter, 1995 (28)	E	2–0 Ethibond	1–2	N.S.
Das and Palmer, 1995 (17)	I	1–0 polyester, bone anchors	1	155
Lam et al., 1995 (29)	I and E	0-Ethibond	2	187 (120–300)
Radomski and Herschorn, 1996 (30)	I	Nonabsorb, braided	2–3	196 (130–300)
Ross, 1995 (16)	I and E	0-Ethibond or 0-Gore-Tex	2	N.S.
Cooper, 1996 (31)	I and E	0-Ethibond or O-Demulon	2	108 (30–320)
Yang, 1995 (32)	E	2–0 Gore-Tex	1	108–121 (57–330)
Theobald, 1995 (33)	E	Nonabsorbable mesh bands	N/A	35
Lobel, 1997 (34)	I	0-polyester or 2–0 Gore-Tex	1–2	190 (120–340)
Papasakelariou, 1997 (35)	E or I	2–0 polypropylene or CV-0 Gore-Tex	2	145–204 (145–330)
Lee, 1998 (36)	E or I	1–0 Ethibond	2	32 (20–90)
Lyons, 1995 (37)	I or E	0-polygalactin or polyester or staples	1–2	N.S.
Lavin, 1998 (38)	E or I	0-PDS	2	80
Saidi, 1998 (39)	E	N.S.	N.S.	49 (28–75)
Miamnay, 1998 (40)	I	0-Ethibond	2	89
Ross, 1998 (41)		0-polydioxanone	2	N.S.

* I, intraperitoneal; E, extraperitoneal; N.S., not stated in paper.
† Mean time in minutes (range).

subjectively and objectively preoperatively and at 6 and 12 months post-operatively. At 12 months, the laparoscopic group lost significantly more urine on a 1-hour pad test (12 g vs 2 g), reported more symptoms of stress incontinence on a visual analogue scale, and recorded more incontinent episodes on a urinary diary (a mean of six leakages per 24 hours compared to two). Objectively, videourodynamics done 12 months postoperatively diagnosed recurrent genuine stress incontinence in eight women in the laparoscopy group, versus one woman in the laparotomy group. The mean urethral closure pressure was also lower at 12 months for the laparoscopic procedure. The author noted that proper assessment would take 5 years and until longer term data were available, recommended that laparoscopic colposuspension be done only if patients were involved in an ongoing clinical trial.

This sentiment was echoed by Lobel, who, on finding that the efficacy of laparoscopic Burch urethropexies was lower at 34 months than at one year post-operatively (69 vs 86%), note "these poor results in the hands of experienced laparoscopists should cause surgeons to reconsider the procedure carefully".

Similar trends have recently been reported for needle suspension procedures and anterior colporrhaphies. During the 1990s, many publications reported success rates exceeding 90% for various modifications of the Pereyra urethropexy.[9] In almost all cases, the follow-up interval was under 12 months. Unfortunately, these excellent results have not held up over time. Several recent reports noted a drop in the success rate to 50% or less by 10 years postoperatively.[10] Thus, while most of the early reports about laparoscopic urethropexy are very encouraging in their high success rates, it would behoove surgeons to remain skeptical until long-term success rates also are shown to be equally high.

While many urogynecologists and other surgeons feel that such reticence is warranted, others are convinced that the laparoscopic approach is superior to that by laparotomy because of the advantages outlined above. Many are also convinced that the efficacy should be identical when the identical procedure is performed and only the exposure route differs. In addition, many are convinced that laparoscopic surgeries carry a lower cost to the hospital, patient, or society than the open approach.

Both proponents and opponents of the laparoscopic Burch procedure for stress urinary incontinence cite cost as a deciding factor in the selection of procedure. The assumption was initially made that the shorter hospital stay required for the laparoscopic procedure would be advantageous. However, depending upon the variables of cost included in the analysis, the final outcomes vary between studies. For example, Kung and colleagues[11] used a historical cohort followed for 1 year to assess their primary outcome, cost/cure ratio. The total cost of the procedure was divided by the percentage of patients cured. Cure, defined as subjective and objective lack of incontinence, was reported for 97% of women who underwent a laparoscopic Burch procedure and for 90% cure who underwent an open Burch procedure. The costs to cure ratios were significantly different, as the decreased hospital stay for the laparoscopic procedure yielded greatly decreased costs. The cost analysis used included personnel, hospital, nursing (including overtime), drugs, and investigative. One interesting finding from their study was that the average hospital stay for the laparoscopic approach was 3.6 days (range 2–6 days), and for the abdominal, 11.2 days.

Most of the studies comparing cost between the two procedures cite expensive equipment, additional operating theater time, personnel, equipment charges, and a steep learning curve as important factors in the cost of the laparoscopic procedure. In a retrospective case-control study, Loveridge[12] found that the greatly decreased stay required for laparoscopic cases accounted for overall comparable costs in performance of the two procedures. However, in another cost study, Kohli and colleagues[13] found that the cost of the laparoscopic equipment and longer operating times outweighed the cost of the decreased hospital stay, resulting in significantly higher hospital charges for the laparoscopic procedure. The authors noted that they were unable to assign a cost benefit to variables such as decreased postoperative pain, shorter hospitalization, or smaller incisions. Overall, studies attempting to assess cost disagree in the most significant variables to use in calculation. Procedure complications, hospital stays and operating costs vary so between institutions that a clear cost–benefit analysis will be difficult to apply to all health care systems. This difference is especially noted between different health care systems and delivery models. The final decision of which procedure to perform should continue to rely upon operator experience, outcome evaluations, patient satisfaction, and informed consent. Cost can be factored into the decision after individual hospital and provider analysis to give the patient full information.

In Table 12-1, the specific techniques used by each of these authors, as well as their listed operating times, is summarized. It is somewhat difficult to compare operating room times. Some surgeons consider only the actual time spent surgically performing the procedure, while others include the time required to set up the instrumentation, which can be considerable, and a few even include anesthetic induction time. Table 12-2 summarizes the published data at the time of this writing on laparoscopic urethropexies, and lists complications and follow-up. It should be noted that follow-up is rarely objective and often the precise criteria for success are not listed.

While there is, as noted, a paucity of prospective data comparing the two approaches, there are several reports in which the laparoscopic procedure is compared with other procedures retrospectively. McDougall and coworkers[14] compared laparoscopic urethropexy with a Stamey needle suspension. Polascik and colleagues[15] and Ross[16] compared the laparoscopic approach with historical controls who underwent an open Burch urethropexy. Das and Palmer[17] compared the laparoscopic approach with both an open procedure and with a needle suspension procedure. In all of these retrospective comparisons, the success rates were similar. However, of interest, Das[18] subsequently published follow-up at 3 years and found a marked drop in efficacy for both procedures with continence rates of 50% for open Burch procedures and 40% for the laparoscopic one.

Table 12-2. Results of laparoscopic retropubic colposuspension

Author (ref.)	No. subjects	Intraoperative complications	Postoperative complications*	F/U interval mo.	Results†
Vancaille and Schuessler (21)	9	Cystotomy-1, technical difficulty-1		3 weeks	100% cure
Albala et al. (22)	22 MMK 10 Burch	Cystotomy-1, technical difficulty-2	Retention-2	7–12	100% cure
Ou et al. (23)	40			6	
Liu (24)	58	Cystotomy-1, SP catheter site bleed-1	None	6–22	Negative standing stress test in all, urge incontinence in 3
McDougall et al. (14)	19	Cystotomy-1	Retropubic bleed, transfusion-1	3–12	7/9 dry at 12 mo.
Polascik et al. (15)	12	Cystotomy-2	Retention-1, Enterococcus umbilical site infections	20 (8–29)	83% continent; of these, 25% have urgency
Langebrekke et al. (26)	8	Subcutaneous emphysema	Retention-1, *de novo* DI-1	3	7/8 dry by stress test
Wallwiener (27)	20	Stich in bladder	Retention-1, DI-1	2–12	92% cured
Das and Palmer (17)	10		Transient bilateral femoral neuropathy	10	90% success
Lam et al. (29)	15	Inf. epigastric injury-1	None	1.5–9	All continent
Radomski and Herschorn (30)	46	12 converted to open, intraoperative hypotension‡	Hematoma-2, enterocoele-1, uterine prolapse-1, Retention-1	17 (12–26)	29/34 dry
Burton (8)	30			12	22/30 cured per urodynamics (see text)
Ross (16)	32	Hernia-1, epigastric injury-1	UTI-1, detrusor a instability-1	12	30/32 cured by cough stress test
Theobald (33)	72	Cystotomy-2	Retention-1 Pelvic pain-1	24 mo (efficacy reported for 37 women only)	70% cured 16% improved

Author (ref)	N	Intraoperative complications	Postoperative complications	Follow-up	Success
Lobel (34)	35	Cystotomy-1, Retropubic bleed-1	Vulvar hematoma-1, Vaginal granulation tissue-5, Retropubic abscess-1, Enterocoele-2, Retention-1, Incisional hernia-1, Suture in bladder-1	3 mo, 1 yr, 34 mo	89%, 86%, 69%
Papasakelariou (35)	32	None	None	2 yrs	91%
Lee (36)	48	Cystotomy-1, Inferior epigastric injury-1	Detrusor instability-2, Voiding difficulties-8, Wound infection-3, Trocar hematoma-3, Vesicocutaneous fistula-1	12–26 mo	94% "satisfied"
Cooper (31)	113	Cystotomy-10, Vaginal tear-1	Retropubic hematoma-2	8.4 mo	87% subjective improvement
Yang (32)	79	Cystotomy-2, Inferior epigastric injury-4	Pulmonary edema-1, pulmonary embolus-1, urinary retention-8	6 mo	90%
Miannay (40)	72	Cystotomy-1, Hemorrhage-1	Wound infection-1, Voiding dysfunction-2	17 mo	72%
Saidi (39)	70	Cystotomy-1	Trocar site infection-1	13 mo	91% free of pads
Lyons (37)	18	Cystotomy-1	Voiding dysfunction-1	12 mo	90% dry with Valsalva
Lavin (38)	139	Cystotomy-6	De novo DI-3	6 mo, 2 yrs	71% cure, 91% improvement; 58% cure, 77% improvement
Ross (41)	48	Inferior epigastric injury-1, Cystotomy-1	Vaginal cuff hematoma-1	6 weeks, 1 year, 2 years	98%, 93%, 89%; Success confirmed during urodynamic testing

* Retention = urinary retention; in no case did this exceed 4 weeks.
† Most articles do not state parameters by which cure or success were determined.
‡ Occurred with insufflation pressures of 15 mm during extraperitoneal approach and resolved when insufflation pressure was maintained below 11 mm.

One of the major purported benefits of the laparoscopic retropubic colpo-suspension is that it allows patients to resume normal activities and work much sooner. In none of the articles listed was this evaluated in any rigorous fashion. For example, Liu noted that all patients were allowed to drive and return to work after 1 week, but it was not stated how many actually did. Polascik noted that the subjective response to the amount of time needed before returning to normal activities varied from 2 to 30 days. Carter stated that "on average, they returned to their normal nonstrenuous activities within one week of discharge," but it is unclear whether this could also include normal child care or work, both of which can be strenuous. Lamb stated, "most women were able to return to normal activities within one to two weeks". Ross was more specific, noting that the return to work for women in his laparoscopic group ranged from 2.5 to 4 weeks, while for the laparotomy group, none returned before 6 weeks.

At the American Urogynecologic Society Annual Meeting in 1994, a vigorous debate ensued about the appropriateness of laparoscopic urethropexy. One point consistently raised was that the surgeons would still prohibit any heavy lifting or straining after a laparoscopic urethropexy on the theory that this would jeopardize the actual colposuspension sutures similar to the open procedure. Another point raised by this large group was the prolonged and very steep learning curve. It was the general consensus of the group that approximately 50 procedures needed to be done before the learning curve plateaued. While very experienced laparoscopic surgeons may be successful in performing the procedure in minimal time after only several procedures have been done, this is unlikely to be true for, for example, experienced urogynecologists who have no laparoscopic experience.

One way to help less experienced laparoscopic surgeons obtain the necessary monitored education for safely performing these procedures may be in the form of telerobotic-assisted laparoscopic surgery. Kavoussi and collaborators[19] reported on a bladder suspension procedure as well as other laparoscopic procedures performed by a team using a robotics system controlled by an experienced surgeon from a remote site. The procedures were all successfully completed without complications, and the authors concluded that current technology is available to successfully allow for telerobotic-assisted surgery. Advantages of telepresent surgical interaction includes improved utilization of surgical specialists, as well as the ability for the surgical manipulations to be performed with minimal risk to surgical specialists in hazardous environments, such as the battlefield. Another use for robot-assisted laparoscopic surgery was described by Partin and associates[20] in providing robotic assistance, thereby potentially decreasing the costs needed for human assistance.

In conclusion, laparoscopic urethropexies can be accomplished and may provide equal success rates as the open procedure by laparotomy. This will remain unknown until further randomized prospective long-term trials are available. Patients should be informed that no information is available at this time as to whether the laparoscopic procedure carries an equivalent long-term success rate. In addition, it is our opinion that if untested modifications of the procedure are done through the laparoscope, each patient should be informed preoperatively about the experimental nature of her surgery and given the ability to make an informed decision about whether she chooses these modifications. While we must continue to strive to improve our surgical technique and outcomes for our patients, we must also hold tightly to the basic ethical principles involved in informed consent and medical decision making.

REFERENCES

1. Bergman A, Ballard CA, Koonings PP. Comparison of three different surgical procedures for genuine stress incontinence: prospective randomized study. *Obstet Gynecol* 1989; **160**: 1102–1106.
2. van Geelen JM, Theeuwes AGM, Eskes TKAB, Martin CB. The clinical and urodynamic effects of anterior vaginal repair and Burch colposuspension. *Am J Obstet Gynecol* 1988; **159**: 137–144.
3. Kil PJM, Hoekstra JW, van der Meijden APM, Smans AJ, Theeuwes AGM, Schreinemachers LMH. Transvaginal ultrasonography and urodynamic evaluation after suspension operations: Comparisons among the Gittes, Stamey and Burch suspensions. *J Urol* 1991; **146**: 132–136.
4. Harewood LM. Laparoscopic needle colposuspension for genuine stress incontinence. *J Endourol* 1993; **7**: 319–322.
5. Knapp PM, Siegel YI, Lingeman JE. Laparoscopic retroperitoneal needle suspension urethropexy. *J Endo Urol* 1994; **8**: 279–284.
6. Flax S. The gasless laparoscopic Burch bladder neck suspension: early experience. *J Urol* 1996; **156**: 1105–1107.
7. Smith ML, Perry C. Simplified visual preperitoneal access to the space of Retzius for laparoscopic urethrocolpopexy. *J Amer Assoc Gynecol Laparoscopists* 1996; **3**: 295–298.
8. Burton G. A randomized comparison of laparoscopic and open colposuspension. *Neurourol Urodyn* 1994; **13**: 497–498.
9. Karram MM, Bhatia NN. Transvaginal needle bladder neck suspension procedures for stress urinary incontinence: A comprehensive review. *Obstet Gynecol* 1989; **73**: 906–914.
10. Leach GE, Trockman BA, Hamilton J, Sakamoto M, Santiago L, Zimmem PE. Modified Pereyra bladder neck suspension: Mean 10 year follow-up in 125 patients. *Neurourol Urodyn* 1995; **14**: 493–494.
11. Kung RC, Lie K, Lee P, Drutz H. The cost-effectiveness of laparoscopic versus abdominal Burch procedures in women with urinary stress incontinence. *J Amer Assoc Gynecol Laparoscopists* 1996; **3**: 537–544.
12. Loveridge K, Malouf A, Kennedy C, Edgington A, Lam A. Laparoscopic colposuspension: is it cost-effective? *Surg Endosc* 1997; **11**: 762–765.
13. Kohli N, Jacobs PA, Sze EHM, Roat TW, Karram MM. Open compared with laparoscopic approach to Burch colposuspension: a cost analysis. *Obstet Gynecol* 1997; **90**: 411–415.
14. McDougall EM, Kloutke CG, Cornell T. Comparison of transvaginal versus laparoscopic bladder neck suspension for stress urinary incontinence. *Urology* 1995; **45**: 641–646.
15. Polascik TJ, Moore RG, Rosenberg MT, Kavoussi LR. Comparison of laparoscopic and open retropubic urethropexy for treatment of stress urinary incontinence. *Urology* 1995; **45**: 657–652.

16. Ross JW. Laparoscopic Burch repair compared to laparotomy Burch for cure of urinary stress incontinence. *Int Urogynecol J* 1995; **6**: 323–328.
17. Das S, Palmer JK. Laparoscopic colpo-suspension. *J Urol* 1995; **154**: 1119–1121.
18. Das S. Comparative outcome analysis of laparoscopic colposuspension, abdominal colposuspension and vaginal needle suspension for female urinary incontinence. *J Urol* 1998; **160**: 368–371.
19. Kavoussi LR, Moore RG, Partin AW, Bender JS, Zenilman ME, Satava RM. Telerobotic assisted laparoscopic surgery: Initial laboratory and clinical experience. *Urology* 1994; **44**: 15–19.
20. Partin AW, Adams JB, Moore RG, Kavoussi LR. Complete robot-assisted laparoscopic urologic surgery. A preliminary report. *J Am Coll Surg* 1995; **181**: 552–557.
21. Vancaillie TJ, Schuessler W. Laparoscopic bladder neck suspension. *J Laparoendosc Surg* 1991; **3**: 169–173.
22. Albala DM, Schuessler WW, Vancaillie TG. Laparoscopic bladder suspension for the treatment of stress incontinence. *Semin Urol* 1992; **10**: 222–226.
23. Ou CS, Presthus J, Beadle E. Laparoscopic bladder neck suspension using hernia mesh and surgical staples. *J Laparoendosc Surg* 1993; **3**: 505–508.
24. Liu CY. Laparoscopic retropubic colposuspension (Burch procedure): A review of 58 cases. *J Reprod Med* 1993; **38**: 526–530.
25. Seman E, O'Shea RT. Laparoscopic Burch colposuspension: A new approach for stress incontinence. *Med J Austral* 1994; **160**: 42–43.
26. Langebrekke A, Dahlstrom B, Eraker R, Umes A. The laparoscopic Burch procedure: A preliminary report. *Acta Obstet Gynecol Scand* 1995; **74**: 153–155.
27. Wallwiener D, Grischke EM, Rimbach S, Maleika A, Bastert G. Endoscopic retropubic colposuspension: "Retziusscopy" versus laparoscopy: A reasonable enlargement of the operative spectrum in the management of recurrent stress incontinence? *Endosc Surg* 1995; **3**: 115–118.
28. Carter JE. Laparoscopic bladder neck suspension. *Endosc Surg* 1995; 81–86.
29. Lam AM, Jenkins GJ, Hyslop RS. Laparoscopic Burch colposuspension for stress incontinence: Preliminary results. *Med J Austral* 1995; **162**: 18–21.
30. Radomski SB, Herschorn S. Laparoscopic Burch bladder neck suspension: Early results. *J Urol* 1996; **155**: 515–518.
31. Cooper MJW, Cario G, Lam A, Carlton M. A review of results in a series of 113 laparoscopic colposuspensions. *Aust NZ J Obstet Gynecol* 1996; **36**: 44–46.
32. Yang S, Park D, Lee J, Graham R. Laparoscopic extraperitoneal bladder neck suspension for stress urinary incontinence. *J Korean Medical Science* 1995; **10**: 426–430.
33. Theobald P, Guillaumin D, Levy G. Laparoscopic preperitoneal colposuspension for stress incontinence in women. *Surg Endosc* 1995; **9**: 1189–1192.
34. Lobel RW, Davis GD. Long-term results of laparoscopic Burch urethropexy. *J Amer Assoc Gynecol Laparoscopists* 1997; **4**: 341–345.
35. Papasakelariou C, Papasakelariou B. Laparoscopic bladder neck suspension. *J Amer Assoc Gynecol Laparoscopists* 1997; **4**: 185–189.
36. Lee C, Yen C, Wang C, Huang KG, Soong YK. Extraperitoneal colposuspension using CO_2 distension method. *Int Surg* 1998; **83**: 262–264.
37. Lyons TL, Winer WK. Clinical outcomes with laparoscopic approaches and open Burch procedures for urinary stress incontinence. *J Amer Assoc Gynecol Laparoscopists* 1995; **2**: 193–198.
38. Lavin JM, Lewis CJ, Foote AJ, Hosker GL, Smith ARB. Laparoscopic Burch colposuspension: a minimum of 2 years' follow up and comparison with open colposuspension. *Gynaecol Endoscopy* 1998; **7**: 251–258.
39. Saidi MH, Sadler RK, Saidi JA. Extraperitoneal laparoscopic colposuspension for genuine urinary stress incontinence. *J Amer Assoc Gynecol Laparoscopists* 1998; **5**: 247–251.

40. Miannay E, Cosson M, Lanvin D, Querleu D, Crepin G. Comparison of open retropubic and laparoscopic colposuspension for treatment of stress urinary incontinence. *Europ J Obstet Gynecol and Reproduc Biol* 1998; **79**: 159–166.

41. Ross JW. Multichannel urodynamic evaluation of laparoscopic Burch colposuspension for genuine stress incontinence. *Obstet Gynecol* 1998; **91**: 55–59.

CHAPTER 13

The climacteric bladder: the role of estrogen

MARIE-ANDRÉE HARVEY AND EBOO VERSI

Menopausal age has remained, unlike the menarche, fixed since the Middle Ages. However, due to increasing life expectancy, the proportion of time spent in that life period has steadily increased. Where life expectancy was 23 years old in the Roman Empire, now the disease-free life expectancy reaches 80.5 years and the disability-adjusted life expectancy, 73.9 years in women of established market economies in 1997.[1] Consequently, women will spend over a third of their life-span in the postmenopausal state. In parallel, due to the post-war "baby boom", a large proportion of the population is entering the climacteric age group. Indeed, in western countries, over 30% of women were menopausal or postmenopausal[2] in 1991. Lower urinary tract dysfunction is common at the time of the menopause[3] and is thought to increase in prevalence thereafter. Consequently, many physicians will be faced with urologic complaints if they care for a middle-aged population as those complaints are no longer accepted as normal part of aging.

The menopause can result in early or late symptoms. Vasomotor instability, loss of libido, sleep disturbance and mood changes are examples of early symptoms. Well-recognized late manifestations include cardiovascular disease and osteoporosis. However, often neglected are symptoms of lower urinary tract dysfunction. They include incontinence, irritative syndromes and voiding dysfunction. It is not clear whether this symptomatology is the result of estrogen deprivation, estrogen flux, the aging process or combination of all of the above.

This chapter will attempt to consolidate the available evidence on the role played by sex steroid hormones, mainly estrogen, in the pathophysiology and treatment of urinary disorders of the climacteric bladder. The clinical entities of stress and urge incontinence, urgency-frequency syndrome as well as the evaluation of the incontinent female will not be covered here as they have been discussed in Chapter 4 and Parts IV and V.

EPIDEMIOLOGY

Epidemiologic surveys have revealed a high prevalence of symptoms around the time of the menopause, but the data do not consistently support the proposition that menopause itself is responsible for this morbidity. It is known that most women relate the onset of their symptoms to the climacteric period,[4] but the prevalence of incontinence was shown to be proportional to aging.[5] The only study analysing both urinary symptoms and urodynamic findings amongst climacteric women was carried out in a menopause clinic in London.[6] We reported on 285 patients (mean age 50.2 years), not primarily complaining of urinary problems. They exhibited a high prevalence of symptomatology of stress incontinence (53%) and urge incontinence (26%), frequency (29%), urgency (51%) and nocturia (27%). A surprisingly large proportion (41%) of the group studied had abnormal urodynamic evaluation (by pad test, videocystourethrography, cystometry and urethral pressure profilometry): genuine stress incontinence was present in 29%, detrusor instability in 10%, voiding dysfunction in 7% and sensory urgency in 4% (some patients had two diagnoses). No correlation was seen in any of the variables with timing of the menopause except for the symptoms of frequency and nocturia (Figure 13-1), which increased 2 years after the menopause ($p<0.05$).

The overall prevalence of incontinence rises with age,[5,7] which is also the pattern followed by urge incontinence after the age of 50.[8] In contrast, the prevalence of stress incontinence peaks at 45–54 years of age and thereafter

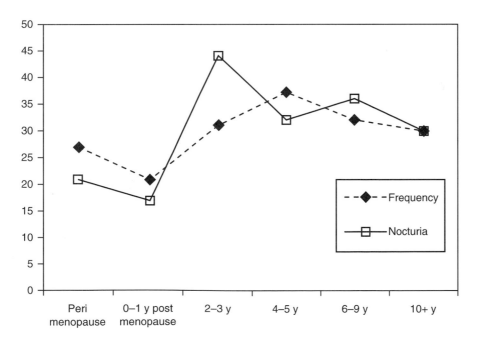

Figure 13-1. Prevalence of urinary frequency and nocturia with advancing menopausal age. The increase in rates 2 years after the menopause is significant ($p<0.05$). (from Versi E, Cardozo L, Studd J, Brincat M, Cooper D. Urinary disorders and the menopause. *Menopause* 1995; **2:** 89–95, with permission).

declines.[9] It is possible that this decrease in prevalence of stress incontinence may be a reflection of the level of activity of the older women; however no existing studies correlate incontinence with age having accounted for activity level.

Molander and colleagues[7] reported a correlation of increased frequency of urinary infection with increasing age. The prevalence of the urethral syndrome (association of dysuria, frequency and urgency with sterile urine) is less clear, ranging from 2%[6] to 23–30%.[10] Symptomatic voiding dysfunction, which can be due to detrusor failure or outflow obstruction, was found to be around 10–15%[6] of a general population of women with climacteric complaints.

Bladder and urethral functions become less efficient with age. Malone Lee[11] has shown that elderly women have *1)* a reduced urinary flow, *2)* increased residual urine, *3)* higher end-filling cystometric pressures, *4)* reduced bladder capacity and *5)* lower maximum voiding pressure. Others[12] also found a decreased urethral closure pressure and functional urethral length.

BIOLOGICAL EFFECTS OF ESTROGEN ON THE LOWER URINARY TRACT

The components of the lower urinary tract, namely the bladder trigone and urethra, share an embryologic origin with the vagina,[13] in that they all evolve from the urogenital sinus. As a result, estrogen receptors are present in those tissues, as shown through the work of Ingelman-Sundberg and colleagues[14] and Iosif and colleagues.[15] Hypoestrogenism was shown to affect the sensory threshold of the bladder, leading to earlier first sensation and decreased capacity volume, with estrogen improving frequency and nocturia.[16] As a consequence of this hormonally receptive milieu, the urethral mucosa is expected to thicken under the influence of estrogen, as does the vaginal mucosa. Indeed, urethral mucosal cytology does show a correlation with vaginal cytology after the menopause.[17] Similarly, the bladder exhibits cytologic changes with the menstrual cycle and menopause.[18]

Continence is assured in part through the coaptation of the urethral mucosa that provides a passive watertight seal.[19,20] Coaptation is thought to be created by the thickness of the mucosa and its softness, probably under the influence of estrogens.[21] Similarly, the submucosal vascular plexuses, as identified by Huisman,[22] play a role in the continence mechanism. In the rabbit, urethral blood flow was shown to increase in response to estrogens.[23] It is hypothesized that these plexuses function as an "inflatable cushion" as, when filled, they distend the area underneath the mucosa at rest and help in creating a hermetic seal.[24] Indeed, Rud and coworkers[25] demonstrated that the vascular bed had a critical role in the maintenance of intraurethral pressure, and we have shown that urethral vascular pulses are under the influence of estrogen activity.[26]

Continence is also assured via a proper interrelationship between the urethra and its support, the muscles and the connective tissue of the fascia and ligaments. As eloquently described in the anatomical studies of DeLancey,[24] the distal urethra is fixed to the pubic bones as is passes through the perineal membrane. The proximal urethra and the bladder are mobile and are supported as in a hammock by the pubocervical/pubourethral fascia. The endopelvic fascia attaches the urethra and anterior vagina to the arcus tendineus fascia pelvis. The arcus tendineus lies on the fascia of the obturator internus muscle and goes from the symphysis pubis to the ischial spine. The levator ani sling (pubovaginalis—anterior part of the puborectalis) provides the muscular support and is attached to the arcus tendineus. The levator tone maintains the retropubic position of the bladder neck at rest and diminishes descent during strain. Prior to micturition, the pelvic floor muscles relax and the bladder neck is allowed to descend. When a sudden increase in abdominal pressure occurs, the levators reflexively contract and the "hammock" is tented, thus compressing the urethra against the underlying endopelvic fascia; this squeeze maintains continence.

This brief review was necessary to understand the importance of connective tissue, which links the urethra, the bladder and the striated muscle (levator ani) to the pelvic bones, as well as interlaces between the muscular fibers within the striated and smooth muscles. The levator ani contain estrogen receptors in the nuclei of their connective tissue cells, the fibroblasts,[27–29] as well as in the striated muscular cells.[27,28] The pelvic fascia is constituted of different types of collagen, mainly type I and III. A change in the ratio in favor of the weaker type III has been demonstrated by Norton and colleagues[30] to be occurring in patients with inguinal hernias, and similar findings have been found in patients with pelvic organ prolapse.[31] This supports the finding of a significant and exponential decrease in skin collagen content 2–4 years after the menopause, which is restored with estrogen replacement therapy.[32–35] Subsequently, a significant correlation between skin collagen content and urethral pressure profile has been found.[36]

Two other muscles are important: the urethral striated and smooth sphincters. The first, a rabdomyosphincter, located in the middle third of the urethra, consists of fast- and slow-twitch striated fibers, and contributes to the resting tone but like the levator ani, it reflexly contracts with sudden increases in abdominal pressure. It can also be made to contract consciously to inhibit micturition. The second, a smooth muscle sphincter, stretches the entire length of the urethra, but at the bladder neck it is poorly developed in women (in contrast to men). Moreover, this smooth muscle has been shown to contain a substantial quantity of estrogen receptors.[37] The urethra is rich in adrenergic receptors and their effect is recognized in potentiation of the proximal urethral tone under the influence of estrogens.[38] Another smooth muscle component is the longitudinal muscle that functions to shorten the urethra during micturition.

Finally, the effect of estrogen on recurrent urinary tract infection must be considered. Under the stimulation of estrogen, the muscosal cells of the vagina produce glycogen (the main substrate of lactobacilli), which favors the growth of these bacteria. The latter generate, through the metabolism of glycogen, lactic acid that lowers the vaginal pH. This low pH decreases the colonization rate, thus decreasing the chance of lower urinary tract infection. Furthermore, certain strains of lactobacilli have been shown to produce hydrogen peroxide, which acts as an antimicrobial agent against uropathogens.[39]

The effects of estrogens are summarized in Table 13-1.

Table 13-1.   Summary of action of sex hormones on the lower urinary tract and pelvic floor support

	Estrogens	*Progestogens*
Urethra	↑ Tone (when used with alpha-adrenergic drug) ↑ Mucosal thickness ↑ Submucosal vascular plexuses	↓ Tone (probably by stimulation of beta-adrenergic fibers)
Bladder	↑ Sensory threshold ↓ Frequency ↓ Urgency	↑ Contractility (via potentialization of cholinergic effect)
Pelvic floor support	↑ Collagen content	
Vaginal flora	↑ Lactobacilli ↓ pH ↓ Uropathogen	

BIOLOGICAL EFFECTS OF PROGESTERONE ON THE LOWER URINARY TRACT

As cyclical progestogens are often used in conjunction with estrogen replacement therapy, it is important to review their effect on the lower urinary tract (Table 13-1). Progesterone receptors have been detected in the bladder wall and in the trigone[40,41] in women, and in the urethra and bladder of rabbits.[42] Furthermore, research involving muscle fibers from the bladder and the urethra of rabbits has demonstrated that progesterone has a slight effect. It appears to potentiate the sensibility to parasympathomimetics, and slightly increases the contractile responsiveness of the bladder to bethanechol[43] (a parasympathetic agent, causing detrusor contraction).

Youssef[44] noted an increased bladder capacity in pregnant women. This change had also been demonstrated,[45] although with controversy,[46] during the luteal phase of the cycle and following administration of exogenous gestagen. With regards to the urethra, progesterone was found in dogs to increase the response of beta-receptors, hence promoting relaxation of the smooth muscle sphincter.[47] van Geelen and coworkers[48] found no correlation between the fluctuation of hormone levels and urethral pressure profile measurements at 8, 16, 28, or 36 weeks of pregnancy and 8 weeks post-partum. Similarly, Rud,[49] when comparing incontinent and continent women, found no change in maximal urethral pressure profile with the use of a gestagen, but did find a decrease in urethral pressure transmission during the cough profile. Benness and colleagues[50] evaluated 14 postmenopausal women on continuous estrogen and cyclical progestogen and in 10 patients noted increased incontinence by pad testing during the progestational phase of the cycle. Eight of their patients had genuine stress incontinence, and in seven of these, urethral sphincter incompetence was worse when the patient took progesterone. In summary, the clinical effect of progesterone on the urinary tract awaits further evaluation, and no firm conclusion can be drawn about its effect in humans.

ANDROGENS AND THE LOWER URINARY TRACT

There are few data regarding the presence of androgen receptors in the urinary tract, especially in humans. Rosenzweig and colleagues[37] found androgen receptors in high concentration in the urethral and trigonal epithelium of nonestrogenized rabbits, in moderate concentration in the smooth muscle of the bladder and urethra, and in low concentration in the smooth muscle of the detrusor. Similarly, Kimura[51] found androgen receptors in the vesical smooth muscle of human bladder.

The clinical effect of androgens is poorly understood. Castrated female baboons, following testosterone treatment, showed an augmentation of their urethral pressure profile, which was similar but less profound than following treatment with estrogen.[52] In contrast, Iosif and coworkers[53] found a modest decrease in urethral closure pressure and pressure transmission ratio after danazol therapy, with no subjective symptoms. However it should be appreciated that danazol is an androgenic progestagen.

There is a need for further clinical investigation of both progesterone and androgen effects on the lower urinary tract.

CLINICAL PRESENTATION OF THE CLIMACTERIC BLADDER

Lower urinary tract dysfunctions present as stress incontinence, urge incontinence, urgency, dysuria, frequency, recurrent urinary tract infections and voiding difficulties. As most of these issues have been reviewed elsewhere in this text (Chapter 4 and Parts IV and V), we will limit this discussion to the latter two.

Urinary tract infections (UTI), should be considered separately from asymptomatic bacteriuria. Urinary tract infection is a symptomatic state in patients whose urine culture grows >10^5 colony forming units (cfu/ml) of a single organism and is often associated with pyuria. Asymptomatic bacteriuria is defined by the recovery of >10^5 cfu/ml of a single bacterium in the absence of clinical symptoms. The long-term effect of asymptomatic bacteriuria is unknown, but no association with renal pathology has been found except in pregnancy. Indeed, two studies[54,55] comparing treatment with placebo showed a spontaneous clearance in 60–80% in both groups. Recurrent infections are defined as symptomatic UTI occurring more than twice a year. Causes of recurrent UTI are multiple and are listed in Table 13-2.

Table 13-2.   Causes of recurrent urinary tract infection (UTI)

High postvoid residual (voiding dysfunction, prolapse)
Systemic diseases (diabetes, peripheral vascular diseases)
High vaginal pH (postmenopausal)
Atrophic urothelium (postmenopausal)
Altered immune system (deficiencies, aging)
Impaired mobility (decreases in hydration and delays in micturition → urine stagnation)

The spectrum of voiding dysfunction progresses from incomplete emptying to retention. Symptoms can be nonspecific, but may include hesitancy, weak stream, straining to void, incomplete emptying and frequency. Table 13-3 summarizes the International Continence Society classification[56] of voiding phase anomalies. Causes are varied and extend beyond the scope of the present chapter, but they include those listed Table 13-4. These causes can be related to aging, but can also be attributed to estrogen deficiency.

Table 13-3.   International Continence Society classification of voiding phase dysfunction

Detrusor function during voiding
1. Normal
2. Underactive
3. Acontractile

Urethral function during voiding
1. Normal
2. Obstructive
   • Overactive
   • Mechanical

(From Abrams P, Blaivas JG, Stanton SL, Anderson JT. The standardization of terminology of lower urinary tract function. *Br J Obstet Gynecol* (Suppl. no. 6 1990; **97**: 14–15, with permission)

ESTROGEN TREATMENT

Stress Incontinence and Estrogens

The use of estrogen alone in the treatment of stress incontinence has yielded inconsistent results. Uncontrolled studies showed improvement with estrogen

Table 13-4. Etiologies of voiding phase anomalies (examples are noted in parentheses)

Neurologic diseases multiple sclerosis
Medications (anti-histamines, anti-cholinergic)
Infective causes (UTI, herpes simplex)
Obstructive causes (prolapse)
Over-distension
Endocrine (diabetes)
Psychogenic
Constipation

---

therapy; however, because lower urinary tract symptoms are susceptible to placebo effect, no conclusion should be drawn without controlled data. Four placebo-controlled trials have used oral estrogen[16,57–59] for a period of 6 months or less. However, only one[59] demonstrated a significant subjective and objective improvement in stress incontinence and this has not been replicated. A long-term study of climacteric patients treated with estradiol implants (50 mg) for 1 year with videourodynamic assessment before and after treatment revealed improved urethral pressures at rest (but no change in the stress profile) and a significant reduction in the degree of cystocele as judged on fluoroscopy.[60]

Nonetheless, when used in combination with alpha-adrenergic agents, several trials disclosed a significant improvement with the use of this combination when compared with estrogens alone.[59,61–64] Three studies[59,62,63] performed a placebo-controlled comparison of estrogen alone or in combination with an alpha-stimulant, and found a subjective and an objective amelioration of the stress incontinence, but only in the combined group.

The results of studies evaluating the impact of the use of estrogen on the urethral pressure profile have been inconsistent.[16,59,60,61,65–71] However, the validity of urethral pressure measurement is debated,[72] since both the trans-mission pressure ratio[73] and the urethral pressure profile[74] show a wide overlap between normal women and those suffering with genuine stress incontinence. This limits its use as a diagnostic tool for stress incontinence, let alone for treatment evaluation of the latter.

Urge incontinence and estrogens

In contrast to stress incontinence, the use of estrogen yields more consistent results for urge incontinence. Subjective improvement was noted in three randomized, placebo-controlled studies,[57,67,75] while objective improvement was not significant. However, a significant placebo effect was also found. The treatment lasted <6 months. Iosif[69] has shown that urogenital atrophy, a late manifestation of estrogen deficiency, is only completely relieved after a year of treatment with 0.5 mg estriol suppositories, and that symptoms recur after discontinuation of therapy. Consequently, the lack of objective improvement may reflect the brief duration of the studies performed to date, or the lack of discrimination from the placebo due to deficient effect.

Recurrent urinary tract infections

Estrogen therapy has been shown to reverse urogenital atrophy and reduce the incidence of postmenopausal urinary tract infections. A randomized controlled trial involving 83 postmenopausal patients, conducted by Raz and Stamm,[76] documented that intravaginal estrogen (estriol) significantly reduced the incidence of urinary tract infections, promoted vaginal colonization by lactobacilli, and lowered pH in postmenopausal patients. Others[77,78] found similar results. These results suggest that estrogens have an important therapeutic role in climacteric and postmenopausal women.

Voiding difficulties

Few investigations have been carried out on this subject, and good controlled data are lacking. Nonetheless, Hilton and Stanton[66] showed a decrease in symptoms of voiding difficulty following the use of vaginal cream, although no statistical significance was found, probably because of the small number of patients.

CONCLUSION

Estrogen is likely to play a role in lower urinary tract function, as supported by the common embryologic origin with the genital tract, the presence of hormonal receptors and its effect on vaginal flora. Whether it is a major or minor participant in climacteric bladder symptomatology remains unknown, as age is a strong confounder.

However, one does recognize the effect of estrogen deprivation on the sensory threshold of the bladder, and it may help the symptoms of urgency, frequency, nocturia and dysuria. For stress incontinence, its use seems better supported when in combination with an alpha-adrenergic agent, but it is unlikely that estrogen alone is effective. Estrogen surely has a role in the management of recurrent urinary tract infection, as it renders the vaginal and perineal milieu more resistant to uropathogens. Furthermore, not to be neglected, is the use of estrogen preoperatively when planning a vaginal or retropubic procedure as this is likely to improve tissues, and possibly adding to the success of surgery as well as decreasing technical difficulties and complications. However, evidence-based validation is awaited.

Further studies will be necessary to define the effect of progesterone on the lower urinary tract as well as the most beneficial use of estrogen. Estrogen undoubtedly has a place in the armamentarium of the physician for management of the climacteric and postmenopausal states for its other well-recognized properties, but there are little data to justify its use purely for lower urinary tract dysfunction.

REFERENCES

1. Murray CJL, Lopez AD. Regional patterns of disability-free life expectancy and disability-adjusted life expectancy: Global burden of disease study. *Lancet* 1997; **349**: 1347–1352.
2. Central Statistical Office Annual Abstract of Statistics. No 127. London: Her Majesty's Stationery Office, 1991.
3. Versi E. The bladder in menopause: Lower urinary tract dysfunction during the climacteric. In: *Current Problems in Obstetrics, Gynecology and Fertility*. Barbieri RL, Berek JS, Creasy RK, DeCherney AH, Ryan KJ (eds) St. Louis: Mosby Year Book; 1994; **17**: 204–205.
4. Iosif CS, Bekassy Z. Prevalence of genitourinary symptoms in the late menopause. *Acta Obstet Gynecol Scand* 1984; **63**: 257–260.
5. Thomas TM, Plymat KR, Blannin J, Meade TW. Prevalence of urinary incontinence. *Br Med J* 1980; **281**: 1243–45.
6. Versi E, Cardozo L, Studd J, Brincat M, Cooper D. Urinary disorders and the menopause. *Menopause* 1995; **2**: 89–95.
7. Molander U, Milsom I, Ekelund P, Mellström D. An epidemiological study of urinary incontinence and related urogenital symptoms in elderly women. *Maturitas* 1990; **12**: 51–60.
8. Kondo A, Saito M, Yamada Y, Kato S, Hasegawa S, Kato K. Prevalence of hand-washing urinary incontinence in healthy subjects in relations to stress and urge incontinence. *Neurourol Urodyn* 1992; **11**: 519–523.
9. Jolleys JV, Reported prevalence of urinary incontinence in women in a general practice. *Br Med J* 1988; **296**: 1300–1302.
10. Scotti RJ, Ostegard DR. Urethral syndrome. In: *Urogynecology and Urodynamics: Theory and Practice*. Ostegard DR, Bent AE (eds). Baltimore: Williams and Wilkins; 1996: 340.
11. Malone-Lee JG, Wahedna I, Characterisation of detrusor contractile function in relation to old age. *Br J Urol* 1993; **72**: 873–880.
12. Susset J, Plante P. Studies of female urethral pressure profile. Part II: Urethral pressure profile in female incontinent. *J Urol* 1980; **123**: 70–74.
13. Gosling JA. Anatomy. In: Stanton SL (ed). *Clinical Gynecologic Urology*. St. Louis: CV Mosby; 1984: 3–12.
14. Ingelman-Sundberg A, Rosén J, Gustafsson SA, Carlström K. Cytosol estrogen receptors in the urogenital tissues in stress incontinent women. *Acta Obstet Gynecol Scand* 1981; **60**: 585–586.
15. Iosif CS, Batra S, Ek A, Åstedt B. Estrogen receptors in the human female lower genitourinary tract. *Am J Obstet Gynecol* 1981; **141**: 817–820.
16. Fantl JA, Wyman JF, Anderson RL, Matt DW, Bump RC. Postmenopausal urinary incontinence: Comparison between nonestrogen-supplemented and estrogen-supplemented women. *Obstet Gynecol* 1988; **71**: 823–828.
17. Smith P. Age changes in the female urethra. *Br J Urol* 1972; **44**: 667–676.
18. McCallin PF, Taylor ES, Whitehead RW. A study of the changes in the cytology of the urinary sediment during the menstrual cycle. *Am J Obstet Gynecol* 1950; **60**: 64–74.
19. Zinner NR, Sterling AM, Ritter RC. The role of urethral softness in urinary continence. *Urology* 1980; **16**: 115–117.

20. Zinner NR, Sterling AM, Ritter RC. Evaluation of inner urethral softness. *Urology* 1983; **22**: 446–468.

21. Versi E. Incontinence in the climacteric. *Clin Obstet Gynecol* 1990; **33**: 392–398.

22. Huisman AB. Aspects on the anatomy of the female urethra with special relation to urinary continence. *Contrib Obstet Gynecol* 1983; **10**: 1–31.

23. Batra S, Bjellin L, Sjögren C Iosif S, Widmark E. Increases in blood flow of the female rabbit urethra following low dose estrogens. *J Urol* 1986; **136**: 1360–1362.

24. DeLancey JOL. Anatomy of the female bladder and urethra. In: *Urogynecology and Urodynamics: Theory and practice.* Ostergard DR, Bent AE (eds). Baltimore: Williams and Wilkins; 1996; 8.

25. Rud T, Andersson KE, Asmussen M, Hunting A, Ulmsten U. Factors maintaining the urethral pressure in women. *Invest Urol* 1980; **17**: 343–347.

26. Versi E, Cardozo LD. Urethral vascular pulsations. In: *International Continence Society, Proceedings: 15th Annual Meeting*, London, 1985: 503.

27. Smith P, Heimer G, Norgren A, Ulmsten U. Localization of steroid hormones receptors in the pelvic muscles. *Euro J Obstet Gynecol* 1993; **50**: 83–85.

28. Smith P, Heimer G, Norgren A, Ulmsten U. Steroid hormone receptors in pelvic muscles and ligaments in women. *Gynecol Obstet Invest* 1990; **30**: 27–30.

29. Stumpf WE, Sar M, Joshi SG. Estrogen target cells in the skin. *Experimentia* 1974; **30**: 196–198.

30. Friedman DW, Boyd CD, Norton P, et al. Increases in type III collagen expression and protein synthesis in patients with inguinal hernias. *Ann Surg* 1993; **218**: 754–760.

31. Norton P, Boyd C, Deak S. Collagen synthesis in women with genital prolapse or stress urinary incontinence. *Neurourol Urodyn* 1992; **11**: 300–301.

32. Brincat M, Versi E, O'Dowd TM, et al. Skin collagen changes in postmenopausal women receiving oestradiol gel. *Maturitas* 1987; **9**: 1–5.

33. Brincat M, Moniz CJ, Studd JWW, Darby A, Magos A, Emburey G, Versi E. Long-term effects of the menopause and sex hormones on skin thickness. *Br J Obstet Gynaecol* 1985; **92**: 256–259.

34. Brincat M, Moniz CF, Kabalan S, et al. Decline in skin collagen content and metacarpal index after the menopause and its prevention with sex hormone replacement. *Br J Obstet Gynaecol* 1987; **94**: 126–129.

35. Brincat M, Versi E, Moniz CF, Magos A, de Trafford JC, Studd JWW. Skin collagen changes in postmenopausal women receiving different regimens of estrogen therapy. *Br J Obstet Gynaecol* 1987; **70**: 123–127.

36. Versi E, Cardozo L, Brincat M, Cooper D, Montgomery J, Studd J. Correlation of urethral physiology and skin collagen in postmenopausal women. *Br J Obstet Gynaecol* 1988; **95**: 147–152.

37. Rosenzweig BA, Bolina PS, Birch L, Moran C, Marcovici I, Prins GS. Location and concentration of estrogen, progesterone and androgen receptors in the bladder and urethra of the rabbit. *Neurourol Urodyn* 1995; **14**: 87–96.

38. Schreiter F, Fuchs P, Stockamp K. Estrogenic sensitivity of α-receptors in the urethra musculature. *Urol Int* 1976; **31**: 13–19.

39. Klebanoff SJ, Hillier SL, Eschenbach DA, Waltersdorph AM. Control of the microbial flora of the vagina by H_2O_2-generating lactobacilli. *J Infect Dis* 1991; **164**: 94–100.

40. Wolf H, Wandt H, Jonat W. Immunohistochemical evidence of estrogen and progesterone receptors in the female lower urinary tract and comparison with the vagina. *Gynecol Obstet Invest* 1991; **32**: 227–231.

41. Pacchioni D, Revelli A, Casetta G, et al. Immunohistochemical detection of estrogen and progesterone receptors in the normal urinary bladder and in pseudomembranous trigonitis. *J Endocrinol Invest* 1992; **15**: 719–725.

42. Batra SC, Iosif CS. Progesterone receptors in the female lower urinary tract. *J Urol* 1987; **138**: 1301–1304.

43. Ekström J, Iosif CS, Malmberg L. Effects of long-term treatment with estrogen and

progesterone on in vitro muscle responses of the female rabbit urinary bladder and urethra to autonomic drugs and nerve stimulation. *J Urol* 1993; **150**: 1284–1288.

44. Youssef AF. Cystometric studies in gynecology and obstetrics. *Obstet Gynecol* 1956; **8**: 181–188.
45. Gitsch E, Brandstetter F. Phasen spinktero-zystometrie. *Zentralbl Gynakol* 1954; **76**: 1746–1754.
46. Sørensen S, Knudsen UB, Kirkeby HJ, Djurhuus JC. Urodynamic investigations in healthy fertile females during the menstrual cycle. *Scand J Urol Nephrol* (Suppl.) 1988; **114**: 28–34.
47. Raz S, Ziegler M, Caine M. The effect of progesterone on the adrenergic receptors of the urethra. *Br J Urol* 1973; **45**: 131–135.
48. van Geelen JM, Lemmens WA, Eskes TK, Martin CB Jr. The urethral pressure profile in pregnancy and after delivery in healthy nulliparous women. *Am J Obstet Gynecol* 1982; **144**: 636–649.
49. Rud T. The effects of estrogens and gestagens on the urethral pressure profile in urinary continent and stress incontinent women. *Acta Obstet Gynecol Scand* 1980; **59**: 265–270.
50. Benness C, Gangar K, Cardozo LD, Cutner A, Whitehead M. Do progestogens exacerbate incontinence in women on HRT? *Neurourol Urodyn* 1991; **10**: 316–318.
51. Kimura N, Mizokami A, Oonuma T, Sasano H, Nagura H. Immunocytochemical localization of androgen receptor with polyclonal antibody in paraffin-embedded human tissues. *J Histochem Cytochem* 1993; **41**: 671–678.
52. Bump RC, Friedman CI. Intra-luminal urethral pressure measurements in the female baboon: Effect of hormonal manipulation. *J Urol* 1986; **136**: 508–511.
53. Iosif S, Forman A, Jeppson S, Mellqvist P, Rannevik G, Ulmsten U. The effect of danazol on the human female urethra. *Zentralbl Gynakol* 1981; **103**: 1344–1348.
54. Guttmann D. Follow up of urinary tract infection in domiciliary patients. In: Brumfitt W, Asscher AW (eds). *Urinary Tract Infection*. London: Oxford University Press; 1973: 62.
55. Mabeck CE. Treatment of uncomplicated urinary tract infection in non-pregnant women. *Postgrad Med J* 1972; **48**: 69–75.
56. Abrams P, Blaivas JG, Stanton SL, Anderson JT. The standardization of terminology of lower urinary tract function. *Br J Obstet Gynaecol* (Suppl. no 6) 1990; **97**: 14–15.
57. Samsioe G, Jansson I, Mellström D, Svanborg A. Occurrence, nature and treatment of urinary incontinence in a 70 years old female population. *Maturitas* 1985; **7**: 335–342.
58. Wilson PD, Faragher B, Bulter B, Bu'lock D, Robinson EL, Brown ADG. Treatment with oral piperazine oestrone sulphate for genuine stress incontinence in post-menopausal women. *Br J Obstet Gynaecol* 1987; **94**: 568–574.
59. Walter S, Kjaergaard B, Lose G, et al. Stress urinary incontinence in postmenopausal women treated with oral estrogen (estriol) and alpha adrenoreceptor—stimulating agent (phenylpropanolamine): a randomized double blind placebo controlled study. *Int Urogynecol J* 1990; **1**: 74–79.
60. Versi E, Cardozo L, Studd J. Long term effect of estradiol implants on the female urinary tract during the climacteric. *Int Urogynecol J* 1990; **1**: 87–90.
61. Beisland HO, Fossberg E, Sander S. On incompetent urethral closure mechanism: treatment with estriol and phenylpropanolamine. *Scand J Urol Nephrol* (Suppl.) 1981; **60**: 67–69.
62. Kinn AC, Lindskog M. Estrogens and phenylpropanolamine in combination for stress urinary incontinence in postmenopausal women. *Urology* 1988; **32**: 273–280.
63. Ahlström K, Sandahl B, Sjöberg B, Ulmsten U, Stormby N, Lindskog M. Effect of combined treatment with phenylpropanolamine and estriol compared with estriol treatment alone, in post-menopausal women with stress urinary incontinence. *Gynecol Obstet Invest* 1990; **30**: 37–43.

64. Ek A, Andersson K-E, Gullberg B, Ulmsten U. Effects of oestradiol and combined norephedrin and oestradiol treatment on female stress incontinence. *Zentralbl Gynakol* 1980; **102**: 839–844.
65. Faber P, Heidenreich J. Treatment of stress incontinence with estrogen in post menopausal women. *Urol Int* 1977; **32**: 221–223.
66. Hilton P, Stanton SL. The use of intravaginal oestrogen cream in genuine stress incontinence. *Br J Obstet Gynaecol* 1983; **90**: 940–944.
67. Walter S, Wolf H, Barlebo H, Jansen HK. Urinary incontinence in postmenopausal women treated with estrogens: a double blind clinical trial. *Urol Int* 1978; **33**: 135–143.
68. Beisland HO, Fossberg E Moer A, Sander S. Urethral sphincteric insufficiency in post-menopausal females: Treatment with phenylpropanolamine and oestriol separately and in combination. *Urol Int* 1984; **39**: 211–216.
69. Iosif CS. Effects of protracted administration of estriol on the lower genitourinary tract in postmenopausal women. *Arch Gynecol Obstet* 1992; **251**: 115–120.
70. Karram MM, Yeko TR, Sauer MV, Bhatia NN. Urodynamic changes following hormonal replacement therapy in women with premature ovarian failure. *Obstet Gynecol* 1989; **74**: 208–211.
71. Langer R, Golan A, Neuman M, Pansky M, Bukovsky I, Laspi E. The absence and effect of induced menopause by gonadotrophin releasing hormone analogs on lower urinary tract symptoms and urodynamic parameters. *Fert Steril* 1991; **55**: 751–753.
72. Rai RS, Versi E. Urethral pressure profilometry. *Int Urogynecol J* 1991; **2**: 222–227.
73. Versi E, Cardozo L, Cooper DJ. Urethral pressures: Analysis of transmission pressure ratios. *Br J Urol* 1991; **68**: 266–270.
74. Versi E. Discriminant analysis of urethral pressure profilometry data for the diagnosis of genuine stress incontinence. *Br J Obstet Gynaecol* 1990; **97**: 251–259.
75. Eriksen PS, Rasmussen H. Low-dose 17 β-estradiol vaginal tablets in the treatment of atrophic vaginitis: a double blind placebo controlled study. *Eur J Obstet Gynecol Reprod Biol* 1992; **44**: 137–144.
76. Raz R, Stamm WE. A controlled trial of intravaginal oestriol in postmenopausal women with recurrent urinary tract infection. *N Engl J Med* 1993; **329**: 753–756.
77. Kirkengen AL, Andersen P, Gjersoe E, Johannessen GA, Johnsen N, Bodd E. Oestriol in the prophylactic treatment of recurrent urinary tract infections in post menopausal women. *Scand J Prim Health Care* 1992; **10**: 139–142.
78. Brandberg A, Mellstrom D, Samsioe G. Peroral estriol treatment of older women with urogenital infections. *Lakartidningen* 1985; **82**: 3399–3401.

CHAPTER 14

Management of urogenital organ injury sustained during urethropexy procedures

MICHAEL E. MAYO

Injury to the pelvic organs during incontinence procedures is less common than those sustained in the course of other pelvic procedures, particularly abdominal hysterectomy. However, complications do arise from damage to the bladder, ureter, urethra, and, less commonly, to the peritoneum, bowel, and nerves in the pelvic sidewall. This chapter discusses the risk factors and prevention of injuries; their assessment and management if recognized at the time of surgery; and those presenting in the postoperative period.

RISK FACTORS AND PREVENTION

The best management of surgical complications is their prevention. Although knowledge of the anatomy, both normal and pathologic, and the selection of the correct procedure are essential, all are beyond the scope of this chapter. Women who have had prior pelvic or vaginal procedures, radiation, and who are obese are at increased risk. If possible, open retropubic dissection should be avoided in favor of needle suspensions in those patients. However, a narrow introitus or vagina would be a contraindication to the needle suspensions or other vaginal procedures. Having selected the right patient for surgery and the right procedure for that patient, there are measures that can be taken during the surgery itself to improve exposure and vascular control.

An extended lithotomy and Trendelenberg position would improve vaginal exposure, but care must be taken to avoid vascular and neurologic compromise in the groin, which is more likely, again, in obese patients. Suturing the labia minora out laterally, correct retraction, good lighting, and infiltration of the vaginal wall with saline, are all important. For suprapubic approaches mild hyperextension of the hips and the Trendelenberg position both help exposure. The legs should be abducted enough to allow access to the vagina, which should have been prepped. Hemorrhage, more common with the retropubic approaches, can always be controlled by vaginal pressure while suture-ligating the vessel. Indeed the chance of organ injury during pelvic procedures is increased in the presence of excessive bleeding, as not only are tissue planes obscured, but attempts to control the bleeding with sutures may include the bladder, ureter, or urethra.

Serious infection may occur after organ injury, especially in the presence of a pelvic hematoma. A sterile preoperative urine and careful skin and vaginal preparation with antibacterial soaps are recommended. Antibiotic coverage against gram-negative, gram-positive, and anaerobic organisms should be started at the time of surgery and continued for 24 hours. A broad-spectrum oral antibiotic may be continued for 5 to 7 days after surgery, especially in those patients at increased risk due to obesity, diabetes, radiation, or pelvic hematoma.

ASSESSMENT AND MANAGEMENT OF INJURIES RECOGNIZED DURING URETHROPEXY

See Table 14-1.

Hemorrhage

A careful history will usually uncover any bleeding diathesis. Although coagulation screening tests are commonly done during preoperative blood draws, a bleeding time would probably be the best single test if it was not so

Table 14-1. Organ injury and complications of urethropexies

Procedure	Complications
Suprapubic	
General	Hemorrhage, peritoneotomy, and bowel injury more common after previous surgery
Specific	
Marshall-Marchetti-Krantz	Urethral obstruction and damage
	Bladder injury (anterior)
	Osteitis pubis
Burch	Bladder injury (base)
	Ureteral ligation
Vaginal (with retropubic dissection)	
Raz	Hemorrhage
Slings	Hemorrhage
	Urethral obstruction
	Detrusor instability
	Erosion and infection (synthetic slings)
Vaginal (needle suspension)	
Pereyra, Stamey, Gittes	Bladder suture, stone, and urinary tract infection
and Benderev	Ilioinguinal nerve injury (except with bone fixation)
	Infection due to Dacron pledgets (Stamey)

labor-intensive. If there is concern for a possible coagulation defect a thrombo-elastogram should be ordered. All patients should be instructed to stop aspirin 10 days and other nonsteroidal antiinflammatory agents 5 days before surgery.

Hemorrhage is more common with the open retropubic procedures than the needle suspensions, particularly if there has been prior surgery. Having access to the vagina is essential, as it allows control with finger compression as described.

Venous hemorrhage also occurs with vaginal procedures, and again is more common when there has been prior surgery. The plane under the vaginal mucosa should be bloodless and infiltration with saline before starting will assist the surgeon in finding it. It is also important to break through the endopelvic fascia right on the ischiopubic ramus when entering the retropubic space from below.[1] The source of bleeding at this point cannot be seen and ligated directly, but can usually be controlled with a sponge while the other side is dissected. When the suture or sling is passed on the side that is bleeding, it must be done carefully to prevent injury to the bladder or bladder neck, but quickly to minimize blood loss. Most venous hemorrhage will be well controlled once the urethropexy is completed and a firm vaginal pack inserted. The use of a Foley catheter inside a gauze pack has been advocated.[2] All visible vaginal bleeding should be controlled by the vaginal packing before the patient leaves the operating room, and vital signs and serial hematocrits followed carefully in the immediate postoperative period.

Bladder Injury

Indications that the bladder has been entered during a urethropexy, either by the suprapubic or needle suspension methods, are often subtle. A copious amount of clear fluid in the operative field is obvious, but smaller quantities may be obscured if there is marked blood loss. If the Foley catheter is plugged during the surgery it should be periodically released and injury suspected if the urine is obviously bloody. If there is doubt direct injection of methylene blue solution through the Foley should be diagnostic.

Bladder injury may be more common in the open retropubic urethropexy than the needle suspensions, and in particular when there has been prior surgery.[3] In this situation the bladder is often firmly attached to the periosteum of the pubis. Thus injury may occur during initial mobilization and it is usually easy to repair in two layers using absorbable suture material. Sequelae are uncommon unless the tear has extended into the bladder neck mechanism. Potentially more serious damage may occur at the base in a Burch or colposuspension when the bladder is being dissected off the anterior vaginal wall.[4] Bleeding and poor tissue planes may make this maneuver more difficult and the surgeon should consider doing a formal cystotomy in the dome of the bladder to visualize the trigone and assess and repair any injury. Before putting in sutures to repair the base of the bladder, it is essential to protect the ureters even if the ureteral orifices look as if they are well away from the injury. To do this a 5 Fr catheter or pediatric feeding tube can be passed before the repair is done, or indigo-carmine given and efflux observed from the ureteral orifices after suturing the defect. A recent prospective study of 97 consecutive patients, who had a Burch urethropexy alone or in combination with other pelvic surgery, revealed no intraoperative injuries to the bladder or ureters. The authors concluded that routine intraoperative cystocopy was not necessary.[5]

Bladder injuries may also occur in the retropubic dissection from below during the needle suspension procedures. If the bladder base is injured, it may be possible to expose it well enough from below, otherwise a tear in the anterior bladder will be better repaired from above with a formal retropubic approach. Again, before repairing the bladder base, the ureteral orifices must be protected by cystoscopy and passage of a ureteral catheter on that side, or by observing the efflux from the orifice after the repair has been completed. The repairs themselves should be performed with an absorbable suture. My preference is for a 3.0 synthetic adsorbable suture, either monofilament or braided, with the inner mucosa and half the muscle layer closed with a running suture, and the outer layer of muscle and adventitia if present, closed with an inverting interrupted suture. The vaginal wall closure forms a third layer. The tissue should be under no tension, the bladder drained for at least 7 days, and a cystogram performed before removing the catheter.

Injuries to the bladder with a needle during the needle suspension procedures are common, particularly if the retropubic space is not finger dissected. All these procedures must be combined with cystoscopy to rule out this complication. It is usually enough to remove the needle or suture, repass it correctly, and drain the bladder with a catheter for a few days.

Urethral Injuries

Urethral injuries are rare but may occur in both retropubic and needle suspension procedures, and, as noted before, prior surgery is a significant risk factor. The original description of the Marshall-Marchetti-Krantz urethropexy described the placing of suspension sutures in the urethral and bladder neck muscle.[6] However, those surgeons performing this procedure now use the adjacent anterior vaginal wall. This reduces the risk of damage to the intrinsic mechanism and the chance of bladder neck obstruction. The use of a midline vaginal incision instead of an inverted U or two lateral incisions for needle suspension procedures may more likely result in urethral injury. Injuries recognized at the time should be carefully repaired in two layers and if the tissues are compromised by radiation, scarring, or attenuation of the muscle, a vascularized labial fat pad (Martius graft) should be mobilized and used to cover the repair before closing the vaginal mucosa. Prolonged catheter drainage is recommended for at least 10 to 14 days, and the catheter removed only after demonstration on a cystourethrogram that the injury is healed.

Ureteral Injuries

The incidence of ureteral injuries in routine gynecological surgery is estimated at 0.2% to 2.5%,[7] and these usually occur with a hysterectomy or ovariectomy.

Urethropexy procedures by themselves are a rare cause but certainly have been described,[8,9] and these may be found more commonly if routine upper tract imaging is performed after surgery. The suprapubic procedures are more likely to cause ureteral obstruction, due to either the hemostatic or suspension sutures being passed through the trigone and obstructing the ureterovesical junction.[10] In the vaginal approach, repairs or injuries to the trigone may result in compromise to the intramural ureter. Injuries sustained by suprapubic procedures rather than the needle suspension are likely to be missed, as most surgeons performing the latter will check the patency of the ureters with indigo-carmine. When injuries are detected at the time of surgery the repair should be taken down and the sutures removed sequentially until a guidewire or contrast can be introduced through the damaged area. A double J stent should be then be passed and left in for at least 3 weeks. If the ureter cannot be stented, suprapubic ureteroneocystostomy will have to be performed. As the damage is low down, there should be no need for a bladder flap or psoas hitch.

Damage to Peritoneum and Bowel

Urethropexies performed by the needle suspension technique without other vaginal wall repair or gynecologic procedures are very unlikely to cause injury to the peritoneum or bowel, as the needle and sutures are passed low down right over the pubic bone. However, during insertion of a suprapubic catheter by a blind technique, peritoneum and bowel may be entered when previous lower abdominal surgery has fixed these structures down so that they will not ride up as the bladder is distended.

The suprapubic procedures commonly result in peritoneotomies. Obtaining adequate mobilization of the peritoneum from the underside of the rectus muscle and transversalis fascia may be very difficult in the presence of scarring from previous surgery. Often it is easier and quicker to make a formal opening in the peritoneum and dissect away adherent bowel and get into the correct retroperitoneal piane. Having achieved this and having mobilized the peritoneum so that there is no tension, it can be then closed without difficulty before inserting the self-retaining retractors for the urethropexy procedure. If an omental wrap is being used to reinforce bladder or bladder-neck repairs, or in patients with bladder-neck obstruction from prior urethropexies, the peritoneum should be opened transversely on the left side. Bowel injuries are very rare and can easily be repaired with interrupted inverting 3.0 silk sutures. Resection of bowel should be unusual and only necessary if a large portion of the wall or the mesenteric vessels are damaged.

Repair of large bowel injuries above the peritoneum reflection should probably be protected by a proximal colostomy. A large bowel injury below the peritoneal reflection, a rare complication in a urethropexy, may be repaired without a colostomy. The operative field in all cases of bowel injuries should be irrigated copiously with antibiotic solution.

INJURIES AND COMPLICATIONS PRESENTING IN THE POSTOPERATIVE PERIOD

Clinical Presentation and Evaluation

Hemorrhage and Hematoma

In the absence of visible vaginal blood loss, hypotension, tachycardia, low urine output and a falling hematocrit after adequate fluid replacement in the post-operative period suggests retroperitoneal bleeding. Venous bleeding will usually tamponade, especially after vaginal surgery, and therefore arterial hemorrhage is the most likely cause for continuing blood loss. Early exploration if the situation does not stabilize after replacement of 2 to 3 units is therefore recommended. At the time of exploration and vascular control the hematoma can be drained, which will avoid the possibility of this large hematoma becoming infected.

Wound Infection and Abscess

Wound infections are probably more common after open retropubic procedures, particularly with diabetes, obesity, or hematoma as risk factors. Although the vagina is potentially contaminated, it is rare for infection to follow the vaginal urethropexies; an incidence as low as 3% has been reported.[1] However, late infections have been reported with pledgets used to bolster the vaginal suture in the Stamey type of needle suspension.[11] Other non-absorbable materials caused late infections after both retropubic and vaginal urethropexy.[12] These presented with a painful lump in the anterior vaginal wall that may discharge sponta-neously and not heal until the foreign material has been removed. Slings made of nonabsorbable material are also more likely to form a vaginal sinus or erode into the urethra. Although generally replaced by autologous fascia, their use has recently been readvocated.[13]

Flank Pain and Ileus

Flank pain and ileus is the classical presentation of a ureteral injury that has produced obstruction and/or extravascation. If obstruction is suspected an excretory urogram is still probably the best radiologic study, but in the presence of a pelvic collection a computed tomography (CT) scan with contrast may be better. Ultrasound imaging in the first day or two after obstruction may not show much dilation, particularly if obstruction is complete, and it is not recommended as a screening test. See Figure 14-1.

Incontinence

The differential here lies between true incontinence (continuing stress, overflow, or urgency) and false incontinence (fistula from the ureter, bladder, or bladder neck). Occasionally copious vaginal discharge due to vaginitis will be reported

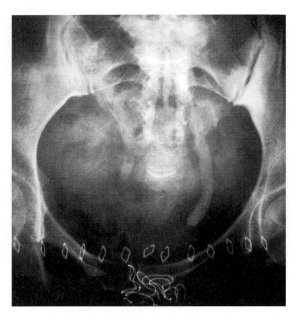

Figure 14-1. Ureteral obstruction: a pelvic film taken 6 hours after intravenous contrast given 24 hours following a hysterectomy and Burch urethropexy. The patient was anuric. The right ureter is obstructed in the midpelvis as a result of the hysterectomy and the left ureter at the ureterovesical junction due to the Burch urethropexy suture.

as urinary leakage. Urinary infection will exacerbate urgency incontinence and is usually associated with retention and overflow. Physical examination, urinalysis and measurement of postvoid residual, by catheter or dedicated ultrasound machine, will often yield a diagnosis. It is important to find the fistula early so that it can be properly managed. Stress and urgency incontinence are often treated empirically with medication early in the postoperative period and re-evaluation with urodynamics postponed for 2 to 3 months until surgical induration has resolved. If a ureteral or bladder fistula is suspected tampon tests after pyridium by mouth or bladder instillation of methylene blue may be tried initially. However, excretory urography, cystography, cystourethroscopy, vaginoscopy, and retrograde pyelography may all be necessary to completely evaluate the site of the fistula. Even if damage to the bladder is confirmed, appropriate studies should be performed to rule out concomitant injury to the ureter and vice versa. See Figure 14-2.

Persistent stress incontinence suggests that either there was a technical error or that tissue or suture failure occurred. Alternatively the perioperative studies may not have identified that the patient had some degree of intrinsic sphincter deficiency. Detrusor instability and urgency incontinence may be transitory in the first few weeks and in many patients it may resolve with healing. *De novo* instability may be the result of obstruction of the bladder neck and is discussed

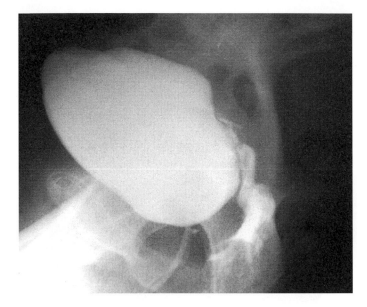

Figure 14-2. Vesicovaginal fistula. A lateral view cystogram shows a large vesicovaginal fistula.

in the next section. However, stress incontinence will probably not improve with time and reevaluation with videourodynamics can reasonably be undertaken earlier than in those patients with symptoms of urgency.

Difficulty Voiding

Some degree of difficulty is common in the first few weeks especially after a compressive procedure such as a fascial or *in situ* sling. If the patient had a high postvoid residual before the procedure, it is much more likely she will have chronic retention afterward. These patients should be fully evaluated preoperatively with videourodynamics and the majority will be found to have hypocontractility due to myogenic failure or possibly occult neuropathy. These women should be counseled to expect a long period of temporary or even permanent retention and undergo the procedure with the probability that intermittent self-catheterization will be necessary. It is generally believed that a women who voided with a low postvoid residual preoperatively should be able to establish satisfactory voiding afterward. Those that fail to do so are thought to be obstructed. However, it is possible that very low outflow resistance, almost certainly associated with intrinsic sphincter deficiency, may allow complete emptying by straining and that these patients are in fact truly noncontractile and are at risk for retention after successful urethropexy. Any history or evidence of intermittency, straining, and increased postvoid residual should be thoroughly evaluated preoperatively, so that a persistent retention state after surgery can be anticipated.

Obstruction after urethropexy is usually due to overcorrection but circumferential scarring may occasionally be a contributing factor. It may present with retention and/or overflow incontinence, and in some cases with persistent detrusor instability that was either not present preoperatively, or became worse after the surgery. Obstruction is said to be commoner with the Marshall-Marchetti-Krantz procedure,[14,15] although, since the sutures have no longer been placed through the bladder neck, the risk of this complication may have decreased. It has been shown to occur early on after the Stamey procedure, but the obstructive phenomena decreased with time.[16] It is important to evaluate for obstruction urodynamically as urethrolysis in the presence of a noncontractile detrusor is much less likely to be successful. Also urethrolysis performed for instability alone without some degree of retention or demonstrable obstruction may be successful but the outcome is less certain.

Pain

Nerve entrapment may occur with any of the procedures but the obturator is at most risk with the retropubic procedures, particularly the Burch. The ilio-inguinal nerve may also be involved in the needle suspensions when the suture is placed too far laterally.[17] This can be avoided if fixation to the pubic bone is used.[1]

Pain in the pubis with contraction or stretching of the adductor muscles is typical of osteitis pubis. This rare complication is said to be commoner with the Marshall-Marchetti Krantz[18,19] technique but may also occur with any procedure in the retropubic area even when the pubic bone or symphyseal cartilage are not used for suture anchorage.[20] In the past the diagnosis was difficult to confirm by plain tomography but, today, computed tomographic and bone scans should show bony changes and increased uptake, respectively, in the area of symphysis pubis. Osteomyelitis of the symphysis has been described and if the osteitis pubis fails to respond to the usual measures, bone biopsy and culture, and even open exploration and biopsy, may necessary for a diagnosis.[21]

Urinary Tract Infection

Bacteriuria is common after urethropexy and the incidence rises with the length of catheterization. Treatment with antibiotics is probably only indicated if the patient is symptomatic. Treatment should also be considered even if the bacteriuria is asymptomatic for those women emptying incompletely in the initial period after catheter removal. Bacteriuria is likely to resolve spontaneously in those emptying well. If the patient is in enough retention to justify self-catheterization bacteriuria should probably only be treated if causing symptoms.

It the patient continues to get bacteriuria with or without symptoms later on, an underlying problem should be suspected. This is more likely if the bacteria each time are the same type and antibiogram suggesting a relapsing rather than reinfection. In this situation an intravesical suture perhaps associated with a stone should be suspected and cystoscopy performed.[22]

Management

General management strategies for hemorrhage, pelvic infection, and urinary tract infection have already been covered. This section discusses the management of specific complications of organ injuries sustained during urethropexy procedures.

Vesicovaginal Fistula

Conservative management with catheter drainage is reasonable for a period of 3 to 4 weeks. There is no clear advantage to the type of catheter drainage, urethral, suprapubic, or both, but the patient must understand the importance of having the drainage bag below the bladder at all times. She should use a leg bag in the day and a standard drainage bag hanging below the level of the mattress overnight. If the fistula tract is small and appears to be epithelialized, an unlikely situation with a recent fistula, removal of the epithelium either mechanically with a screw, or electrosurgically with the bovie has been advocated but there is little evidence that this is helpful.

After 3 or 4 weeks of bladder drainage open repair should be considered. The timing of this is still being debated. There is now a consensus that early repair, even if it means a suprapubic approach rather than a vaginal one, is preferable to a long waiting period with incontinence and social isolation.[23,24] However, the fistula repair should not be attempted until the inflammatory reaction has resolved, but waiting several more months for the area around the fistula to lose its induration and become supple will probably not improve the results. The only exception to this is in women who have had radiation. In these a period of 6 months with biopsy of the fistula tract prior to repair is recommended.

Surgical approach should be individualized. Generally vaginal repair is less morbid and is preferred unless there are contraindications. These include an inability to position the patient due to reduced range of motion of the hips and knees; inadequate vaginal access because of a narrowed introitus or a small vagina that will, after further vaginal surgery, be too small for intercourse; and factors relating to the fistula itself. The latter include a large fistula, one that is too close (<1 cm) to the ureters, and a fistula associated with a lot of induration (2 cm or more).[24] Patients requiring a concomitant abdominal procedure such as a ureteral reimplant or an augmentation cystoplasty will obviously have a fistula repaired transabdominally.

The principles of fistula repair are an adequate mobilization of tissues for a multilayered tension free closure, the use of vascularized tissue to buttress the repair if there is any doubt that it will heal (omental flap, labial fat pad, or gracilis muscle), and excellent drainage of the bladder. The latter can be achieved by both suprapubic and urethral indwelling catheters, although some authors recommend removing the urethral catheter as soon as hematuria has cleared so that nothing rests on the site of the repair. With either approach the ureters must be protected with ureteral catheters or stents passed at cystoscopy for vaginal repairs, or via cystotomy for suprapubic procedures. In the vaginal repair an inverted U-shaped anterior vaginal wall flap is raised with the tip just proximal to the fistulous opening. This flap should be mobilized so that it will cover the area of the repair after the margins of the fistula have been excised. Dissecting the bladder wall around the fistula is aided by traction on a Foley catheter placed through the tract. The tract, the margins of the anterior vaginal wall mucosa, and indurated tissue should be excised and the defect closed in at least two layers with interrupted inverting sutures of absorbable suture material with knots placed on the outside. Before closing anterior vaginal wall, a Martius flap can be raised through a separate vertical incision over the labium major on one side. The fibrofatty tissue is mobilized from the pubic symphysis and based with blood supply anteriorly. It is tunneled under the vaginal mucosa and sutured over the repair. If one flap is insufficient a second one can be raised from the other labium.

In the suprapubic repair the fistulous tract and bladder wall are dissected in a similar manner with the aid of Foley catheter traction, via a cystotomy after suitable retraction of the bladder wall. If the bladder is too small or the fistula very large and complicated the bladder wall can be split down to the fistula. This will considerably improve access and allow excellent separation and closure of the vaginal wall. Mobilization of an omental flap should be considered if there is any doubt about the repair even if it means extending the incision and mobilizing the omentum from the stomach. Although the vascular arrangement can vary, the right gastroepiploic artery is usually better than the left, and the omentum can normally be swung down to the pelvic floor without tension by dividing the short vessels to the stomach from the gastroepiploic. The stomach has ample alternative blood supply and its vascularity is never in question. Drainage of the bladder after either approach should be continued for at least a week and most authors advocate 2 or 3 weeks with a cystogram or dye and tampon test to confirm that the repair is sound before removing the catheter.

Urethrovaginal Fistula

Conservative management for 3 to 4 weeks again should be enough time for spontaneous healing to occur. Repair can be undertaken when the acute inflammatory response and at least some of the induration has resolved. If the fistula involves the bladder-neck sphincter, in addition to closure and reconstruction of the area, compression with a fascial sling will almost certainly be necessary for adequate continence. The fistula should almost always be accessible for repair from below. A Martius fibrofatty flap under the sling has been recommended to decrease the risk of the sling eroding through the compromised tissue.[25]

Ureteral Injuries

At the time of diagnosis in the postoperative period an attempt should be made at cystoscopy to get a stent across the injured segment unless the patient is not stable enough for this procedure. In the latter situation a percutaneous nephrostomy can usually be placed under local anesthetic to decompress the upper tract and divert the urine. If the retrograde catheter cannot be passed, an antegrade approach via a percutaneous nephrostomy may be successful. With recent advancement in endourological techniques, unless there is extensive loss of tissue (>2 cm), most ureteral injury problems will be resolved without resorting to open surgery. The key is to get a double J stent across the injured segment.[26–28]

Open repair may be necessary but the timing is still being debated. Except for patients who have had radiation, repair is generally recommended as soon as the patient is fit enough.[23] However, the acute infective complications in the pelvis must have been resolved with percutaneous nephrostomy drainage of urine and percutaneous or open drainage of any pelvic abscess. Depending on the site of injury and with the urethropexy procedures it is likely to be low down, a simple ureteroneocystostomy should be successful. If there is insufficient length, a psoas hitch or Boari flap can be used. For radiated patients tissue viability is always a problem, and if the latter procedures are not possible, a transuretero-ureterostomy may be necessary as long as the other ureter is normal and there is not too much discrepancy in size between the two.

Nerve Entrapment

Before considering exploration and removal of sutures it is essential to obtain evidence from EMG, nerve conduction studies, or nerve blocks that there is indeed nerve entrapment. Exploration and release of sutures in the groin for ilioinguinal problems should be successful and may not lead to recurrence of pelvic floor descensus. If the obturator is involved, exploration, identification, and freeing of the nerve should be undertaken, or the nerve completely divided. Adductor paralysis and sensory impairment are often mild and better tolerated than chronic pain.

Neurologic problems other than pain due to nerve entrapment can result from urethropexy. Vaginal dissection, especially during endoscopic bladder neck suspension, has recently been found to worsen preexisting perineal neuropathy in patients with stress incontinence due to pelvic floor relaxation.[29]

Osteitis and Osteomyelitis Pubis

Osteitis pubis will usually respond to antiinflammatory agents but may take several weeks to do so. A small recently reported series suggests that low-grade osteomyelitis is present in many cases previously described as osteitis.[21] If response to antiinflammatory agents in osteitis pubis is not apparent in 3 to 4 weeks or if there are extensive changes in bone on CT scan, a CT-guided needle biopsy should be considered. The tissue obtained should be cultured anaerobic-ally and aerobically and any organisms grown treated with appropriate antibiotics for at least 4 weeks. If the response to antibiotics is poor or if no organisms are obtained open biopsy and debridement with further cultures has also been recommended.

Bladder Problems

Foreign Bodies and Stones

When a nonabsorbable suture with or without an associated stone is found in the bladder it must be removed. This can sometimes be done using cystoscopic scissors and alligator forceps. If not, and the previous repair was a needle type of urethropexy, the knot on the anterior rectus fascia or on the pubic bone can be found, one end cut, and the whole suture removed. If the urethropexy was an open retropubic procedure and the suture cannot be removed cystoscopically, the retropubic space will need to be explored to find the upper end of the suture, or, alternatively, the bladder can be opened and the suture removed via that route.

Retention

If the patient's bladder is noncontractile and especially if there is a history of voiding difficulties before surgery, the patient should be managed on clean intermittent catheterization. Those patients who do not have clear evidence of obstruction on videourodynamics but who seem to be emptying before surgery, and those definitely obstructed can be offered urethrolysis. However, they should all be counseled that the alternative is self-catheterization with or without medication to control detrusor instability, if present.

Urethrolysis was originally described as a retropubic procedure that allows not only good visualization but also the interposition of omentum in the retropubic space between the mobilized bladder neck and the symphysis. Transvaginal urethrolysis approaching the bladder neck posteriorly and laterally was also successful and less morbid than the retropubic procedure.[30] Recently, a suprameatal or anterior approach has been described in which the anterior attachments of the bladder neck, including the pubourethral ligaments, are divided. The space anterior to the bladder neck can also be filled with a Martius pad which may prevent further scarring and adherence of the bladder neck to the symphisis.[31,32]

Detrusor Instability

The initial approach to urgency, presumably to detrusor instability, in the immediate postoperative period, should be medication with bladder training. If this fails and when the surgical reaction has resolved at 3 months videourodynamic evaluation should be performed. Patients with obstruction can be offered urethrolysis and those with no demonstrable obstruction should probably be counseled to wait to see if further medication trials and the passage of time will lead to resolution of the instability. Eventually these patients may elect to have urethrolysis as well.[14]

Stress Incontinence

Patients with a technical failure and recurrent descensus can be offered a standard urethropexy. However, if there was a failure of the tissues of the pelvic floor, it is likely that further standard repairs will also fail unless new tissue, in the form of a fascial sling, is brought into the area. With intrinsic sphincter deficiency collagen injections can be tried, especially in elderly patients before considering a fascial sling. Collagen can also be offered to those with recurrent descensus before resorting to further urethropexy, as these are procedures with minimal morbidity and may be successful in some patients.

SUMMARY

Injury to adjacent organs is relatively uncommon during standard urethropexies, with the bladder and urethra being the commonest organs involved. Careful preoperative evaluation and planning, good access, meticulous dissection, and control of hemorrhage, and an awareness during surgery of possible injury to adjacent organs will avoid most of these complications. Postoperatively early evaluation and treatment will mitigate much of the morbidity of those injuries not found during surgery.

In the past 5 years "laparoscopic" urethropexies[33] have been described both via intraperitoneal and retroperitoneal approaches.[34] As with all procedures of this type there has been a long learning curve, and a number of complications have been reported in addition to an increased failure rate. Whether this approach has clear advantages over the minimal invasive needle suspensions and fascial slings will have to be determined by well-controlled trials.

REFERENCES

1. Kelly MJ, Zimmern PE, Leach GE. Complications of bladder neck suspension procedures. *Urol Clin North Am* 1991; **18**: 339–348.
2. Schmidbauer CP, Hadley HR, Staskin DR, Zimmern P, Leach GE, Rax S. Complications of vaginal surgery. *Semin Urol* 1986; **4**: 51–62.
3. Parnell JP, Marshall VF, Vaughan ED. Management of recurrent urinary stress incontinence by the Marshall-Marchetti-Krantz vesicourethropexy. *J Urol* 1984; **132**: 912–914.
4. Webster GD. The urethra. In: Paulson DF (ed). *Genitourinary Surgery* Vol. 2. New York: Churchill Livingstone, 1984; 399–583.
5. Klutke JJ, Klutke CG, Hsieh G. Bladder injury during the Burch retropubic urethropexy: is routine cystoscopy necessary? *Tech Urol* 1998; **4**: 145–147.
6. Marshall VF, Marchetti AA, Krantz KE. The correction of stress urinary incontinence by simple vesicourethral suspension. *Surg Gynecol Obstet* 1949; **88**: 509–518.

7. Giberti C, Germinale F, Lillo M, Bottino P, Simonato A, Carmignani G. Obstetric and gynaecological ureteric injuries: Treatment and results. *Br J Urol* 1996; **77**: 21–26.
8. Virtanen HS, Kiilholma PJA, Måkinen, Nurmi MJ, Chancellor MB. Ureteral injuries in conjunction with Burch colposuspension. *Int Urogynecol J* 1995; **6**: 114–118.
9. Neale R. Complications of urogynaecological surgery. *Curr Opin Obstet and Gynecol* 1995; **7**: 400–403.
10. Schoenwald MB, Orkin LA. Bilateral intravesical ureteral ligation: Complication of Cooper's ligament suspension. *Urology* 1974; **3**: 787–789.
11. Knispel HH, Klän R, Siegmann K, Miller K. Results with the Stamey procedure in 251 consecutive patients with genuine urinary stress incontinence. *J Urol* 1995; **153**: 431A.
12. McIntosh LJ, Mallett VT, Richardson DA. Complications from permanent suture in surgery for stress urinary incontinence. A report of two cases. *J Reprod Med* 1993; **38**: 823–825.
13. Chin YK, Stanton SL. A follow up of Silastic sling for genuine stress incontinence. *Br J Obstet Gynaecol* 1995; **102**: 143–147.
14. Webster GD, Kreder KJ. Voiding dysfunction following cystourethropexy: Its evaluation and management. *J Urol* 1990; **144**: 670–673.
15. Nitti VW, Raz S. Obstruction following anti-incontinence procedures: Diagnosis and treatment with transvaginal urethrolysis. *J Urol* 1994; **152**: 93–98.
16. Mundy AR. A trial comparing the Stamey bladder neck suspension procedure with colposuspension for the treatment of stress incontinence. *Br J Urol* 1983; **55**: 687–690.
17. Miyazaki F, Shook G. Ilioinguinal nerve entrapment during needle suspension for stress incontinence. *Obstet Gynecol* 1992; **80**: 246–248.
18. Lentz SS. Osteitis pubis: a review. *Obstet Gynecol Surv* 1995; **50**: 310–315.
19. Kammerer Doak DN, Cornella JL, Magrina JF, Stanhope CR, Smilack J. Osteitis pubis after Marshall-Marchetti-Krantz urethropexy: a pubic osteomyelitis. *Am J Obstet Gynecol* 1998; **179**: 586–590.
20. Wheeler JS. Osteomyelitis of the pubis: Complication of a Stamey urethropexy. *J Urol* 1994; **151**: 1638–1640.
21. Sexton DJ, Heskestad L, Lambeth WR, McCallum R, Levin LS, Corey GR. Postoperative pubic osteomyelitis misdiagnosed as osteitis pubis: Report of four cases and review. *Clin Infect Dis* 1993; **17**: 695–700.
22. McIntosh LJ, Mallett VT, Richardson DA. Complications from permanent suture in surgery for stress urinary incontinence: A report of two cases. *J Reprod Med* 1993; **38**: 823–825.
23. Blandy JP, Badenoch DF, Fowler CG, Jenkins BJ, Thomas NWM. Early repair of iatrogenic injury to the ureter or bladder after gynecological surgery. *J Urol* 1991; **146**: 761–765.
24. Blaivas JG, Heritz DM, Romanzi LJ. Early versus late repair of vesicovaginal fistulas: Vaginal and abdominal approaches. *J Urol* 1995; **153**: 1110–1113.
25. Blaivas JG. Treatment of female incontinence secondary to urethral damage or loss. *Urol Clin North Am* 1991; **18**: 355–363.
26. Dowling RA, Corriere JN, Sandler CM. Iatrogenic ureteral injury. *J Urol* 1986; **135**: 912–915.
27. Kramolowsky EV, Tucker RD, Nelson CMK. Management of benign ureteral strictures: Open surgical repair or endoscopic dilation? *J Urol* 1989; **141**: 285–286.
28. Selzman AA, Spirnak JP, Kursh ED. The changing management of ureterovaginal fistulas. *J Urol* 1995; **153**: 626–628.
29. Zivkovic F, Tamussino K, Ralph G, Schied G, Auer-Grumbach M. Long-term effects of vaginal dissection on the innervation of the striated urethral sphincter. *Obstet and Gynecol* 1996; **87**: 257–260.
30. McGuire EJ, Letson W, Wang S. Transvaginal urethrolysis after obstructive urethral suspension procedures. *J Urol* 1989; **142**: 1037–1039.

31. Raz S, Stothers L, Broseta E, Chopra A. The Martius flap technique to correct iatrogenic urinary obstruction following anti-incontinence procedures. *J Urol* 1996; **155**: 588A.
32. Petrou SP, Brown JA, Blaivas JG. Suprameatal transvaginal urethrolysis (STU): A simple, efficacious technique for treating bladder outlet obstruction after anti-incontinence procedures. *J Urol* 1966; **155**: 589A.
33. Radomski SB, Herschorn S. Laparoscopic Burch bladder neck suspension: Early results. *J Urol* 1996; **155**: 515–518.
34. Wallwiener D, Grischke EM, Rimbach S, Maleika A, Bastert G. Endoscopic retropubic colposuspension: "Retziusscopy" versus laparoscopy: A reasonable enlargement of the operative spectrum in the management of recurrent stress incontinence? *Endosc Surg Allied Technol* 1995; **3**: 115–118.

CHAPTER 15

Persistent or recurrent urinary incontinence

CINDY A. AMUNDSEN, R. DUANE CESPEDES AND EDWARD J. McGUIRE

BACKGROUND

Late failure of an operation to cure stress incontinence permanently is not uncommon, and although immediate failure of operative procedures to cure incontinence is less common, it also occurs. Most stress urinary incontinence (SUI) operations are designed to correct anatomic malposition of the urethra, an abnormality most commonly determined by measurement of the posterior urethrovesical angle. This condition, characterized by urethral hypermobility, is typified by incontinence that occurs with increases in abdominal pressure. Patients with persistent or recurrent incontinence after surgical procedures may describe an incontinence pattern that is identical to that which bothered them preoperatively, or the incontinence may be entirely different in character. Some patients may complain of incontinence associated with urgency and frequency, symptoms that may have been present before surgery or developed *de novo*. Patients with persistent incontinence have never received any benefit from the operative procedure, and as soon as the catheter is removed, such patients are as incontinent, or more incontinent, than they were preoperatively. Patients with recurrent incontinence have achieved continence for a period of time after a surgical procedure and resumption of urinary leakage is therefore considered a new problem.

The incidence of recurrent incontinence after a procedure for urethral hypermobility varies from 10% to 40%.[1] Failure can occur as a result of a lack of precise diagnosis of the etiology of the incontinence preoperatively, which results in selection of an improper operative procedure. Failure of an operative procedure may also be due to tissue factors, suture material breakdown, the persistence of detrusor instability, or the *de novo* development of that problem postoperatively. In addition to these rather common causes for failure, some other unusual urinary tract problems may cause incontinence:

1. Urethral causes
   a. Anatomic incontinence (recurrent hypermobility)
   b. Intrinsic sphincter deficiency
   c. Mixed: anatomic and intrinsic sphincter deficiency

2. Bladder causes
    a. Sensory/motor urgency
    b. Decreased compliance
    c. Hypocontractility (areflexia)
3. Other causes
    a. Fistulae: vesicovaginal, urethrovaginal, ureterovaginal
    b. Ectopic ureter
    c. Urethral diverticulum
    d. Detrusor hyperreflexia (neuropathy)

Patients with recurrent or persistent incontinence are a clinical problem in that the first repair is generally recognized to be the most successful, and subsequent repairs are often considered more difficult or thought to have poorer outcomes than the primary repair. The precise diagnosis of the exact cause of the incontinence and tailoring treatment to fit that cause is obviously essential to achieve the desired outcome.

ETIOLOGIES

Uncommon Problems

Although very uncommon, an ectopic ureter, a urethral diverticulum, a urinary tract fistula, or some neurologic disease may cause incontinence after urethral suspension surgery. Ectopic ureters are rare and are diagnosed by intravenous urography or other retrograde radiographic maneuvers. A urethral diverticulum, or more commonly bilateral diverticula, are uncommon problems after urethral suspension surgery. However, there are descriptions of pseudodivertula arising from sloughing of the periurethral fascia associated with sutures placed for Kelly plications, as part of needle urethral suspensions, or during the performance of retropubic operative procedures. The diagnosis of a diverticulum is made on voiding urethrography and cystoscopy. These diverticula are commonly bilateral and are associated with very wide mouth openings entering into the proximal urethra.

Urinary fistulae can be associated with previous urethral suspension and are more common following retropubic procedures than any other. They are, nevertheless, very rare causes of persistent incontinence. Fistulae are generally diagnosed by cystography or voiding cystoureterography. Occasionally, urethral fistulae are found in association with diverticula formation apparently as a result of penetration of the urethral mucosa by the suspension suture material.

Occasionally, a subtle neurologic disease may be associated with persistent incontinence. Neurologic diseases include: disc disease resulting in detrusor areflexia with overflow incontinence, multiple sclerosis with detrusor sphincter dyssynergia or hyperreflexic detrusor dysfunction, or cerebrovascular disease resulting in uninhibited bladder contractility. The diagnosis of these abnormalities is made on the basis of a neurologic and urodynamic evaluation.

Abnormalities of Detrusor Control Not Associated With Neurogenic Dysfunction

As many as 16% of patients who fail stress incontinence surgery will do so as a result of "sensory or motor urge incontinence".[2] Various studies report a 2% to 20% incidence of "detrusor instability" in the immediate postoperative period following bladder suspension surgery.[3,4] Iatrogenic causes of detrusor-related incontinence are commonly associated with *overt* motor urge incontinence. A cystometrogram will demonstrate an uninhibited contraction. Iatrogenic conditions include intravesical sutures, intravesical foreign bodies, and perivesical or periurethral granulomatous processes resulting from the urethral suspension. Diagnosis of foreign bodies in the bladder or urethra can be made on careful cystoscopy. The usual position for such foreign bodies is anterior at the bladder neck or superior in the dome of the bladder. As many as 5% of patients following suspension procedures, at least in the short term, will have some degree of voiding dysfunction. This includes overflow incontinence related to persistent urethral obstruction and motor urge incontinence directly related to urethral obstruction without overt urinary retention.[5]

Operative Failure

Most stress incontinence procedures fail because of recurrence of urethral hypermobility or intrinsic sphincter dysfunction (ISD) even if motor urge incontinence is also present. In the case of the anterior colporrhaphy or needle suspension procedures, the 45% to 70% incidence of recurrent hypermobility may be due to suture material tearing through the vaginal and endopelvic fascia.[2] Factors which predispose to an unsuccessful repair, putatively include: the type of suture used, placement vis-à-vis the urethrovesical junction and/or unusually severe physical stress such as a chronic cough associated with asthmatic bronchitis or obstructive pulmonary disease or very strenuous physical activity. In addition, the quality of the tissue incorporated into the suture suspension may be related to failure. This may be due to the composition of collagen in the support structures which affects the durability of the urethral suspension.[6] Development of vaginal prolapse following a suspension, particularly a large cystocele, can directly contribute to failure of a repair. In addition, urethral hypermobility may coexist with intrinsic sphincter deficiency. The latter is a definite cause of failure of stress incontinence operations. McGuire[2] showed that patients were twice as likely to have intrinsic sphincter dysfunction (or poor urethral function) following failure of incontinence surgery than those who presented with primary stress incontinence having never had an incontinence procedure. His study found a 27% incidence of intrinsic sphincter dysfunction after one failed operative procedure and a 75% incidence after failure of two or more such procedures. Clearly, the misdiagnosis of pure or mixed intrinsic sphincter dysfunction as pure hypermobility can result in a high failure rate. Whether the appearance of intrinsic sphincter dysfunction in patients who fail one or more operative procedures is a reflection of the preoperative presence of this condition, or if it is the operative procedure itself, is currently unknown. It seems likely that both etiologies are involved. In addition to idiopathic ISD, there are known causes for the condition. For example, the 50% failure rate of bladder-neck suspensions after a radical hysterectomy is due to a peripheral neuropathy which leads to urethral dysfunction and very severe intrinsic sphincter dysfunction.[7] Such patients are not suitable candidates for suspension procedures. The etiology of their incontinence is related to poor proximal urethral closing function and not hypermobility.

EVALUATION

Evaluation of patients with persistent or recurrent incontinence after stress incontinence procedures should include a history, physical examination, urinalysis, and a urine culture. The underlying purpose of the evaluation is to determine which of the two major causes of persistent or recurrent incontinence is present: a detrusor abnormality or a urethral abnormality.

Even if the exact etiology of the incontinence was precisely determined preoperatively, repeat studies are necessary. The symptoms relayed by the patient and the pattern and character of her incontinence are important. These suggest additional studies which may be required, including pressure flow studies, cystometry, cystourethroscopy, and/or videourodynamics. Grading the amount of urinary leakage by a pad test or some other method gives the examiner an idea of the significance of the problem. The incontinence grades are as follows:

Grade I: Patient loses urine only with sudden severe increases in abdominal pressure, but never at rest or in the supine position.
Grade II: Incontinence with minimal to moderate degrees of physical stress such as walking or changing to a standing position, but not while supine.
Grade III: Severe incontinence without significant relationship to physical activity or position.

The physical examination should include a brief directed neurologic examination and a very extensive pelvic examination. Perineal sensation and sacral reflex integrity can be evaluated with the patient in the pelvic examination position. Decreased sensation in the perineum or a lack of volitional or reflex contractility of the pelvic floor musculature and/or anal sphincter suggests a sacral or peripheral nerve injury. Careful examination of the vagina is useful to assess areas of vaginal prolapse. The anterior, posterior, and superior vaginal walls should be inspected first with the patient in the supine position and then with the patient in the upright position with one foot on a stool.

DIAGNOSIS

Uncommon Causes of Incontinence

Ectopic ureters with openings into the urethra associated with incontinence enter at a level distal to the continence mechanism. About one-third of extraurinary ureteral orifices open in the vaginal vestibule adjacent to the external urethral meatus.[8] An intravenous pyelogram, as mentioned above, is the best way to make the diagnosis of this problem. Almost all ectopic ureters are associated with duplication of abnormalities of the upper urinary tract.

A urethral diverticulum presents with an anterior vaginal wall mass with or without urethral tenderness, postvoid dribbling, dysuria, or dyspareunia. The diagnosis can be made on the basis of voiding cystourethrogram and sometimes on a urethral endoscopic evaluation. Diverticula may have been present pre-operatively, but they can also develop, as mentioned above, as a result of a surgical injury to the urethral fascia, creating a large mouth pseudodiverticulum. Patients with such diverticula have a very high rate of persistent incontinence related to intrinsic sphincter dysfunction that appears to be related to the diverticula. Such patients require a combined repair of their diverticulum and a pubovaginal sling procedure. That method is reported to achieve a 77% cure rate.[9]

Looking for an obvious vesicovaginal fistula along the vaginal cuff, anterior vaginal wall or periurethral area is important. The fistula should be suspected as an extraurethral etiology of continuous incontinence in cases where a hysterectomy was performed at the time of the incontinence procedure or the incontinence operation was complicated by a bladder injury. However, unrecognized entry of suture material into the urinary tract may also result in fistula formation. Thus, the known lack of any overt bladder injury is not a factor which "rules" out the presence of a fistula. Moreover, fistulae are not always so easily diagnosed, and when a fistula is suspected or even remotely considered, a cystogram, and/or the intravesical administration of dye with placement of a vaginal tampon will often make the diagnosis. Direct cystoscopic evaluation can usually localize the fistula once one knows it is present. Ureterovaginal fistulae are occasionally involved in persistent incontinence and these can be suspected if the tampon test is negative and intravenous injection of dye material produces a positive tampon test. In cases of ureteral fistulae, intravenous pyelography will often demonstrate partial ureteral obstruction and usually extravasation is visible. However, retrograde studies are often necessary to anatomically localize the defect. It should be kept in mind that some patient have both a vesicovaginal and ureterovaginal fistula. Urethrovaginal fistulae are particularly difficult to diagnose and these require voiding cystourethrogram, cystourethroscopy, and sometimes vaginoscopy or vaginograms for a precise diagnosis.

Abnormalities of Detrusor Control

Urgency, frequency, and nocturia suggests motor urge incontinence. Neurologic disorders should, as far as possible, be ruled out in such patients. A history of Parkinson's disease, multiple sclerosis, spinal cord injury, disc surgery, or disc disease as well as pelvic extirpative surgery for rectal or cervical carcinoma should prompt a thorough urodynamic evaluation. In neurogenic conditions, cystometric findings include bladder contractions which occur in a regular, reproducible fashion at a specific volume which the patient cannot control (Figure 15-1). Neurologic causes of persistent incontinence following stress incontinence surgery are unusual and more commonly patients are considered to have "idiopathic" urge incontinence or "detrusor instability" if they complain of urgency and urge incontinence following the operation. In the latter group, a cystometrogram (CMG) is not diagnostic of the precise bladder condition even in grossly symptomatic patients, since only 40% of neurologically intact patients with motor urge incontinence will have a positive CMG.[10] The CMG is used rather, to detect altered detrusor compliance and to assign patients to two broad groups within the category of those with motor urge incontinence. These groups are 1) patients with urge incontinence and a positive cystometric response that is, a bladder contraction on a CMG, which cannot be inhibited (Figure 15-2), and 2) patients with urge incontinence, but a negative "normal" cystometrogram. Group 1 patients respond predictably to drug therapy, group 2 patients do not. Group 2 patients appear to suffer from a poor detrusor monitoring and warning system, and a lack of subconscious neural modulation of reflex bladder contractility, *on occasion*, a condition that responds better to behavioral therapy than to drugs.

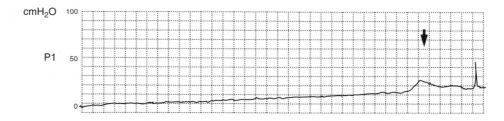

Figure 15-1.   A 35-year-old man with a T5–T6 spinal cord injury. A cystometrogram study revealed a neurogenic bladder with an uninhibited coordinate bladder contraction at a bladder volume of 250 mlH$_2$O. (*arrow*).

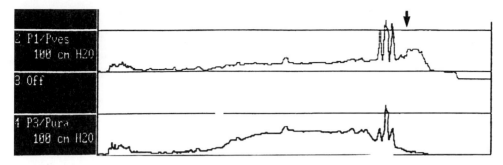

Figure 15-2. An 81-year-old woman who complained of sudden, episodic incontinence. A urodynamic study revealed an uninhibited detrusor contraction occurring at 183 mlH$_2$O. (*arrow*) Pves, intravesical pressure; Pura, urethral sphincter pressure.

Abnormal Compliance

Inability to store urine at low pressure (poor compliance) is related to neuro-genic obstructive uropathy, structural obstructive uropathy, or direct injury, such as, radiation therapy. Detrusor "hypertonicity" may also follow a radical hyster-ectomy when pelvic neural injury occurs or with long-term catheter drainage. The inability of the bladder to store urine at a low pressure causes severe "stress" incontinence as well as upper urinary tract damage. A cystometrogram is a sensitive indicator of a lack of normal bladder storage activity (Figure 15-3). If this abnormality is diagnosed, treatment must be directed at the detrusor and not at the urethra, since incontinence is related to the lack of detrusor compliance.

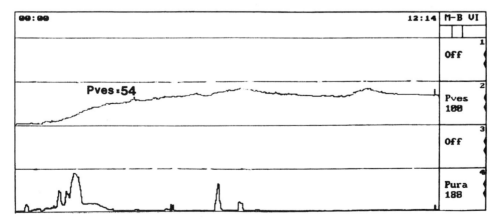

Figure 15-3. A 54-year-old woman after a radical hysterectomy and an indwelling catheter for 14 months. Abnormal compliance was demonstrated by a sustained intravesical pressure of >40 cmH$_2$O. A renal ultrasound revealed bilateral renal pelvis dilatation. Pves, intravesical pressure.

Stress Incontinence and Motor/Sensory Instability

As many as 65% of patients who present with primary, recurrent, or persistent stress incontinence, will have symptoms of both stress and urge incontinence at the time of presentation. Generally, 70% to 80% of such patients will resolve their urge incontinence symptoms after successful correction of the stress incontinence problem.[11,12] These two conditions then commonly occur together, and the putative identification of motor urge incontinence in no way rules out stress incontinence.

Obstructive Uropathy

Hesitancy of urination, incomplete bladder emptying, unusual positions adopted for voiding, and a slow urinary stream after an incontinence procedure are a signs of urethral obstruction and/or poor detrusor function. These symptoms may be present in women with large cystoceles and other genital prolapse, where the obstructive uropathy is relative to the malposition of the bladder and the relative normal position of the urethra. A postvoid urine volume of 20% of the amount voided is considered elevated.[13] If outlet obstruction with resulting voiding dysfunction, including urge incontinence, overflow incontinence, urgency, and frequency is suspected, a vaginal examination may reveal evidence of relative urethral hypersuspension. In cases where true obstruction is present, the urethra can usually be found densely adherent to the posterior surface of the symphysis in a very high retropubic position. However, to prove urodynamically that patients are obstructed is often difficult. There are no normative data for urinary flow rates or pressure flow data for women segregated by age. The classic findings of high detrusor pressure and simultaneous poor urinary flow are not always seen in a study setting.[14] In the urodynamic laboratory, patients may be unable to generate a detrusor contraction and this finding does not by itself imply detrusor dysfunction. Some investigators have reported no difference in outcome in patients who did not exhibit detrusor contractility at the time of the urodynamic study when compared to those in whom a contraction was provoked when a urethral suspension was taken down.[15] This is an important finding because up to 50% of patients may not be able to generate a detrusor contraction during a cystometrogram. It should also be noted that lack of a bladder contraction cannot be used to establish the presence of a poor detrusor preoperatively.[16] The best single evaluation for urethral obstruction or poor detrusor function is probably videourodynamics.[17] In that study, the proximal urethra can be visualized to determine if there is a component of obstruction at that level during a bladder contraction. The fluoroscopic picture generally reveals poor opening of the bladder neck during a sustained detrusor contraction of at least $30\,cmH_2O$ (Figure 15-4). If an areflexic bladder is seen on a cystometrogram, it is difficult to differentiate myogenic, neurologic, or psychogenic etiologies. Neurologic etiologies for detrusor areflexia include cauda equina lesions and peripheral neuropathy. The

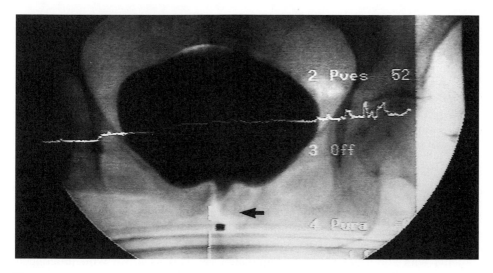

Figure 15-4. A 77-year-old woman with a previous Marshall-Marchetti-Krantz procedure for stress incontinence. A fluoroscopic evaluation showed poor urethral opening distal to the proximal urethra (arrow) during a detrusor contraction of 52 cmH$_2$O. Pves, intravesical pressure; U.S., urethral sphincter.

latter abnormalities can be related to diabetes or previous radical pelvic surgery. During a urodynamic study, patients who cannot relax their external sphincter may have a psychogenic component to their urinary retention. However, a lack of afferent excitation of the cortical and reflex centers involved in bladder contractility may also be the underlying abnormality and a lack of relaxation of the urethral or anal sphincter is not an exclusive indication of psychogenic retention. Finally, patients with a relative urethral hyper-suspension associated with a high residual urine and difficulty voiding in the normal position, particularly if these abnormalities are associated with motor urge incontinence, should be presumed to have urethral obstruction and offered takedown of the urethral suspension as a solution to their problem.

Recurrent Urethral Hypermobility and ISD

Urethral mobility can be grossly assessed by performing a vaginal examination and semiquantified with a "Q-tip" test. The Q-tip test involves placing a cotton swab in the urethra and noting the degree of mobility of the tip of the Q tip during a Valsalva maneuver. A 30-degree rotation is suggestive of gross urethral hypermobility.[18] Obviously, the Q-tip test depends on the character and strength of the Valsalva maneuver thus a perceived lack of mobility cannot by itself be used to establish the presence of some other abnormality like intrinsic sphincter dysfunction. In patients with genital prolapse, it is possible that incontinence may not be demonstrated until the prolapse is reduced.[19] In general, the upright position is ideal to examine patients suspected of recurrent hypermobility or urethral dysfunction characterized by intrinsic sphincter deficiency. The best test of urethral function is abdominal leak point pressure. Maximum urethral closing pressure profile values have been used to determine if an intrinsic sphincter deficiency exists. Maximum urethral closing pressures, however, measure urethral closing forces at the voluntary external sphincter area, an area that does not correlate well with intrinsic sphincter deficiency when the latter is documented by videourodynamics.[20,21] Furthermore, urethral pressure measurements have a very poor correlation with the presence of continence or incontinence. For example, periurethral collagen injections improve continence by increasing urethral coaptation and dramatically increasing abdominal leak point pressures. However, collagen injections do not change urethral pressure profile values even in patients who become "dry" with treatment. An abdominal leak point pressure is performed during a routine cystometrogram. The cystometrogram is used to evaluate bladder compliance. Patients with abnormal bladder compliance, as well as those with unreduced genital prolapse, are unsuitable for leak point pressure testing. If the increase in pressure during filling is largely due to a detrusor component, the urethra looks worse than it actually is. Abnormal compliance results in achievement of an isobaric bladder and proximal urethra at some volume, but the isobaric condition is related not to malfunction of the urethra, but to the increase in bladder pressure, which gradually overwhelms urethral resistance. ISD exists when intravesical and proximal urethral pressures are equal due to a poorly functioning proximal urethra.

To perform a leak point pressure, the patient's bladder is slowly filled to 200 ml. The patient is placed in the upright position and the pressure transducer adjusted for the height of the pubic symphysis. The patient is asked to perform a slow, progressive increase in abdominal pressure until leakage occurs. The point of leakage can be visualized fluoroscopically or visualized by careful inspection of the external urethra meatus. If no leakage occurs with several attempts to do so by straining and pressures in the range of $120-130$ cmH$_2$O are achieved, then coughing must be used to induce leakage. An abdominal leak point pressure of 100 cmH$_2$O water or more is generally associated with urethral hypermobility and thus such patients are suitable candidates for urethral suspension procedures. Intermediate values between 60 and 100 cmH$_2$O of water generally are associated with both urethral hypermobility and some degree of intrinsic sphincter dysfunction. Patient with abdominal leak point pressures <60 have overt intrinsic sphincter dysfunction and such patients are completely unsuitable for standard operative procedures. The reproducibility of abdominal leak point pressure testing is very high when the test is performed in the standardized fashion described.[22] Fluoroscopic evaluation of proximal urethra is also helpful in those patients with severe prolapse (Figure 15-5). Intrinsic sphincter dysfunction is very common in the elderly population, where as many as 50% will have intrinsic sphincter dysfunction, even those who have never had any prior pelvic surgery or radiation.[2]

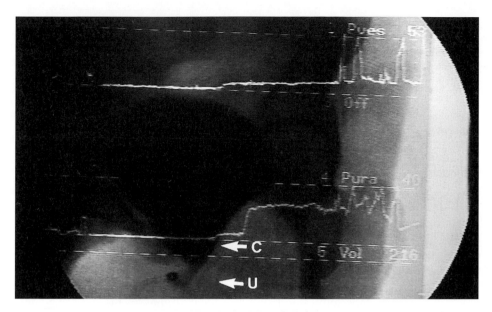

Figure 15-5. A 46-year-old woman with stress incontinence and a cystocele. An oblique fluoroscopic view, during an ALPP assessment, demonstrated posterior rotational descent of the urebra and visible urinary leakage. C, cystocele; U, urethra.

TREATMENT

Unusual Conditions

Fistulae, ectopic ureters, and ureteral diverticula should be repaired in the appropriate manner and these will not be addressed here.

Motor Urge Incontinence

In those patients with motor urge incontinence related to a neurologic impairment or those with detrusor hyperreflexia, pharmacologic therapy will generally be successful. Commonly used agents include imipramine hydrochloride, hyoscyamine sulfate, and oxybutynin chloride. Patients may need to practice timed interval voiding as well. In situations where the cystometrogram detects abnormal compliance, treatment of the detrusor is usually mandatory. Sustained intravesical pressures above $40\,cmH_2O$ are associated with a 100% risk of damage to the upper urinary tract.[23] Moreover, patients with poor compliance generally are incontinent as a result of that problem and the incontinence will not respond until the detrusor abnormality is corrected. Treatment in such instances involves bladder enlargement, either by drugs or surgery.

Urge Incontinence Related to Iatrogenic Conditions

When urge incontinence is related to sutures or other foreign bodies in the bladder, appropriate treatment of these abnormalities should eliminate the irritative focus and eliminate the urge incontinence.

Idiopathic Motor and Sensory Instability

In patients with idiopathic motor or sensory instability, behavioral therapy or bladder retraining in the form of timed voiding can have up to an 80% success rate.[24] These patients have unreliable bladder sensations and they may need to void according to a present interval starting at one hour and then working up gradually to 3-hour intervals. Anticholimergic medications do not by themselves change the patient's ability to sense bladder events, but such medication may delay the bladder contraction. However, unless a conscious cortical effort is made with timed voiding, urge incontinence will continue to occur generally in a random pattern. In Europe, electrical stimulation has been performed for urge incontinence with reportedly good success. Most studies in the United States, however, have been more variable with respect to subjective and objective results.[25,26] In cases where behavioral therapy and medication have not improved urge incontinence, a peripheral bladder denervation (a modified Ingelman-Sundberg procedure) may be tried.[27,28] This minimally invasive procedure has been reported to have a 64% to 72% 1-year cure rate and should be considered before other surgical options such as partial detrusor mymectomy or augmentation cystoplasty are performed.

Urethral Obstruction

Patients with partial or complete urinary retention after a vesical urethral suspension procedure can be managed initially with intermittent self catheterization. Milder degrees of urethral obstruction generally resolve within 3 to 6 months without further surgical therapy. However, if significant obstruction continues, and/or videourodynamic evaluation is suggestive of that problem, transvaginal urethrolysis has been reported to have a 65% to 92% rate with a very rare development of recurrent stress incontinence.[16,29,30] Webster and Kreder[14] described a retropubic urethrolysis procedure that involved complete mobilization of the anterior vaginal wall. They used an omental pedicle placed around the urethra in the retropubic space to prevent further scarring. The success rate with their procedure was reported to be 93%. A suprameatal transvaginal urethrolysis has also been reported which involves dissection anterior to the urethra, but medial to the arcus tendineous fasciae pelvis. This allows the urethra to be freed from the symphysis pubis. Early reports claimed excellent results.[31] Cutting urethral suspension sutures alone is beneficial only if done before permanent fibrosis has occurred. This is rarely the case, since generally several weeks are allowed to elapse before patients are considered for take down of the urethral suspension.

Recurrent Urethral Dysfunction

Urethral causes of incontinence after urethral suspension may be related to anatomical hypermobility, intrinsic sphincter deficiency or both. If the leak point pressure is greater than 100 cmH$_2$O the patient may benefit from a repeat bladder suspension procedure. However, patients who have failed previously performed needle or retropubic suspension procedures should probably be considered for slings. Moreoever, the incidence of intrinsic sphincter deficiency is 27% after one failed procedure and 75% after two or more failed procedures and, in these cases, it is prudent to use slings.[2] Pubovaginal slings designed to increase proximal urethra coaptation when that area no longer functions as a sphincter also are very effective in the prevention of urethral hypermobility. In cases where hypermobility and ISD occur together, for example, those patients without prolapse who leak at abdominal pressures of 60–100 cmH$_2$O, a sling is probably the best overall procedure. The McGuire modification of the pubovaginal fascia sling was first employed in patients with documented pure ISD. It has since been applied to patients with combined ISD and hypermobility as well as those with hypermobility only.

Other workers have used nonautologous material such as Marlex or Gore-Tex for slings and these have been associated with good results, but up to a 20% incidence of erosion and fistula formation has been reported.[32] Because autologous fascia is never associated with erosion or fistula formation, currently, the most popular sling material is rectus abdominis or fascia lata. McGuire and Blavias,[33,34] in independent series, reported 82% to 91% long-term cure rates with this procedure. The most common complications of sling procedures are urinary retention and bladder instability which seem to be associated with placing too much tension on the sling at the time of surgery. When looser slings are employed, the incidence of permanent retention is less than 3% in neurologically intact women. Transient urinary symptoms still will occur in up to 14% of such patients, but these numbers are not significantly different from the same symptoms occurring after needle suspension or retropubic suspension.[15,34,35] More recently, slings have been developed using vaginal mucosa as a source of the sling material. Raz and colleagues[36] described use of an island of anterior vaginal wall which creates a sling underlying the bladder neck and urethra. The technique is a modification of the Pereyra suspension. The procedure involves permanent sutures placed at the bladder neck incorporating the underlying fascia and the vaginal mucosa is used as a sling. Two additional sutures are placed distally at the other two corners of the mucosal flap. Ligature carriers are passed through the retropubic space to pick up the sutures and allow the sutures to be tied over the rectus fascia. Using this procedure, the *de novo* detrusor instability rate was reported to be 15%, the long-term intermittent self-catheterization rate was reported at 5.5%, and the cure rate was reported to be 95% with respect to stress incontinence. Other workers using the same or similar technique have reported a 67% and 68% cure rate long term.[37,38] This procedure may have less morbidity than a pubovaginal sling, but that remains to be determined. Patients with a foreshortened vagina from previous surgery may not be good candidates and patients with poorly estrogenized vaginal tissue may not have sufficient tissue strength to permit use of that material as a sling.

An additional method designed to treat intrinsic sphincter dysfunction and combined urethral hypermobility employs a Stamey bolster type procedure in conjunction with insertion of a Martius fat pad.[39] An inverted U-shaped incision is made in the anterior vaginal wall and a vaginal flap is created at the proximal urethra and bladder base, a paravaginal tunnel is then developed under the labia minora. A pedical fat graft is brought into the vaginal wound and laid outside the silastic bolsters used for the Stamey ligature suspension. The Stamey procedure is then completed as originally described. The symptomatic success rate was 91% over a 13-month period of follow-up.[39]

Shull[40] and Richardson[41] have each described paravaginal repair techniques designed to correct cystourethroceles resulting from lateral vaginal wall suspension defects not repaired by standard retropubic suspension procedures. Their patient populations included 12% to 23% with persistent or recurrent incontinence after a prior procedure. Both workers reported a 90% success rate in the cure of stress incontinence, but they did not distinguish primary repair patients from secondary repair patients.[40,41] In summary, the pubovaginal sling procedure probably remains the procedure of choice in patients with intrinsic sphincter deficiency or recurrent or persistent incontinence following previous operative procedures. Newer procedures will need long-term follow-up to assess durability.

Other Urethral Procedures

Patients with ISD and minimal hypermobility may be candidates for periurethral injection of glutaraldehyde crosslinked bovine collagen. This product is easy to inject due to relatively low viscosity and there is no particle migration. It is relatively stable to degradation by collagenases as a result of its glutaraldehyde crosslinking. Collagen appears to work by inducing urethral coaptation that measurably improves the efficiency with which the urethra resists abdominal pressure. Voiding pressures and urethral pressure profile values are not changed by the agent, even in those patients cured of their incontinence.[43] Use of collagen requires skin testing to determine antigenicity, but after a negative skin test the material is injected transurethrally into a submucosal plane at the 4 and 8 o'clock positions proximal to the external sphincter just distal to the bladder neck. One study reported at 16 months after the last injection, 68% of patients were cured and 20% improved. In the latter group, pad usage decreased from an average of five to 10 per day to one to two pads per day. The mean number of treatments was 1½ with a mean total of 9.1 ml of collagen used. Late outcome data suggest that 20% of patients who are dry or improved may need a booster injection at 6–18 months after their initial treatments because of decreased efficacy.[44] The degree of worsening recorded by these patients was subjective and was relatively minimal. Collagen did not induce permanent urinary retention and no allergic reactions to the material were encountered. Cost is less than that related to sling procedures as collagen injections are performed under local anesthesia in an out-patient setting.[44]

This procedure then is an excellent choice for patients with minimal mobility and ISD, conditions frequently encountered in the elderly who are not candidates for more extensive operative procedures.

Finally, a last-resort surgical procedure that is certainly applicable to the management of recurrent incontinence is the artificial urinary sphincter (AUS). This prosthesis may be implanted transvaginally or abdominally. The sphincter cuff is placed at the bladder neck. That placement is technically difficult, particularly after multiple procedures for incontinence. Sphincters are left in the deactivated state for 6 weeks to allow tissue healing. Early reports of a 30% urethral erosion rate appear to be related to patient selection, lack of delayed activation, and infection.[45] While current results are much better, there remains a potential for mechanical failure and for erosion after implantation of these devices. However, most reports note a 68% to 80% cure rate of incontinence.[46,47] Webster noted that 92% of his 25 patients were satisfied after a mean period of follow up of 2.6 years.[48] At the present time, artificial sphincters are considered the last resort option in the neurologically intact female.

CONCLUSION

Persistent or recurrent incontinence after a stress incontinence procedure can be very discouraging for the surgeon and frustrating for the patient. In the majority of the cases, recurrent urethral hypermobility is the reason for the incontinence, but urodynamics are usually required to precisely determine the etiology. If a patient has recurrent hypermobility and a high aLPP, they may qualify for a repeat retropubic suspension or bladder neck suspension. Nevertheless, one should consider these questions: Why did urethral hypermobility recur and does the patient continue to have those same risk factors? Does the tissue have poor vascularity and a collagen composition that may affect the long-term success? Was the repair subjected to chronic stresses such as recurrent vaginal prolapse, physical activity or a pulmonary condition? The autologous graft pubovaginal sling is the procedure of choice in patients with evidence of ISD and urethral hypermobility or patients that have recurrent urethral hypermobility and it is suspected that the same operation or a similar one will fail again. Patients with ISD without urethral hypermobility can be treated with a pubovaginal sling or collagen injections. The AUS is only rarely the preferable method in the neurologically intact woman.

In most cases urge incontinence can be treated conservatively with behavioral therapy and medication, reserving surgery for the most refractory of cases. Often the symptoms are transient, but an intrinsic etiology should always first be ruled out. Even though urethral obstruction with or without detrusor decompensation is difficult to precisely diagnosis preoperatively, the clinical scenario should aid one in deciding if a urethrolysis will regain normal voiding.

It is most important for the physician to obtain a precise diagnosis for the persistent or recurrent incontinence before any further procedure or treatment is offered. The history and physical examination should guide the examiner as to which specific diagnostic tests are necessary to accomplish this task.

REFERENCES

1. Schaeffer AJ. Treatment of recurrent urinary incontinence. *Clin Obstet Gynecol* 1984; **27**: 459.
2. McGuire EJ. Urodynamic findings in patients after failure of stress incontinence operations in female incontinence, In: *Female Incontinence*. New York: Wiley-Liss. 1981: 351–360.
3. Steel SA, Cox C, Stanton SL. Long term followup of detrusor instability following the colposuspension operation. *Br J Urol* 1986; **58**: 138.
4. Cardozo LD, Stanton SL, Williams JE. Detrusor instability following surgery for genuine stress incontinence. *Br J Urol* 1979; **51**: 204.
5. Juma S, Sdrales L. Etiology of urinary retention after bladder neck suspension. *J Urol* 1993; **149(Part 2)**: 401A.
6. Norton P. Pelvic floor disorders: The role of fascia and ligaments. *Clin Obstet Gynecol* 1996; **36**: 926.
7. Scotti RL, Bergman A, Bhatia NN, et al. Urodynamic changes in urethrovesical function after radical hysterectomy. *Obstet Gynecol* 1986; **68**: 11.
8. Glassberg RL, Braven V, Duckett JW, et al. Suggested terminology for duplex systems, ectopic ureters and ureterocele. *J Urol* 1984; **132**: 1153.
9. Bass JS, Leach GE. Surgical treatment of concomitant urethral diverticulum and stress incontinence. *Urol Clin North Am* 1991; **18**: 365.
10. McGuire EJ. Idiopathic bladder instability, In: ED Kursh and EJ McGuire (eds.), *Female Urology*. Philadelphia: JB Lippincott; 1994: 95–102.
11. McGuire EJ, Savastano JA. Stress incontinence and detrusor instability/urge incontinence. *Neurol Urodyn* 1985; **4**: 313.
12. Ghoriem GM, Gamasy AN. Outcome of the treatment of mixed incontinence with modified pubovaginal sling. *J Urol* 1996; **55**: 577A.
13. Starrey TA. Stress urinary incontinence. In: Harrison, JM, Glitter RF, and Dettritter AP (eds). *Campbell's Urology*. Philadelphia: WB Saunders, 1979: 2272–2280.
14. Webster GD, Kreder KJ. Voiding dysfunction following cystourethropexy: Its evaluation and management. *J Urol* 1990; **144**: 670.
15. McGuire EJ, Letson W, Wang S. Transvaginal urethrolysis after obstructive urethral suspension procedures. *J Urol* 1987; **142**: 1037.
16. Foster ME, McGuire EJ. Management of urethral obstruction with transurethral urethrolysis. *J Urol* 1993; **150**: 1448.
17. Blaivas JG. Multichannel urodynamic studies. *Urology* 1984; **23**: 421.
18. Karram MM, Bhatia NN. The Q tip test standardization of the technique and its interpretation in women with urinary incontinence. *Obstet Gynecol* 1988; **71**: 807.
19. Rosenzweig BA, Pushkin S, Blumenfeld D, Bhatia NN. Abnormal urodynamic test

results in continent women with severe genitourinary prolapse. *Obstet Gynecol* 1992; **79**: 539.

20. McGuire EJ. Combined radiographic and manometric assessment of urethral sphincter function. *J Urol* 1977; **118**: 632.
21. McGuire EJ, Fitzpatrick CC, Wan J, et al. Clinical assessment of urethral sphincter function. *J Urol* 1993; **150**: 1452.
22. Song JT, Campo R, Chai TC, et al. Observer variability and stress leak point pressure measurement using flurourodynamics. *J Urol* 1995; **153**: 492A.
23. McGuire EJ. Interaction of bladder filling behavior and urethral function. *World J Urol* 1990; **8**: 194.
24. Fantl JA, Hurt WG, Dunn LJ. Detrusor instability syndrome. The use of bladder retraining drills with and without anticholinergics. *Am J Obstet Gynecol* 1981; **140**: 885.
25. Caputo RM, Benson JT, McClellan E. Intravaginal maximum electrical stimulation treatment of urinary incontinence. *J Reprod Med* 1993; **35**: 667.
26. Stein M, Discippio W, Davia M, Taub H. Biofeedback for the treatment of stress and urege incontinence. *J Urol* 1995; **153**: 641.
27. Cespedes RD, Cross CA, McGuire EJ. Modified Ingelman-Sundberg bladder denervation procedure for refractory urge incontinence. *J Urol* 1996; **156**: 1744–1748.
28. Wan J, McGuire EJ, Wang SE, et al. Ingelman-Sundberg bladder denervation for detrusor instability. *J Urol* 1991; **145**: 358A.
29. Nitti V, Raz S. Obstruction following anti-incontinence procedures: Diagnosis and treatment with transvaginal urethrolysis. *J Urol* 1994; **152**: 93.
30. Zimmern PE, Hadley HR, Leach GE, Raz S. Female urethrol obstruction after Marshall-Marchetti-Krantz operation. *J Urol* 1987; **138**: 517.
31. Petrou SP, Brown JA, Blaivas JG. Suprameatal transvaginal urethrolysis: A simple, efficacious technique for treating bladder outlet obstruction after anti-incontinence procedures. *J Urol* 1996; **155**: 589A.
32. Blaivas JG. Pubovaginal slings. *AUA Update Ser* 1992; **11**: 282.
33. McGuire EJ, Bennett CJ, Konnak JA, Sonda P, Savastano JA. Experience with pubovaginal slings for urinary incontinence at the University of Michigan. *J Urol* 1987; **138**: 525.
34. Blaivas JG Jacobs BZ. Pubovaginal fascial sling for the treatment of complicated stress urinary incontinence. *J Urol* 1991; **145**: 1214.
35. Mason C, Roach M. Modified pubovaginal sling for treatment of type III stress urinary incontinence. A review of 78 cases. *J Urol* 1996; **155**: 700A.
36. Juma S, Little N, Raz S. Vaginal wall sling: Four years later. *Urology* 1992; **39**: 424.
37. Litwiller SE, Nelson RT, Fore PD, Sone AR. Vaginal wall sling: Long term outcome analysis of factors contributing to patient satisfaction and surgical success. *J Urol* 1996; **155**: 538A.
38. Pidutti RW, George SW, Morales A. Correction of recurrent stress urinary incontinence by needle urethropexy with a vaginal sling. *Br J Urol* 1994; **73**: 418.
39. Ganabathi K, Abrams P, Mundy AR, et al. Stamey-Martius procedure for severe genuine stress incontinence. *Br J Urol* 1992; **69**: 34.
40. Shull B, Baden W. A six year experience with paravaginal defect repair for stress urinary incontinence. *Am J Obstet Gynecol* 1990; **160**: 1432.
41. Richardson A, Edmonds P, Williams N. Treatment of stress urinary incontinence due to paravaginal fascial defect. *Obstet Gynecol* 1981; **57**: 357.
42. Appell RA. Collagen injection therapy for urinary incontinence. *Urol Clin North Am* 1994; **21**: 177.
43. Hershchorn S, Radomski SB, Steele DJ. Early experience with intraurethral collagen injections for urinary incontinence. *J Urol* 1992; **148**: 1797.
44. Cross CA, Cespedes RD, O'Connell HE, McGuire EJ. Long term follow up of transurethral collagen injection therapy for urinary incontinence in women. *J Urol* 1996; **155**: 537A.

45. Light JK, Scott FB. Management of urinary incontinence in women with the artificial urinary sphincter. *J Urol* 1985; **134**: 476.
46. Donovan MG, Barrett DM, Furlow WL. Use of the artificial urinary sphincter in the management of severe incontinence in females. *Surg Gynecol Obstet* 1985; **161**: 17.
47. Scott FB. The use of the artificial sphincter in the treatment of urinary incontinence in the female patient. *Urol Clin North Am* 1985; **12**: 305.
48. Webster GD, Perez LM, Khoury JM, Timmons SL. Management of type III stress urinary incontinence using artificial urinary sphincter. *Urology* 1992; **39**: 499.

PART V

FREQUENCY, URGENCY, AND URGE INCONTINENCE

CHAPTER 16

Urinary frequency and urgency

TAMARA G. BAVENDAM

Millions of women present to health care providers each year with symptoms of irritation and/or discomfort associated with lower urinary function.[1] The etiology of these symptoms ranges from acute bacterial cystitis to spasm and dysfunction of the pelvic floor muscles. Sensations arising from pelvic organs and the supporting musculoskeletal system are poorly localized and travel via common pathways to the central nervous system. Consequently, afferent nerve impulses originating in any of the pelvic organs, the bony pelvis with its supporting muscle and fascial attachments or the peripheral nerves themselves can generate impulses that can be perceived as originating in the bladder and/or urethra and are often misdiagnosed as urinary tract infections.

In this chapter, the lower urinary tract (LUT) is defined as the bladder and the bladder outlet, which includes the pelvic floor support. Symptoms of urinary frequency, urgency, and discomfort before, during, or after the act of urination are commonly perceived by patients and health care providers as being generated by the bladder and/or the urethra. The most common cause is assumed to be bacteria requiring antibiotics for symptom improvement. While bacterial bladder infections can cause all of these symptoms, so can many other conditions.

The phrase "lower urinary tract hypersensitivity" (LUTH) is used as the global category for this spectrum of symptoms and allows the transition from assuming symptoms are related to specific diseases to thinking about symptoms as a result of abnormalities of function of the LUT. Viewing symptoms associated with LUT as dysfunctions rather than necessarily caused by a specific disease liberates the provider from establishing a specific diagnosis and "cure" for each and every symptom. After obvious treatable causes are eliminated (bacterial cystitis, pelvic mass, vaginitis, perianal pathology), the patient and provider are able to utilize a problem-solving approach to symptom management. Once patients are appropriately reassured that there is nothing seriously wrong, for example, cancer, their main goal is to feel better irrespective of the source of their symptoms. The severe end of the spectrum of irritable bladder symptoms is a clinical syndrome commonly referred to as "interstitial cystitis," which is also discussed in this chapter.

This chapter will provide a broader perspective for thinking about frequency and urgency of urination with a common sense strategy for the evaluation and treatment of these symptoms. The evaluation and management strategy presented here should be useful for all providers caring for women with symptoms perceived as arising from the pelvis. The goal is for all providers to be comfortable taking a quick, but thorough history in women who present with symptoms of bladder irritation. Based on this target history, appropriate tests and examination will be performed. Women who do not have evidence of a bacterial cystitis will be confidently treated with behavior recommendations rather than the reflex decision of antibiotics for infection. The current pattern of over-diagnosis of "cystitis" and inappropriate treatment with antibiotics and unnecessary dependence on the health care profession for treatment of symptoms can be avoided.

LOWER URINARY TRACT FUNCTION

The female lower urinary tract consists of the bladder detrusor muscle and mucosa, the bladder-outlet (bladder-neck muscle, urethral smooth and striated muscle, urethral mucosa and submucosa), the myofasical elements of the pelvic floor support as well as an intact nerve and vascular supply. There are three phases of LUT functioning: storage, emptying, and the transition phase between storage and emptying. The goals of LUT function are to provide low-pressure storage of urine in the bladder without involuntary loss of urine (incontinence) as well as rapid, complete low-pressure evacuation of urine from the bladder. Normal functioning of the LUT represents a delicate balance between the bladder and outlet, as well as the facilitory and inhibitory control mechanisms through the autonomic and somatic nerve supply. While the neurologic control of the LUT is incompletely understood, it is generally agreed upon that sympathetic innervation is responsible for urine storage and parasympathetic for evacuation of urine. Somatic innervation, which travels through the pudendal nerve to the pelvic floor muscles and the periurethral striated muscle, is important in all phases of LUT function. The pudendal nerve also provides sensory innervation to the clitoris and perineum.

Sympathetic innervation originates in the thoracolumbar area of the spinal cord and travels in the hypogastric nerve. Sympathetic innervation promotes urine storage by promoting bladder neck closure and inhibiting active detrusor contraction. Parasympathetic innervation, which originates in sacral cord segments 2 through 4 and is carried in the pelvic nerve, is responsible for bladder contraction and emptying. The pudendal nerves provide innervation for the periurethral striated muscle and the entire pelvic floor muscle group. The pudendal nerve also originates in the sacral cord (S1 to S2). Extensive pelvic surgery can damage both the pelvic and pudendal nerves resulting in detrusor, urethral, and skeletal muscle dysfunction.

The bladder acts as a passive storage reservoir during filling and actively contracts during urination. During storage, the bladder outlet must maintain a pressure that exceeds bladder pressure. The role of the bladder neck smooth muscle is to maintain a constant tone or pressure during bladder filling (storage phase). With bladder muscle contraction during the emptying phase, the bladder neck muscle relaxes, which decreases the outlet resistance and promotes emptying.

The urethra itself has important functions in maintaining continence (intrinsic urethral factors). The urethral mucosa normally has abundant folds, which provide complete apposition or a mucosal seal. This is supplemented by the rich vascular supply of the submucosa. Normal estrogen levels are important to maintain the folds of the mucosa and the rich vascular network. In addition, there are smooth and skeletal muscle fibers in the wall of the urethra.

The skeletal muscle of the external sphincter mechanism is made up of the periurethral and urethral muscular systems. The urethral striated muscles are circularly arranged fibers that maintain a state of constant tone. The periurethral muscle provides urethral closure through its resting tone and reflex active contraction, which results in increased urethral closure during increases in intra-abdominal pressure. The periurethral skeletal muscle is an extension of the levator musculature. The entire pelvic floor muscle group supports the bladder and proximal urethra and augments the external sphincter mechanism. Voluntary contraction of the pelvic floor muscles can be an important adjunct to the reflex (involuntary) contraction that occurs at times of increased intraabdominal pressure (cough, sneeze, lift). Pelvic muscle contraction is also important in delaying the onset of urination or urinary incontinence. During a strong urge to urinate any increase in the detrusor pressure can be inhibited by voluntary contraction of the pelvic muscles.

All of the anatomic and neurologic forces which promote continence during the storage phase must be reversed to empty. The coordination between the bladder and outlet mechanisms in the transition phase between storage and emptying is poorly understood and difficult to evaluate in humans because of the significant voluntary (inhibitory and facilitory) influences involved in LUT function. Recognizing the delicate balance between bladder storage and emptying is crucial to understanding the symptoms associated with LUTH and how seemingly innocuous occurrences unrelated to the urinary tract can contribute to its dysfunction.

Normal bladder capacity is considered to be in the range of 400 to 600 ml. Normally, an initial sense of bladder awareness would occur around 150 to 300 ml, with gradually increasing awareness of fullness/urge with progressive filling. In general, the urge to urinate can be postponed indefinitely and the bladder should never empty without permission. Urge is delayed through central and peripheral mechanisms. Central mechanisms diminish awareness of bladder sensations while peripheral involuntary and voluntary contraction of pelvic muscles increase "outlet pressure" opposing any small increases in bladder pressure that occur during filling. Pelvic muscle contraction also reflexively inhibits parasympathetic activity necessary for bladder contraction.

Once the appropriate destination for bladder emptying is reached, the outlet must relax and stay relaxed while the detrusor is generating and maintaining a contraction. When the volume in the bladder is <200 to 300 ml, the bladder may have difficulty generating and sustaining a contraction. Without a detrusor contraction, the outlet has difficulty maintaining relaxation. When there is a source of irritation in or around the LUT, the urge to urinate may occur at very low volumes (30–100 ml). At this low volume, coordinated detrusor contraction/outlet relaxation may not occur and urination may be hesitant; slow, or interrupted with a sense of incomplete emptying. This can become exacerbated when the sense of urge is intense or painful at low volumes. The intensity of the urge will elicit increased pelvic muscle activity to prevent incontinence which further exacerbates the difficulty of initiating and sustaining coordinated urination with a low bladder volume. Typically, the inability to void despite a strong painful urge leads to straining to initiate urine flow. Unfortunately, using the Valsalva maneuver to assist with voiding is only effective when outlet relaxation is maintained. Chronic straining against "contracted" pelvic muscles can further contribute to the voiding dysfunction. In summary, increased bladder sensitivity can become quickly associated with a voiding dysfunction. Irrespective of what may have caused the irritation initially, the resulting voiding dysfunction can be responsible for chronically maintaining the symptoms.

In general, most women with LUTH note increased frequency of urination compared to their previous habits. While urinating every 3 hours is not excessive, for someone who used to urinate every 4 to 6 hours it may be very bothersome. The key is to determine what bladder volumes signal the urge to urinate and what happens if the signals are ignored. A voiding diary of time and volume of urination over several days and nights in invaluable. A bladder that can hold 600 ml at night but only holds 100 to 300 ml during the day suggests "hypersensitivity" of LUT. Likewise, a woman who gets out of bed to urinate several times with very small volumes after initially lying down but is able to hold her urine all night once she falls asleep is different from someone who gets up every 2 hours to urinate 100 ml.

The reasons women choose not to ignore the signals of urgency are important to understanding the etiology of the problem. There is the fear of being incontinent; putting off the urge may be associated with severe pain, aching, or cramping and most commonly the urge sensation is "annoying" enough to impair concentration on current vocational or recreational tasks (but the urge can be ignored without fear of leakage or pain). Women may also void frequently because they have been told never to "hold" their urine after an urge is felt because "holding" can cause bladder infections. This behavior change can lead to voiding in progressively smaller volumes out of habit.

When fear of urinary incontinence is a woman's main reason for frequent voiding, underlying involuntary detrusor activity is probable. Young women with normal anatomic support may feel a pain/discomfort sensation during an *involuntary detrusor contraction* (with actual bladder-neck opening observed on video urodynamic evaluation) yet never experience incontinence. This is possible because voluntary contraction of the pelvic floor muscles is stronger than the detrusor contraction and therefore able to prevent leakage. Severe pain with holding is suggestive of the syndrome currently identified as *interstitial cystitis* (IC) as the underlying problem. The "annoying" urgency is most suggestive of a *hypersensitivity* phenomenon.[2]

Pain reported during the act of urination is most consistent with acute bacterial cystitis or urethritis and the urinalysis should demonstrate pyuria. When urine shows no evidence of infection, additional considerations should be vulvo-vaginal inflammation, urethral diverticulum or nonrelaxation of the outlet muscles (bladder-neck and urethral smooth muscle, and urethral and pelvic floor striated muscle). Pain after urination strongly suggests a muscular etiology: the outlet muscles are relaxed during urination (no pain). After urination is complete, total relaxation stops as the muscles return to their baseline, which is an increase in muscle activity and this increased muscle activity can be perceived as increased pain.

Clinical experience suggests multiple internal and external factors can enhance LUT sensitivity and contribute to pain and voiding dysfunction. Due to the poorly localized afferent input from visceral organs, the interplay between the autonomic and somatic nerve supply, and the sociocultural influences on facilitating and inhibiting bladder function, our ability to isolate and evaluate this phase of LUT function with respect to these factors is hampered. Dehydration and fluid restriction result in concentrated urine which many women report increase their symptoms. Certain dietary factors also increase bladder sensitivity. High acid foods and beverages (coffee—even decaffeinated, tea, citrus, cranberry, tomato, chocolate), spicy foods and carbonated beverages are reported by patients to exacerbate bladder symptoms. In many women, symptoms are exacerbated between ovulation and menses. Sexual intercourse is a potent trigger for some women in the absence of evidence of bacterial cystitis. Symptoms may start with the onset of sexual intercourse, with a new partner, a new form of birth control, or after a period of abstinence. Stress and anxiety are also commonly reported to exacerbate symptoms. While it is not always possible to understand or explain why apparent "triggers" should influence LUT symptoms and function, it doesn't mean these "triggers" are not real. Recognition of "triggers" provides a means of helping the patient manipulate internal and external factors to minimize or prevent symptom flares.

CAUSES OF URINARY FREQUENCY AND URGENCY

Acute Bacterial Cystitis

Bacterial cystitis is a common cause of altered voiding and pain associated with the LUT. The pain is typically described as occurring *with* the act of passing urine and is usually associated with frequency and urgency of urination. Gross hematuria may or may not be present. The presentation is usually acute and symptoms usually resolve promptly with hydration and/or appropriate antibiotics. A simple bacterial bladder infection can generally be treated with a single dose or short course of antibiotics—3 to 5 days rather than 7 to 10 days, which has been classically recommended.[3] Short courses of antibiotics decrease the chances of bowel dysfunction and vaginitis associated with longer courses.

A urine culture may not be cost-effective in the face of classic symptoms, but a urinalysis demonstrating pyuria should be the minimum documentation of bacterial cystitis, particularly in women who are seen with recurrent symptoms or symptoms that do not resolve with antibiotic therapy. The classic definition of bacterial cystitis is greater than 100,000 colony-forming units (cfu) of a single organism. Multiple organisms are suggestive of a contaminated specimen and should not be diagnosed as an infection under most circumstances. Colony counts of <100,000 cfu can represent an acute bacterial infection, but only when accompanied by pyuria.[4,5]

Health-care providers should be careful not to make a diagnosis of bladder infection based on symptoms alone. This can lead to much confusion when the culture returns negative or symptoms do not resolve with antibiotics. Using non-specific terminology, such as "symptomatic episode" or "bladder inflammation," when the woman presents with symptoms helps to minimize this confusion. As soon as the word "cystitis" is used, there is an expectation that antibiotics are necessary. Antibiotics commonly improve symptoms even with a negative urinalysis and culture. One explanation for this occurrence is that all bottles of antibiotics instruct the patient to drink "plenty of water". Once antibiotics are completed, fluid intake returns to normal which often includes negligible amounts of noncarbonated water and symptoms may return because of the hypersensitivity phenomenon discussed below.

Lower Urinary Tract Hypersensitivity

"Lower urinary tract hypersensitivity" is used to replace terminology such as urethral syndrome, chronic trigonitis, chronic urethritis, and chronic nonbacterial cystitis.[2] It simply refers to hyperactivity of the afferent sensory nerves of the bladder which can contribute to the cascade of events leading to uncoordinated low volume urination, voiding dysfunction, and eventually to pain before, during, or after urination. Usually, the pain is worse before or after urination, and women will often report that the pain feels different than when they have had a "bacterial cystitis" in the past. Explaining these symptoms as similar to a sensitive stomach or a sore joint, such as tennis elbow, often helps the patient understand that these symptoms do not have to be from an infection. Identifying and eliminating symptom triggers, increasing water intake, eliminating dietary irritants, and learning pelvic muscle relaxation can alleviate symptoms and minimize the number of symptomatic flares. For example, a woman may be able to drink 4 cups of coffee, drink wine, and have a chocolate dessert without triggering symptoms except premenstrually, or on a day when she performs strenuous exercise. Exercise without increased water intake results in

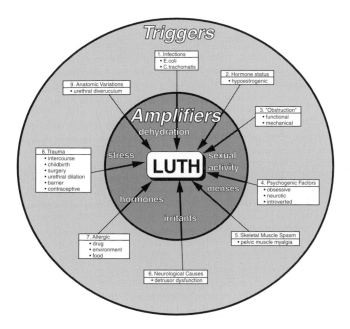

Figure 16-1. Factors triggering lower urinary tract hypersensitivity with potential symptom amplifiers.

dehydration and concentrated urine. For many women, it takes more than one etiologic factor to produce symptoms—a "multiple hit" theory. See Figure 16-1.

Vaginitis

Urinary tract pain in women with vulvovaginal inflammation generally occurs during the act of urination, but typically is felt as the urine contacts the external tissues rather than while passing through the urethra. A history should be specific enough to determine exactly when and where the discomfort urination occurs. Women with vaginitis may not report frequency of urination because woman tend to avoid urinating in order to prevent pain.

Estrogen Deprivation

Atrophic vaginitis/urethritis is another possible cause of LUTH, as it is already known that in postmenopausal women, estrogen deficiency can cause irritative voiding symptoms.[6] It is believed that estrogen has a protective property on the vaginal mucosa, and one study determined that women with documented UTIs had a lower estrogen/progesterone ratio while infected versus noninfected controls.[7] The same research in women with LUTH is not available, but one author points to the possibility of an estrogen–collagen–obstruction relationship in women with urethral syndrome.[8] Other sources note a connection between menses and LUT symptom exacerbation.[9,10]

Allergic Response

Allergies can cause irritation of the mucosa and smooth muscle of the lower urinary tract, just as it does in the upper respiratory tract. A minimal allergic reaction may only cause mild LUT discomfort, whereas a severe reaction may cause sudden, severe bladder pain with increased frequency, urgency, burning and dysuria. In fact, one study reported that over an 11-year period, 900 patients in a urology clinic were found to be "allergic", and 75% those who were initially refractory to treatment had improvement with dietary restrictions (no food or drug allergens) and antihistamine therapy.[11]

Sexually Transmitted Diseases

Chlamydia urethritis should be considered when there is an acutely swollen and tender urethra, urethral discharge, or pyuria, especially in the face of a new sexual partner or recurrent symptoms. Sexual partners must be treated simultaneously. Diagnoses of human papilloma virus (HPV) and herpes simplex should be sought when there are unexplained lesions in the vulvovaginal area. These patients usually present with pain when the urine comes into contact with the affected tissues not as it passes through the urethra.

Chemical Irritation

Cyclophosphamide can be associated with acute lower urinary tract inflammation and hematuria, and chronic voiding disturbances can persist long after the chemotherapy has been completed.[12] While chronic problems are not well-documented, clinical experience identifies problems in women who have been treated with intravenous and oral cyclophosphamide for various periods of time. There are also reports of a small incidence of transitional cell cancers of the bladder following cyclophosphamide treatment.[13] Oxynol-9, found in most contraceptive preparations, can cause local irritation in sensitive women, as well.

Urethral Diverticulum

While fairly uncommon, a diverticulum of the urethra should be considered in women with recurrent lower urinary infections, pain during urination, painful coitus and postvoid dribbling.[14] This constellation of symptoms may not be present in all women with diverticula. On physical examination, there is usually a sense of fullness to palpation of the anterior vaginal wall, suburethral fullness, tenderness and obliteration of the periurethral "gutter". "Milking" of the urethra may produce purulent secretions. The diagnosis can usually be confirmed on voiding cystourethrogram or cystourethroscopy. Occasionally, a urethrogram performed with a special double balloon catheter (an occluding balloon at the bladder neck and urethral meatus allowing contrast to be forcibly injected into the urethra) may be necessary to demonstrate the diverticulum. This test can be very uncomfortable for the patient and is recommended only in hard-to-diagnose cases when suspicion cannot be confirmed on other tests.

Gynecologic Disorders

Endometriosis,[15] pelvic inflammatory disease (PID),[16] pelvic congestion,[17] and vulvar vestibulitis[18] are disorders (usually treated by gynecologists) that can present with symptoms primarily localized to the LUT. Symptoms that are primarily related to menses even if perceived as arising mainly in the urinary tract, should involve gynecologic evaluation with a urological consultation. The common pathway for symptom generation may be through the pelvic muscles, which may be in spasm secondary to an acute inflammatory process or dyspareunia.

Bowel Disorders

Women with symptoms of lower urinary tract pain commonly report disturbances in bowel function. Irritable bowel syndrome is a diagnosis many of these women have when they present with LUT symptoms.[19] Many women report long-standing problems with constipation, which may be an indicator of incomplete or imperfect neurologic structures, which can affect both bowel and bladder function. The act of defecation triggers the symptom complex in some patients. Many treatments for LUTH can increase the possibility of constipation. Therefore, it is essential that nay preexisting bowel dysfunctions are identified and managed aggressively before instituting anticholinergic, antispasmodic, or antidepressant medication. Passing hard stools is associated with the development of hemorrhoids and perianal fissures, which can be quite painful, acting as a source of pelvic floor spasm.

Local Trauma

Local trauma to the lower urinary tract can be caused by sexual activity especially when aggressive, prolonged, or without adequate lubrication. Certain positions may be more or less uncomfortable for some women. It is not unusual to have women report partner-specific factors such as size of phallus, duration of intercourse, or variety of positions associated with their pain. Pain that begins hours to days after intercourse is highly suggestive of myofascial pain. Vaginal deliveries can damage the myofascial support structures and stretch the pudendal nerve, which can contribute to pain symptoms as well as loss of bladder control that we more commonly associate with the childbirth experience. Direct pressure on the bladder/urethra by the contraceptive diaphragm or cervical cap have been reported by patients to be temporally related to the onset of LUT pain. Changing to a smaller size diaphragm may relieve the symptoms, and is recommended particularly in women who are not candidates for other forms of birth control.

Women report onset of symptoms after abdominal or vaginal hysterectomies, bladder neck suspensions, cystocele repairs, as well as posterior repairs and colorectal and perianal procedures. The mechanism for this pain is not well understood, but likely represents some form of disruption to the intact peripheral nerve supply. Urethral dilation(s) represent another form of trauma to the LUT. Urethral dilations have been the standard of practice for many years for the treatment of recurrent urinary tract infections, symptoms of obstructive voiding, frequency and urgency of urination, and urinary incontinence. While there have been no good studies looking at efficacy and potential harm of this form of "treatment", it is commonly accepted by urologists and gynecologists who specialize in disorders of the LUT in women, that the potential physical and emotional harm far exceeds any potential benefit. Many women do report temporary symptomatic relief following the dilation, but they also report significant pain during the dilation. As one of the goals of treating a chronic pain syndrome is putting the patient in charge of pain control and breaking the pain cycle, it makes no sense to rely on a treatment method where the patient is a passive recipient of a painful procedure they have no control over.

Interstitial Cystitis

Women with interstitial cystitis (IC) typically report frequency and urgency of urination (urinating up to every 15 minutes during the daytime and nighttime) as well as suprapubic, perineal, vulvar, or vaginal discomfort before, during, or after urination. Pain during or after sexual intercourse is also commonly reported. The diagnosis of IC is currently made based on symptoms, functional bladder data (cystometrogram), and cystoscopic criteria. There is no specific blood, urine, or bladder biopsy criteria to confirm the diagnosis.[20]

The exact incidence of IC is not known. In the province of Uusimma in southern Finland, the incidence of IC was 103 out of 974,305 adult inhabitants with a prevalence of 10.6 per 100,000.[21] In this series, 9.8% of the patients were men, which is consistent with most other series. In 1987, Held[22] looked specifically at the epidemiology of IC in the United States. They performed a random survey of 127 Board Certified urologists, a survey of 64 IC patients identified by urologists, 902 IC patients who are members of the Interstitial Cystitis Association and 119 "controls" from the general United States population. Held's data suggests the Finnish study underestimates the incidence in the United States by a factor of 4 to 5. In Held's study, the median age of onset symptoms was 40 years old, with 25% of the patients less than 30 years old, which suggests this is not a problem exclusive of older women as it was initially thought.

The social and economic costs of this syndrome are significant. The economic costs include direct medical costs, loss of production due to inability to work, or working at lower wage jobs than the national average for women of similar age and educational background. Even more profound are the social consequences of overall decrease in quality of life, increase in suicidal thoughts, inability to perform functions as a parent and other activities such as exercise and sex, which are important for the overall physical and emotional well-being of the patients.

The etiology is unknown, and there is no known cure. Etiologic concepts currently being considered are infectious, vascular or lymphatic obstruction, psychological, glycosaminoglycan alterations, reflex sympathetic dystrophy, toxic urinary agents, and immunological.[23] With the wide variety of potential etiologic factors, it is not surprising that no intervention is uniformly successful, and often a combination of interventions are required to control symptoms.

Neuropathic Pain

The diagnosis of a neuropathic etiology for symptoms is rarely considered in women who present with LUTH, but should be considered first in women who describe their symptoms as "burning" or an "electric shock-like" sensation. The mechanism of nerve injury may never be known and can be perpetuated by local trauma, pelvic floor spasm and repeated irritation to the peripheral nerves. Trauma to the pudendal nerve has been attributed to vaginal childbirth, horseback riding prolonged cycling etc.[24] Reflex sympathetic dystrophy[25] has been reported in women with chronic bladder symptoms. Exposure of the pelvic organs to radiation can damage the blood supply and the nerves, leading to similar symptoms. While these often debilitating sensations are "external" to the urinary tract, the perception is that they are related to the bladder and/or urethra and often lead to a markedly abnormal voiding pattern.

Musculoskeletal Pain

Musculoskeletal pain is probably the most frequently missed diagnosis in patients who present with pain in the pelvis and an altered voiding pattern. This pain is typically poorly localized, dull, and aching in nature. Providers are not accustomed to thinking of the pelvic musculoskeletal system as being a source of pain when patients attribute it to their internal organs. Musculoskeletal nociceptors are stimulated by mechanical stimuli (compression or stretching), and chemical stimuli, inflammation and metabolic disturbances. Intrapelvic muscle strain, imbalance between the trunk, hip, and abdominal muscles, poor posture, and strain injuries to abdominal, paravertebral and gluteal muscles (by a short leg) can all generate pain localized to the LUT and alterations in voiding function. Abdominal trigger points are believed to arise superficial to the muscles and fascia, but may be influenced by musculoskeletal abnormalities which exist proximal to the trigger point.[26]

Another source of soft tissue pain which can be perceived as originating in the LUT is myofascial pain. This pain is generated in hyperirritable spots located within a tight band of skeletal muscle or fascia.[27] Referred pain, tenderness, autonomic phenomena, and reflex spasm in surrounding muscle groups are associated with these points of pain. Tearing, coryza, dizzy spells and tinnitus are some of the autonomic symptoms that are reported by patients in conjunction with this pain.[23] Muscle pain can lead to inactivity which exacerbates the problem. Triggers for myofascial pain include direct trauma to muscles or joints, chronic muscle strain, chilling of fatigued muscles, acute myositis, arthritis, nerve root injury, or visceral ischemia.[26] Myofascial trigger points in the levator and coccygeus muscles can be associated with symptoms of altered LUT function and pain. It was recognized by Thiele[29] in 1963 that these symptoms are exacerbated before and during menses.

A thorough musculoskeletal examination should be considered in all patients with abdominal and pelvic trigger points. Standard physiotherapeutic techniques such as applying heat, cold, massage, and appropriate muscle stretching, strengthening, and relaxation, can be effective for the pelvic floor of the body as with any other part of the body.

HISTORY

A complete history is the most important aspect of the initial evaluation of the woman. A questionnaire filled out by the patient before seeing the provider is invaluable in helping decipher complex histories and provides the patient with a vehicle to express fear and frustration. Specific questions which need to be asked are:

1. *What are your current symptoms?* It is important to obtain specific answers to daytime frequency, nocturia, an urgency rating on a scale of 0 to 10 and a pain/discomfort rating on a scale of 0 to 10. When symptoms vary, obtain the above information when symptoms are at their best and at their worst.
2. *Are symptoms the same 24 hours a day, seven days a week?* For example, ask if their symptoms vary depending on time of day (morning vs evening), or with physical exercise (vs no exercise)? Identifying what is different between asymptomatic and symptomatic times can lead to an understanding of what precipitates the symptoms and thus strategies for eliminating or minimizing the symptoms.
3. *What were patients bladder habits before this problem started?* If hesitancy, or a poor, interrupted stream were present before the onset of the irritable symptoms, there was probably a voiding dysfunction as the underlying cause for the new onset of frequency and urgency.

4. *Was there a history of infections, frequency, daytime or nighttime inconti-nence as a child? If so, were there any procedures performed meatotomy, urethrotomy, urethral dilation?* A history of these problems suggests that the patient may have a lifelong voiding dysfunction, possibly due to the incomplete maturation of the nerve pathways to the LUT.

5. *Do symptoms vary with menstrual cycle?* Women usually report symptoms are worse between ovulation and menses, which suggest that hormonal fluctations affect symptoms.

6. *Do any of the following exacerbate symptoms?*

    Dehydration   increased physical activity and sweating or decreased fluid intake

    Dietary factors   coffee, carbonation, acidic foods, juices, spicy foods, sugar, Nutrasweet™

    Physical factors   sitting or standing for prolonged periods, car rides, lift-ing

    Emotional factors stress, anxiety, depression, fatigue, etc.

7. *What relieves symptoms?*
    - lying down
    - cold pack
    - antibiotics
    - prescription pain pills
    - increased water intake
    - NSAID
    - antispasmodics
    - changing the diet
    - warm bath/heating pad
    - onset menses
    - phenazopyridine
    - relaxation

8. *What is normal daily fluid intake of the following?* Limited intake of water with the majority of the fluid intake being acidic and potentially irritating to the bladder can have a significant affect of initiating and maintaining the symptoms.
    - coffee (including decaffeinated)
    - tea
    - carbonated beverages (including seltzers, sparkling water)
    - fruit juices (specifically citrus and cranberry)
    - alcohol
    - water
    - milk

9. *How were symptoms affected by pregnancy?* If so, this again suggests hormones have an affect on generating or maintaining the symptoms.

10. *What treatments have been tried and what was the patient's response to treatments?*

- antibiotics
- urethral dilations
- antispasmodics
- bladder instillations
- topical anesthetics
- bladder dilation (office vs under anesthesia)

11. *What was going on in life around onset of symptom complex?*
    - become sexually active
    - hot weather
    - pelvic infection
    - new sexual partner
    - low back or tail bone injury
    - perianal process (fissure, hemorrhoid)
    - new form of birth control
    - pelvic operation
    - minor gynecological procedure

12. *What does the patient think is causing the problem?* Allow the patient to say whatever she believes without discounting anything as ridiculous, impossible, or unimportant.

13. *What is patient's biggest fear about these symptoms?* Typically women identify the following fears: cancer, an infection being passed back and forth with their sexual partner, possible kidney damage from undiagnosed infection, or the fear of never getting better or having a normal sexual relationship again.

14. *Does the patient have a history of significant physical, sexual or emotional abuse that she feels may have some significance to her current symptom complex?* If rapport with the woman has been difficult to establish, it may be best to bring up this issue on a subsequent visit. The fact a woman has a history of significant physical or emotional trauma does not exclude the possibility that strategies directed toward symptom control may not be effective for her in addition to psychological support.

PHYSICAL EXAMINATION

The examination includes palpation of the lower abdomen, lower back, and sacrum for trigger points and ability to reproduce symptoms. If specific trigger points are identified, these can be injected with local anesthetic before proceeding with the pelvic examination. Having the woman positioned and draped in a manner allowing observation of facial expressions is useful. This allows the woman to feel like a participant in the process and allow the provider to observe her face for indications of pain that she may not verbalize. When significant concern about having a pelvic examination is expressed by the woman or she is not able to relax and allow the examination, issues of physical or emotional trauma or discomfort the patient may have experienced need to be addressed before the examination proceeds. The examination may need to be delayed to a subsequent visit when the woman feels more comfortable. Each part of the examination must be explained before it happens.

First, the external genitalia is visually inspected for signs of irritation, discharge, and atrophic changes. When the external part of the examination causes discomfort, ask the patient to relax and take some deep breaths before proceeding. Next, gently introduce one finger through the introitus, keeping pressure against the posterior vaginal wall. Ask the woman to identify when she is having discomfort/urgency and if these symptoms are the same or different than experiences during her symptomatic episodes. Initially, palpate the introital muscles circumferentially, then gently introduce the finger to the level of the cervix or vaginal cuff (keeping pressure posterior). Now gradually palpate the right levator muscles beginning lateral to the sacrum and continuing to the pelvic sidewall (6 to 9 o'clock; then continuing anteriorly following the arc of pubic bone (9 to 11 o'clock), pushing up on the genitourinary diaphragm as it inserts in to the pubis lateral to bladder and urethra. This should be done on both sides, observing for symptom reproduction.

The anterior vaginal wall is now palpated. Begin with the urethra just proximal to the meatus and gently palpate toward bladder neck. The urethra should feel like a midline spongy tube with a "gutter" on either side. These "gutters" may be obscured by a previous anterior colporrhaphy, anterior vaginal wall mass (cyst or infected glands), or urethral diverticulum. Moving superiorly, gently palpate the base of the bladder. A sense of urge is normal, but a sense of pain, burning, cramping, or aching is not normal and is more consistent with a diagnosis of underlying painful bladder syndrome (IC). A bimanual examination is begun by gently putting downward pressure in the suprapubic area while pushing upward on the base of the bladder in the midline with the vaginal finger. Next, move the vaginal finger lateral to the bladder and push up on the pelvic floor support immediately adjacent to pubic bone. Pain and reproduction of a sense of urgency in this area is consistent with myofascial pain or pelvic floor spasm and dysfunction.

A bimanual of the uterus and ovaries is performed, again carefully assessing pain reproduction. When pain is reproduced, repeat the same examination with palpation abdominally and vaginally at different times to determine if pain is generated by abdominal or vaginal trigger points or the tissue in-between. A speculum examination is then performed to look for signs of vaginitis, cervicitis, etc. When there is concern about anatomic support, the examination is best performed with two separated posterior blades of a standard speculum. Initially one blade is introduced posteriorly with gentle downward pressure. The anterior vaginal wall (urethra and bladder) is inspected at rest and during cough and the Valsalva maneuver, observing for rotational descent consistent with weakened anatomic support. The second blade is introduced anteriorly and withdrawn part way. The apex (cervix, vaginal vault) is observed at rest and during straining as is the posterior wall observing for signs of a rectocele. Rectovaginal exam is completed at this point to determine if there is thinning of rectovaginal septum, adequacy of the perineal body, thickening or modularity of uterosacral ligaments and evidence of intrarectal or anal pathology.

The final part of the examination is to assess the patient's ability to contract and relax the pelvic floor muscles. This muscle group should be supple and non-tender at rest. The woman should be able to circumferentially tighten the muscles around the vagina without contracting the buttocks, thigh or abdominal muscles and be able to relax the muscles on command. It may be difficult to feel a voluntary contraction when the muscles are tight and in spasm. Verbal reinforcement to relax or "not hold back" will often initiate relaxation. Once the muscles are relaxed, palpate the tender areas again. Often, there is less sense of urgency and discomfort when the muscles are less tense, which provides immediate feedback to the patient that at least part of the symptoms are related to tension in the pelvic muscles and can be lessened by muscle relaxation.

A voided urinalysis should always be done. Microscopic examination of a spun specimen allows for immediate assessment of hematuria, infection (pyuria), and whether this specimen is a clean enough specimen to culture. If the specimen appears contaminated with squamous epithelial cells, obtaining an immediate catheterized specimen can eliminate confusion about whether culture results are significant or if the identified hematuria is in the bladder urine. Women with complicated histories need specific, accurate information as quickly as possible. Equivocation, mixed messages, and returning for a repeat specimen can increase the patient's anxiety. Routine culture of a urine that is chemically negative for leukocyte esterase, nitrates and blood and shows no evidence of pyuria on microscopic examination is not indicated unless the patient needs the additional reassurance that there is no bacterial infection requiring antibiotics. A catheterized urine specimen collected with a small caliber catheter (12 or 14 Fr) also provides an accurate determination of the postvoid residual (PVR) which is important in patients with urinary frequency and a feeling of incomplete emptying. Alternatively, an ultrasound estimation of PVR can be done.

A voided urine sample for cytology can be sent as an initial screen to rule out carcinoma-*in situ* of the bladder especially in women with a history of tobacco use. When hematuria is present on urinalysis, an upper tract evaluation (intravenous pyelogram, renal ultrasound imaging, or CT scan) is appropriate as well as a cystoscopy to complete the hematuria evaluation. In the absense of hematuria, the importance of office cystoscopy in the evaluation of symptoms is less clear. During a cystoscopy, the woman expects to find out "what is wrong". As cystoscopies rarely pinpoint a specific diagnosis leading to anything more than symptomatic treatment, normal cystoscopic findings may increase anxiety rather than provide reassurance. If everything "looks normal", then why do they have symptoms? Once a rapport has been established, a normal cystoscopy may offer the necessary reassurance for the provider and the patient that there is nothing visible triggering the symptoms. Urethral calibration and/or dilation are not indicated for diagnosis or therapy.

When the initial "symptomatic" management approach is not successful, further diagnostic evaluation includes urodynamics to assess neuromuscular function of the LUT. Uninhibited detrusor contractions will occasionally present with symptoms of bladder irritability without urgency incontinence that usually accompanies involuntary detrusor contractions. Cystoscopy under anesthesia with hydrodistention looking for evidence of IC may be indicated. Hydro-distention brings symptomatic relief in about 30% of the women.[30] When there is cyclic variation in the symptoms, dysmenorrhea or dyspareunia, a simultaneous diagnostic laparoscopy can help to identify potential gynecologic causes of the patient's symptoms, which can be treated appropriately.

DESCRIPTIVE ANALYSIS OF PATIENTS WITH LOWER URINARY TRACT HYPERSENSITIVITY

A retrospective review of 100 women whose main symptoms (and reasons for seeking evaluation) were urinary frequency and urgency was conducted.[31] Of the 100 women, 91 were white, two were African-American, one was Asian. Ethnic data was not available for six women. The age range at presentation for evaluation was 23 to 54 years of age, with a mean age of 39 years and a standard deviation of 8 years (Figure 16-2). The most common age range for the onset of symptoms, according to patient report, was between 18 and 40 years of age.

Results

Sixty-nine percent of the women urinated at intervals less than every 2 hours during the day and 48% had nocturia greater than or equal to two times per

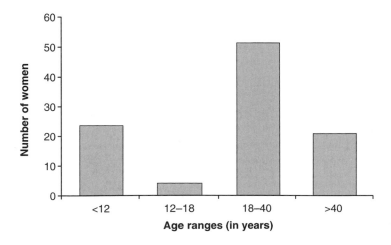

Figure 16-2.

Table 16-1.   Presenting symptoms at initial visit (100 women)

Symptom	Yes (%)	No (%)	No data (%)
Frequency <2 hours daytime	69	29	2
Nocturia ≥2–3 times/evening	48	52	0
Urgency	61	8	31
Pain			
During urination	28	70	2
Before urination	58	41	1
After urination	60	39	1
Quality of stream: strong	70	27	3
Hesitancy	48	50	2
Feeling of incomplete emptying	56	41	3
Incontinence	48	52	0

evening (Table 16-1). Urgency was reported in 61% of the women. Pain during urination was reported in 28% of the women, pain before urination in 58% and pain after urination in 60% of the women. Voiding with a strong urine stream was reported by 70% of the women, while the other 27% had weak or variable streams. Hesitancy of urination was reported by 48%. Fifty-six women had a feeling of incomplete emptying of their bladder either chronically or occasionally. Forty-eight women reported incontinence as a secondary concern to their hypersensitivity symptoms, and 31% of these women had more than one type of incontinence (Table 16-1).

Of these 100 women, 31 had a self-reported positive childhood history of urinary tract problems (Table 16-2). Again by self-report, there were 89% with a history of prior UTI as an adult. The majority of these UTIs (68%) were bladder

Table 16-2.   Past histories (100 women)

History	Yes (%)	Not sure (%)	No (%)	No data (%)
Childhood urinary problems	31	—	66	3
Prior adult infections	89	—	8	3
Low back pain	65	—	34	1
Symptoms cyclic	39	14	33	14
Hormone replacement	9	—	89	2
Dyspareunia	52	—	44	4
Allergies	69	—	31	0
Bowel problems	56	—	44	0
Smoking	38	—	60	2
(currently, 11/38)				
Neurologic disease	7	—	91	2

infections only. Sixty-five had a history of intermittent low back pain. LUT symptoms that exacerbated with menses, or had a cyclic nature, were reported by 39%, while 14% were not sure if there was a correlation. There were 9 women on hormone replacement. Eighty-one of the women replied that they were currently sexually active, and dyspareunia was reported in 52% of the total patient population. Allergies were a problem for 69% of the women, and 56% had reported bowel problems.

Over 70% of this population had been pregnant in the past, and one woman was pregnant during her first visit. Fifty-nine of the women had experienced childbirth, the majority having had vaginal deliveries. Table 16-3 represents the procedures these women reported they had undergone before their presentation to our clinic.

Table 16-3. Prior procedures (100 women)

Procedure	Yes (%)	No (%)	No data (%)
Cystoscopy	41	51	8
Urethral dilation	38	55	7
Antiincontinence surgery	4	87	9
Hysterectomy (5 vaginal; 5 abdominal)	10	87	3

Discussion

The age at presentation to the clinic for LUTH peaked at 31–35 years of age, which corresponds well to the average age at presentation of 37.6 years found by Mabry,[32] and the average range of 25–34 years reported by Brooks.[10] There are several factors unique to this age range that could account for this peak, including onset of sexual activity, beginning college or a career (increased stress), finding partners, and starting families, pregnancies, and deliveries. We found that the next most common age range for initial onset of symptoms was under 12 years old, while the lowest was between 12 and 18 years of age. This finding in LUTH patients complements the existing knowledge that frequent UTIs are common in prepubertal girls, and that at the onset of menses the problem is alleviated, until it reappears with the onset of sexual activity in the late teens and early twenties.[7]

The findings for most common presenting symptoms (Table 16-1) are consistent with what is reported in other articles. Much of the confusion and difficulty in the diagnosis of LUTH is due to the similarity of LUTH symptoms (frequency, urgency, *pain "around" the act of urination*, postvoid fullness) and UTI symptoms (frequency, urgency, *pain during urination*). This confusion may be solely created by the inexact usage of the phrase "painful urination" during history taking, and the assumption that patients mean pain during urination. We found that if patients were asked precisely when they experienced pain (before, during, or after urination), only 28% of the women in this population actually had dysuria in the classic sense (during urination). This simple distinction during the history with a negative urinalysis may be all that is required to distinguish between women with LUTH and UTIs. Pain, discomfort, or a sense of fullness after urination should be considered a common symptom in LUTH.

The finding that 48% of these women had significant nocturia, is higher than previously regarded for this syndrome. Therefore, nocturia should be considered a common presenting symptom in LUTH. This finding is contrary to that of Scotti,[33] who believes significant nocturia is only a problem in severe cases of urethral syndrome or in interstitial cystitis. As women with interstitial cystitis were specifically excluded from this review, nocturia is common in women with LUTH.

The rationale behind treatment of women with LUTH by urethral dilation seems to have been based on the belief that they are "obstructed", which, by definition, should require the symptoms of weak or variable stream, hesitancy, intermittency and incomplete emptying. Only three women reported having all four of these obstructive symptoms, and 70% had strong urinary streams. Other authors have also not found these symptoms to be secondary to an obstructive process—only 1/105 urethral syndrome patients was "obstructed".[31] While only three women were found to have "classic" symptoms of obstruction, 38 had a history of undergoing urethral dilations for their symptoms.

Allergies were reported in the majority of this population. The most commonly reported allergies were drug-related. An interesting question is whether there may be an iatrogenic drug-induced LUTH in women with drug sensitivities, which could be maintained with sensitivities to various other allergens (18% reported more than one type of allergy). As almost 40% of this population reported a past history of smoking, and with the known relationship between tobacco and bladder cancer, aggressive diagnostics (cytology and possibly cystoscopy) are warranted in women with frequency and urgency of urination expecially if there is any indication of hematuria.

It is also noteworthy that over half these women reported bowel problems. Whether this is a cause of LUTH or an effect is not clear, but may be an indication of a more global autonomic dysfunction or autoimmune etiology to their irritable symptoms. Pain with intercourse was reported in over half of this population, which is consistent with pain and spasm in the pelvic floor support.

Summary

Women with LUTH usually present between 31 and 35 years of age, with symptom onset between 18 and 40 years old. They had the common presenting symptoms of frequency (69%), urgency (61%), pain after urination (60%), a feeling of incomplete emptying (56%), low back pain (65%), and dyspareunia

(52%). Only a few women (3%) had symptoms consistent with obstruction, although many of their histories included urethral dilations (38%). Their histories commonly included prior infections as an adult (89%), allergies (69%), bowel problems (56%), past pregnancies (71%) and deliveries (59%).

Based on these findings, there is no rationale for treatment of LUTH in women by urethral dilation, cystoscopy or antibiotics. It is time to consider a new approach which will be discussed below. Rather than feeding the cycle of diagnostic and therapeutic confusion that perpetuates symptoms rather than alleviates them, this approach is aimed at symptom resolution. Improvement is accomplished by using the following behavioral changes: increasing water intake and restricting dietary irritants, and teaching pelvic floor muscle localization, strengthening, and appropriate relaxation.

TREATMENT

General Considerations

Regardless of symptom etiology, treatment always begins with reassurance and education about the structure and function of the lower urinary tract, and the interrelationship with the gynecologic, gastrointestinal, and musculoskeletal systems. Anatomic diagrams can be very helpful in demonstrating the concepts. When possible, intimate partners should be present for the discussion to help dispel any myths or fears they may have. In cases of very long-standing and/or severe symptoms, realistic goals for treatment outcome must be established at the outset. An understanding of the interrelationship between the mind and body needs to be established as the norm for all patients. Therefore, the evaluation and treatment cannot be based solely on the body. Suggesting that her feelings of depression and anxiety are similar to a grief reaction is often helpful. Women grieve the active, symptom-free life they once had and consequently experience a sense of loss in all aspects of their lives. Professional psychological support may be accepted to assist women with feelings of loss and grief.

A partnership for obtaining symptom-control and moving ahead with life needs to be established. When the goal is to "cure" a disease, the patient is at risk for continual disappointment as one treatment after another fails to bring permanent symptom relief. Patients must also be warned that when they do obtain good symptomatic control, they will likely experience a recurrence of symptoms. The first symptom recurrence usually produces significant fear/anxiety that "it is back" and "will not go away this time". Fabricating diagnoses (bad infection, narrow urethra) to satisfy the patient's desire to know what is causing the symptoms should be avoided. Terminology such as "dysfunctions" and "symptomatic episodes" or "flare-ups" are most accurate and do not lead to the expectation that antibiotics will help, as do all words that end with "itis". Ensuring that all of the office personnel having contact with patients (in person or on the phone) must understand the importance of terminology. Getting mixed messages from different personnel fuels fear, frustration and anxiety—a nurse may misinterpret a urinalysis or dipstick as "infection" telling the patient she needs antibiotics and 2 days later after the culture report is back, she is told it was not an infection.

An authoritarian or paternalistic approach to these women is generally not well received. Women want to be viewed as equals with important knowledge about their bodies and which treatments may work best for them. Very few patients are resistant to psychosocial support, or physical therapy evaluation and treatment once they understand the rationale for these recommendations. The cost of psychological support, when not covered by health insurance, can be a limiting factor. When this is the case, an alternative is to schedule short, follow-up visits every 1 to 2 weeks for listening and positive reinforcement.

Behavioral Strategies

Common sense is important in using behavioral recommendations. Using a *bladder diary* to periodically record time and volume of urination can be important in demonstrating objective improvement to the patient. *Increasing the water intake* to dilute the urine and "flush" out the lower urinary tract is important. The optimal volume varies, but starting with 4 to 6 glasses of water per day and gradually increasing seems to work. Urine passed should be pale yellow and the water intake necessary to maintain dilute urine may vary day to day. It is important to inform patients that frequency may actually be worse initially due to the increased intake. Ease of urination (less hesitency and inter-mittency) happens first. As it becomes more comfortable to hold larger volumes of urine in the bladder, the frequency will then decrease. Bladder holding protocols can be helpful in decreasing frequency once pain is less severe.[33,34] Avoiding specific foods or fluids can also relieve the discomfort.[35]

Recognizing the potential of voluntary or involuntary pelvic muscle contraction in symptom generation, perpetuation, or exacerbation is important to the development of self-management strategies. Voluntary pelvic floor relaxation[36] can ease symptoms. Many times patients need instruction in pelvic muscle localization and contraction before they can understand how to relax this muscle group. Anything which promotes generalized relaxation and stress management (aerobic exercise, distraction, etc.) should be utilized whenever possible. In order to be accepted by the patient, these behavioral strategies must be recommended not only as valid, but the best treatment available. When the patients sense that their provider does not take these recommendations seriously, they are not likely to comply with the treatment.

Pharmacologic Management

A variety of medications can be employed in the treatment of LUTH. Often combinations of drugs can be efficacious. Pharmacological management can be used regardless of a confirmed diagnosis of IC. However, in our practice, we do not use DMSO intravesical instillations unless the patient has findings consistent with IC on cystoscopy with hydrodistention under anesthesia. Sodium pentosanpolysulfate (Elmiron)[37,38] has recently received FDA approval for women with the diagnosis of IC which requires the cystoscopy under anesthesia with hydrodistention.

Table 16-4 lists the pharmacologic agents most commonly used, and the symptoms which each agent may be most useful for. Combinations of medications may be appropriate. The use of alpha-blockers (e.g., prazosin) can be helpful in patients with obstructive voiding symptoms that may be secondary to nonrelaxation of the urethral smooth muscle.[39] The listed medications should be viewed as general guidelines. In refractory patients, continuing to try different agents or combinations of drugs may be the key in breaking the pain cycle. Realistic expectations for treatment outcome are necessary, and patients must understand that all medications come with a benefit:side-effect ratio that is not necessarily predictable.

Physiotherapy

The addition of a comprehensive physiotherapy evaluation and treatment regimen to LUTH is invaluable. Initially (10 years ago), our most refractory patients were referred to physical therapists who had a special interest in pelvic floor dysfunction. The success in these very difficult, refractory symptom complexes was surprising and rewarding.[40] Gradually as our confidence grew, women were referred to PT earlier and earlier in our treatment regimen. Currently nearly all patients are referred after their initial visit for physiotherapy assessment. Almost all patients report some, if not total, symptom improvement.

Our practice is to do urodynamic evaluations and cystoscopy with hydrodistention under anesthesia in women who have failed behavioral, pharmacological, and physiotherapy treatments. Since we have been routinely recommending physical therapy, the number of hydrodistention procedures we perform has declined from 2–4 per month to less than 1 per month.[41]

Treatments Specific to Interstitial Cystitis

Even patients presenting with a confirmed diagnosis of IC may respond to some of the simple behavioral strategies. Many provider are not aware of the importance of these simple strategies and concentrate only on the medications or intravesical instillations and are not as helpful to the women as they could be in helping them achieve significant symptomatic relief. The best start in the treatment of IC is to review what the woman knows about IC and the self-help strategies. Ask how successful they have been in incorporating these strategies

Table 16-4. Medications for treatment of LUTH

Medication	Dosage	Symptom	Sign
Tricyclic antidepressants Amitriptyline Doxepin Trazadone Prozac	10–75 mg h.s. 10–75 mg h.s. 50 mg h.s: 20 mg po q.d	Sleep disruption; sharp, burning, shocklike pain; bladder/urethral burning or constant awareness	Increased pelvic muscle tone; painful bladder
Alpha-blockers Terazosin Prazosin Phenoxybenzamine	1–2 mg h.s. (increase to t.i.d. as tolerated and necessary for symptom control)	Hesitancy; slow stream, sense of incomplete emptying; postvoiding pain/spasm	Abnormal uroflow; ± tender pelvic muscles
Antispasmodics Oxybutynin Hyoscyamine Tolteridine	1/2 T po t.i.d. i–ii po t.i.d. i po b.i.d.	Frequency; discomfort with full bladder; severe urgency	Involuntary detrusor contractor on CMG
Skeletal muscle relaxants Carisopradol (Soma) Cyclobenzeprine (Flexaril) Methocarbonol (Robaxin)	i po t.i.d. i po t.i.d. i po t.i.d.	Postvoiding pain; dyspareunia	Increased tone of pelvic muscles; pain reproduction with palpation
Anesthetics Phenazopyridine Lidocaine jelly 2% Lidocaine ointment 5%	100–200 mg po t.i.d.	Hypersensitivity; pain during urination; pain localized to meatal area during urination or intercourse	Tender introital area of perimeatal area

into their day to day existence. Reassure patients (and their families) that most women arrive at a successful treatment strategy by combining behavioral, pharmacologic, and physiotherapeutic techniques. Successful treatment will allow them to have a reasonably functional life. Finding what will be successful for each woman not only takes a significant time commitment, but a willingness to try different approaches, and most of all a positive attitude. Women are fearful that their physician will give up on them if they do not feel better as quickly as the physician has suggested they should.

Current treatment of IC is aimed at symptomatic relief through a variety of means including dietary modification, intravesical instillations of various pharmacologic agents including dimethylsulfoxide (DMSO™) (T. Bavendam, unpublished observations), hydrocortisone, sodium bicarbonate[42] heparin,[43,44] oxychlorosene (Chlorpactin™)[45] lidocaine,[46] doxorubicin,[47] and oral agents such as amitriptyline,[48] hydroxyzine,[49] nifedipine,[50] and sodium pentosanpolysulfate.[37,38] Other modalities used to treat IC include transcutaneous electrical nerve stimulation (TENS),[51,52] neuromodulation (sacral nerve root stimulator)[53] and surgical enlargement of the bladder (augmentation cystoplasty),[54] substitution cystoplasty,[55] or cystectomy with urinary diversion.[56] Some of the many medications prescribed specifically to this patient population are listed in Table 16-5. These drugs are also used for other medical conditions and are thus readily available.

Table 16-5. Medications for treating interstitial cystitis

Medication	Dosage	Proposed action
Amitriptylline	10–75 mg h.s.	Central and peripheral anticholinergic Block reuptake of norepinephrine and serotonin Sedative Analgesic effects
Nifedipine	30 mg q.d. for 2 weeks, gradually increase to 60 mg q.d.	Decrease frequency and strength of visceral smooth muscle contraction Suppressive effect on delay-type hypersensitivity
Hydroxyzine	25 mg h.s. for 1 week, increase to 50 mg h.s. for 1 week, then add 25 mg each morning	Block neuronal activation of mast cells
Pentosanpolysulfate (Elmiron)	100 mg po t.i.d.	Reduce bacterial adherence to bladder epithelial cells Reduce microcrystal adherence Enhance impermeability of epithelium

In general, it is best to prepare patients for a 2- to 3-month trial of any new treatment strategy. It often takes time for improvement to become noticeable to the patient. Keeping accurate accounts of frequency, nocturia, pain, and urgency scores in the patient medical records is important. Improvement may be subtle and gradual over time. Nocturia 8 times per night is not normal, and the woman may feel she is not better. However, if the chart reflects that she reported getting up over 12 times per night at her first visit, the improvement can be stressed to her providing positive reinforcement that this strategy is effective.

As mentioned previously, intravesical therapy has been tried with multiple agents included dimethylsulfoxide, heparin, hydrocortisone, sodium bicarbonate. DMSO is FDA-approved for the treatment of IC. It can be used alone or mixed with the previously mentioned agents. A typical treatment regimen is weekly instillations for 6 to 8 weeks. If good symptom control is achieved, treatment can be restarted when symptoms flare, or, alternatively, a maintenance schedule of instillations every 1 to 2 months can be started. Many patients prefer to learn self-instillations which allows them to do the treatments when they feel they need them rather than when they can schedule an appointment. Most women have no difficulty learning the self-catheterization and -instillation technique. Bladder infections in this patient population are uncommon and have not been a factor in our patients.[57]

CONCLUSION

The evaluation and treatment of women with frequency and urgency of urination is challenging and rewarding. The likelihood of successful symptom management increases exponentially with recognition that the standard biomedical model does not apply to the majority of these women. Awareness that many different organ systems may be involved in generating and amplifying symptoms, establishing a partnership with the women in making decisions about appropriate treatment strategies and early recognition of the psychosocial influences on all chronic conditions is necessary for a successful outcome. The physician is one of the participants involved in successful treatment plans who must be willing to recognize the importance of providers from other disciplines and encourage their participation. A team of providers can provide the best care for women whose complaints of frequency and urgency of urination are certainly not "life-threatening" and often not taken seriously by health care providers, but nonetheless have significant negative impact on women's personal and professional lives.

REFERENCES

1. Krieger J. Urinary tract infections in women: Causes, classification, and differential diagnosis. *J Urol* 1990; **35**: 4.
2. Bavendam T. A common sense approach to lower urinary tract hypersensitivity in women. *Contemp Urol* 1992; **4**: 25.
3. Reid G, Bruce A, Taylor M. Influence of 3-day antimicrobial therapy and lactobacillus suppositories on recurrence of urinary tract infection. *Clin Ther* 1992; **14**: 11.
4. Bruce A, Reid G. Acute and recurrent urinary tract infections in women. *Int Urogynecol J* 1993; **4**: 240.
5. Stamm W, et al. Causes of acute urethral syndrome in women. *N Engl J Med* 1980; **303**: 409.
6. Brubaker LT, Sand PK. Urinary frequency and urgency. *Obste Gynecol Clin North Am* 1989; **16**: 883.
7. Marshall S, Linfoot J. Influence of hormones on urinary tract infection. *Urology* 1977; **9**: 675.
8. Evans AJ. Etiology of urethral syndrome: Preliminary report. *J Urol* 1971; **105**: 245.
9. Eavendam TG. A New Understanding of "cystitis" in women. Part I: Replacing the myths. *Women's Health Forum* 1993; **2**: 1.
10. Brooks DAM. A. Pathogenesis of the urethral syndrome in women and its diagnosis in general practice. *Lancet* 1972; 893.
11. Powell NB, Powell EB, Thomas OC, Queng JT, McGovern JP. Allergy of the lower urinary tract. *J Urol* 1972; **107**: 631.
12. Stillwell T, Benson R. Cyclophosphamide-induced hemorrhagic cystitis: A review of 100 patients. *Cancer* 1988; **61**: 451.
13. Fairchild W, et al. The incidence of bladder cancer after cyclophosphamide therapy. *J Urol* 1979; **122**: 163.
14. Leach G, Bavendam T. Female urethral diverticula. *Urology* 1987; **30**: 407.
15. Ripps B, Martin D. Endometriosis and chronic pelvic pain. *Obstet Gynecol Clin North Am* 1993; **20**: 709.
16. Lipscomb G, Ling F. Relationship of pelvic infection and chronic pelvic pain. *Obstet Gynecol Clin North Am* 1993; **20**: 699.
17. Thomas D, et al. Measurement of pelvic blood flow changes in response to posture in normal subjects and in women with pelvic pain owing to congestion by using a thermal technique. *Clin Sci* 1992; **83**: 55.
18. Goetsch M. Vulvar vestibulitis: prevalence and histologic features in a general gynecologic practice population. *Am J Obstet Gynecol* 1991; **164**: 1609.
19. Rapkin A, Mayer E. Gastrenterologic causes of chronic pelvic pain. *Obstet Gynecol Clin North Am* 1993; **20**: 663.
20. Hanno P, et al. *Interstitial Cystitis*. London: Springer-Verlag, 1990.
21. Oravisto K. Epidemiology of interstitial cystitis. *Ann Chir Gynaecol Fenn* 1975; **64**: 75.
22. Held P, et al. Epidemiology of interstitial cystitis. In: Hanno P, et al. (eds) *Interstitial Cystitis*. New York: Springer-Verlag, 1990: 29.
23. Ratliff T, Klutke C, McDougall E. The etiology of interstitial cystitis. *Urol Clin North Am* 1994; **21**: 21.
24. Turner M, Marinoff S. Pudendal neuralgia. *Am J Obstet Gynecol* 1991; **165**: 1233.
25. Galloway N, Gabale D, Irwin P. Interstitial cystitis or reflex sympathetic dystrophy of the bladder? *Semin Urol* 1991; **9**: 148.
26. Baker P. Musculoskeletal origins of chronic pelvic pain: Diagnosis and treatment. *Obstet Gynecol Clin North Am* 1993; **20**: 719.
27. Travell J, Simons D. *Myofascial Pain and Dysfunction: The Trigger Point Manual*. Baltimore: Williams & Wilkins, 1983.

28. Simons D, Travell J. Myofascial origins of low back pain. *Postgrad Med* 1983; **73**: 66.
29. Thiele G. Coccygodynia: Cause and treatment. *Dis Colon Rectum* 1963; **6**: 422.
30. Hanno P, Wein A. Interstitial cystitis: Part II. *AUA Update Ser* 1987.
31. LaCroix C, Bavendam TG. A Descriptive analysis of women with lower urinary tract hypersensitivity. *J Invest Med* 1995; **43**: 130A.
32. Mabry EW, Carson CC, Older RA. Evaluation of women with chronic voiding discomfort. *Urology* 1981; **18**: 244.
33. Scotti RJ. The urethral syndrome and urethral infections I. Patient evaluation and infectious causes. *Infect Surg* 1989; (March): 102.
34. Blaivas S, Blaivas J. Successful treatment of sensory urgency and interstitial cystitis with behavioral modification. *J Urol* 1986; **135**: 189.
35. Parsons C, Koprowski P. Interstitial cystitis: Successful management by increasing voiding intervals. *Urology* 1991; **37**: 207.
36. Koziol J. Epidemiology of interstitial cystitis. *Urol Clin North Am* 1984; **21**: 7.
37. Phillips H, Fenster H, Samsom D. An effective treatment for functional urinary incoordination. *J Behav Med* 1992; **15**: 45.
38. Mulholland S, et al. Pentosanpolysulfate sodium for therapy of interstitial cystitis: A double-blind placebo-controlled clinical study. *Urology* 1990; **35**: 552.
39. Parsons C, Mulholland S. Successful therapy of interstitial cystitis with pentosanpolysulfate. *J Urol* 1987; **138**: 513.
40. Petersen T, Husted S. Prazosin treatment of neurological patients with lower urinary tract dysfunction. *Int Urogynecol J* 1993; **4**: 106.
41. Bavendam T, et al. Early experience with physical therapy in the management of pelvic pain in female urologic patients. In: *Procedings of the Annual Meeting of American Urological Society, Western Section. Maui, Hawaii, 1992.*
42. Perez-Marrero R, Emerson L, Feltis J. A controlled study of dimethyl sulfoxide in interstitial cystitis. *J Urol* 1988; **140**: 36.
43. Sant G, LaRock D. Standard therapies for interstitial cystitis. *Urol Clin North Am* 1994; **21**: 73.
44. Perez-Marrero R, et al. Prolongation of response to DMSO by heparin maintenance. *Urology* 1993; **41(Suppl)**: 64.
45. Hanno P, Wein A. Conservative therapy for interstitial cystitis. *Semin Urol* 1991; **9**: 143.
46. Wishard W, Nourse M, Mertz J. Use of chlorpactin WCS 90 for relief of symptoms due to interstitial cystitis. *J Urol* 1957; **77**: 420.
47. Asklin B, Cassuto J. Intravesical lidocaine in severe interstitial cystitis: case report. *Scand J Urol Nephrol* 1989; **23**: 311.
48. Khanna O, Loose J. Interstitial cystitis treated with intravesical doxorubicin. *Urology* 1990; **36**: 139.
49. Hanno P, Buehler J, Wein A. Use of amitriptyline in the treatment of interstitial cystitis. *J Urol* 1989; **141**: 846.
50. Theoharides T. Hydroxyzine in the treatment of interstitial cystitis. *Urol Clin North Am* 1994; **21**: 113.
51. Fleischmann J, et al. Clinical and immunological response to nifedipine for the treatment of interstitial cystitis. *J Urol* 1991; **146**: 1235.
52. Fall M, Carlsson C, Erlandson B. Electrical stimulation in interstitial cystitis. *J Urol* 1980; **123**: 192.
53. Fall M. Conservative management of chronic interstitial cystitis: Transcutaneous electrical nerve stimulation and transurethral resection. *J Urol* 1985; **133**: 774.
54. Tanagho E, Schmidt R. Electrical stimulation in the management of the neurogenic bladder. *J Urol* 1988; **140**: 1331.
55. Smith R, et al. Augmentation cystoplasty: A critical overview. *J Urol* 1977; **118**: 35.
56. Webster G, Maggio M. The management of chronic interstitial cystitis by substitution cystoplasty. *J Urol* 1989; **141**: 287.

57. Irwin P, Galloway N. Surgical management of interstitial cystitis. *Urol Clin North Am* 1994; **21**: 145.
58. Whitmore K. Self-care regimens for patients with interstitial cystitis. *Urol Clin North Am* 1994; **21**: 121.

CHAPTER 17

Urinary incontinence due to detrusor overactivity

RAUL YORDAN-JOVET AND L. LEWIS WALL ————————————

Over the past three decades there has been an increasing recognition of the importance of uninhibited contractions of the bladder muscle (*detrusor overactivity*) as a cause of urinary incontinence; however, the etiology of this condition still remains unclear. The importance of detrusor overactivity was first brought to the attention of gynecologists in 1963 by Hodgkinson and associates.[1] Utilizing direct electronic urethrocystometry, these authors found that 64 out of 735 female patients (8.7%) originally thought to have simple stress incontinence instead had uninhibited detrusor contractions as the cause of their incontinence. Based on this finding, these authors concluded that significant numbers of "failures" in surgery for stress incontinence represented preoperative diagnostic failures rather than failures of surgical technique. They recommended preoperative urodynamic testing as a means of eliminating this problem.

Hodgkinson referred to this detrusor muscle overactivity as "dyssynergic waves of detrusor contractions". As a result, the term "detrusor dyssynergia" entered the gynecologic literature, to be joined by many other names over the years: "unstable bladder", "spastic bladder", "hyperreflexic bladder", "hypertonic bladder", "automatic bladder", "systolic bladder", "uninhibited bladder", and so on. The result has been a confusing melange of conflicting and imprecise terminology. Since some estimates place the prevalence of detrusor overactivity as high as 10% of the population,[2] it is important for clinicians who deal with women to understand the terminology, principles of diagnosis, and modes of treatment for this condition, including some appreciation of the contributions that cystometry can make in managing these patients.[3]

DEFINITIONS AND TERMINOLOGY

In order to eliminate confusion and make research reports readily intelligible across the boundaries of both nations and scientific disciplines, the International Continence Society has worked continuously since 1976 to standardize the terminology used in the description of lower urinary tract function and dysfunction.[4] A brief review of this terminology is in order.

"Urinary incontinence" is involuntary loss of urine that is a social or hygienic problem. This loss of urine should be demonstrable by objective testing. Urinary incontinence of any variety may refer to several different things. A symptom reported by the patient, a sign found on physical examination, or a specific diagnosis as determined by urodynamic testing. The sense in which the term is used has very different implications. For example, the term "stress incontinence" may refer to a patient's complaint that she loses urine during periods of increased intraabdominal pressure, or it may refer to the demonstration of such urine loss on physical examination (the "sign" of stress incontinence), or it may refer to a very specific urodynamic diagnosis (genuine stress incontinence). The term "genuine stress incontinence" refers to the specific phenomenon of involuntary loss of urine occurring coincident with a rise in intravesical pressure that exceeds the maximum urethral pressure, in the absence of a detrusor contraction; that is, it refers to a finding made during laboratory urodynamic studies when leakage occurs with a cough pressure spike and a quiescent detrusor.

"Urge incontinence" is most closely associated with detrusor overactivity. Urge incontinence can refer to the patient's complaint of urine loss associated with a strong desire to void, to the demonstration of urine loss associated with urgency during a physical examination or simple bladder filling, or to this finding during urodynamic testing. Demonstrable urge incontinence is usually manifested by the patient's strong protestations of impending leakage followed by obvious urine loss occurring in the absence of any coughing or straining. The specific term "detrusor instability" implies the presence of symptomatic uninhibited detrusor contractions—of any magnitude—during filling cystometry while pressures are being measured. If these contractions provoke a strong desire to void, the condition is called "motor urgency"; if they provoke involuntary urine loss, the condition is called "motor urge incontinence". Strictly speaking, therefore, the term detrusor instability refers to a cystometric diagnosis just as does genuine stress incontinence. Use of either term implies that a urodynamic evaluation has been performed on a patient and that appropriate findings were documented.

"Detrusor instability" is characterized by involuntary detrusor contractions during the filling phase of a cystometrogram. They may be spontaneous or provoked and cannot be completely suppressed while attempting to inhibit micturition. Detrusor instability may be asymptomatic or it may be interpreted as a normal desire to urinate. Its occurrence does not imply the existence of a neurologic disorder. Overactivity due to known a neurologic control disturbance is referred to as "detrusor hyperreflexia". The term "detrusor-sphincter dyssynergia" refers to a neuropathic voiding dysfunction that occurs when the pelvic floor and urethra contract simultaneously with a detrusor contraction. To avoid confusing two very distinct clinical conditions, the use of Hodgkinson's term "detrusor dyssynergia" to refer to uninhibited detrusor contractions should be abandoned. In this chapter we use the term "detrusor overactivity" to refer to the phenomenon of incontinence due to unhibited bladder contractions of any etiology, using "detrusor hyperrelexia" when there is a known, relevant neurological disorder and using "detrusor instability" when we refer to the more common finding of idiopathic detrusor overactivity.

"Urinary frequency" refers to the number of voiding episodes per day. Seven or eight voids with volumes between 200 and 300 ml are considered normal, but this is dependent on fluid intake and environmental temperature, among other factors.[5] More frequent voids may be abnormal, but changes in frequency should always be assessed against prior patient history. Patients with detrusor overactivity often suffer from marked urinary frequency; however, frequency of urination may also be due to causes other than detrusor overactivity.

"Nocturia" refers to the number of times a patient is awakened from sleep with the need to void. To be significant, nocturia should occur on most nights. Nocturia of once per night is considered a normal variant, usually related to fluid intake before sleep. Diurnal regulation of fluid excretion tends to change with age, and increasing nocturia up to twice per night is common in elderly people.[6] "Enuresis" technically refers to any involuntary loss of urine, whereas "nocturnal enuresis" refers to urine loss during sleep. It should be distinguished from "noturnal urge incontinence", which often occurs when the patient is awakened with a strong desire to void, starts to the toilet, but experiences urine loss before the toilet is reached. Nocturia is common in patients with detrusor overactivity, but it is not the sole cause of this symptom.

Three other types of incontinence may be related to detrusor overactivity. "Reflex incontinence" is the loss of urine due to detrusor hyperreflexia, involuntary urethral relaxation, or both in the absence of the sensation usually associated with the desire to void. This condition is seen only in patients with neuropathic bladder or urethral disorders. "Giggle micturition" is an unusual condition found mainly in adolescent girls in which semihysterical laughter results in voiding to completion.[7] This appears to be a true voiding reflex triggered in the cortex by an unknown mechanism that usually disappears spontaneously in early adult life.[8] Patients with this complaint may easily be confused with women complaining of stress incontinence unless a precise history is taken. "Overflow incontinence" is any involuntary loss of urine associated with overdistention of the bladder. In many cases, bladder overdistention triggers a detrusor contraction that results in urine loss.

As will be seen, urodynamic studies are often helpful in understanding the exact pathophysiology responsible for a patient's particular complaint, and several pathophysiologic mechanisms may be present together in the same patient.

PATIENT SYMPTOMS, URODYNAMIC STUDIES, AND DETRUSOR OVERACTIVITY

By definition, the term "detrusor instability" refers to the finding of uninhibited detrusor contractions during cystometry in a patient with no known neurologic disorder. How closely does this urodynamic finding correlate with patient symptoms? To some extent, this depends on the quality of the history taken (as well as the quality of the urodynamic studies). Early publications often reported large discrepancies (25–66%) between symptoms and urodynamic findings with respect to stress incontinence,[9] frequency and urgency,[10] and "recurrent cystitis",[11,12] particularly among elderly women.[13] Cantor and Bates[14] identified three "key" clinical symptoms that were closely associated with the presence of detrusor instability during urodynamic testing: urge incontinence, nocturia, and nocturnal enuresis. In their series of 214 incontinent patients, if one symptom was present, 64% of those studied had detrusor instability; if two symptoms were present the prevalence of detrusor instability rose to 76%, and if all three symptoms were present, 81% had uninhibited detrusor contractions during cystometry. Some of these symptoms may be associated with urethral hyper-sensitivity,[15] but the patient who has frequency and urgency *without inconti-nence*, rarely has detrusor instability as the cause of her symptoms.[16] A number of studies have shown a variable link of detrusor overactivity and the symptom of nocturnal enuresis, with ranges of 15% to 69% having documented detrusor contractions.[17,18] In both daytime and nighttime enuresis is present, the percent-age of overactive bladders on cystometry rises as high as 97%.[19]

Although nocturnal enuresis may be associated with detrusor instability, detrusor instability is not necessarily associated with nocturnal enuresis. Neurologically normal children with a clinical bed-wetting problem showed asymptomatic detrusor instability without incontinence in 15.7% of daytime, and 50% of nighttime, cystometries.[20] This suggests that nocturnal enuresis without associated other urologic complaints is probably due to a defective reflex arc that triggers normal voiding by a sustained detrusor contraction during sleep once the daytime cystometric capacity is reached. A similar process is probably involved in the phenomenon of giggle micturition, in which uncontrollable laughter leads to an uncontrollable detrusor contraction. Urodynamic studies in such patients is generally unrewarding. Fortunately, this problem usually disappears with further maturation of the nervous system.[8,21]

Several studies have shown that detrusor instability may be present in women without the "key" symptoms of urgency, frequency, and urge incontinence. Independent studies by Webster[22] and Korda[23] discovered detrusor instability during cystometry in 31% and 36% of patients who had been suspected clinically of having only stress incontinence. Sand and colleagues[24] found the symptoms of urgency and urge incontinence to have a sensitivity of 78% and a specificity of 39% in detecting detrusor instability among 175 women who com-plained of stress incontinence. Similar findings have been reported by others.[25–28] In elderly women, analysis of symptoms is even more difficult, due to decreased mental acuity, disorientation and concurrent medical problems that may contribute to incontinence.[13,29–31]

Attempts have been made to refine the utility of the patient's history by employing detailed questionnaires in advance of complete urodynamic evaluation. Bergam and Bader[32] found such structured questionnaires to have a positive productive value of 80% for genuine stress incontinence, but only 25% for detrusor instability. An examination history showing false positive results of stress incontinence could be caused by detrusor instability or a urethral diverticulum. A history of false positive indications for detrusor instability could be caused by urethritis, vaginitis, polyuria, or an unstable urethra. Similar findings were reported by Hausler and coworkers,[33] using the Gaudenz Incontinence Questionnaire. The protean manifestations of detrusor instability and the inconstant relationship between symptoms and urodynamic findings led Turner-Warwick to conclude that[34] "no single symptom is particularly helpful in distinguishing between the stable and unstable detrusor". Others have held similar opinions.[35] Although we appreciate the background against which such statements have been made, we believe that this represents an excessively gloomy view of urogynecologic diagnosis, for many patients can be helped to overcome their symptoms without the necessity for a full urodynamic investigation; however, in order to understand those situations in which urodynamic testing may be omitted, it is first necessary to understand what urodynamic testing can tell us about bladder function.

ROLE OF CYSTOMETRY IN DIAGNOSING DETRUSOR OVERACTIVITY

Cystometry is the technique with which the pressure/volume relationship of the bladder is measured. In clinical practice, the goal of cystometry is to correlate changes in the pressure/volume relationship of the bladder with the patient's symptoms. Detrusor overactivity produces symptoms related to bladder storage, and therefore the cause of these symptoms is most likely to be uncovered by filling cystometry. Since the detrusor muscle in normal individuals should only contract volitionally, there should be no detectable detrusor activity during bladder filling. The detrusor should remain relaxed and quiescent until a socially acceptable time and place for bladder emptying, at which time the detrusor should contract in conjunction with voluntary relaxation of the pelvic floor, and that contraction should be sustained until the bladder is completely empty.

The pressure/volume relationship of the bladder is the scientific foundation upon which clinical cystometry rests. It can be represented as a filling and emptying cycle during which changes in volume and pressure occur (Figure 17-1). After the completion of a filling and emptying cycle, the empty bladder begins to refill as the next cycle begins. As it begins to fill, the bladder should increase in volume without an appreciable rise in bladder pressure (Figure 17-1, point 1). This occurs because the smooth muscle of the bladder relaxes to accommodate the increasing volume. As the bladder fills, tension-stretch receptors in the bladder wall signal the first conscious desire to void, usually at a volume between 150 and 250 ml (Figure 17-1, point 2). If a socially acceptable time and place is not present, the cerebral cortex is able to signal the detrusor to remain relaxed, blocking initiation of a micturition reflex (Figure 17-1, point 3). Such cortical suppression continues until bladder capacity is reached, usually between 350 and 650 ml for women. Then, when circumstances are appropriate

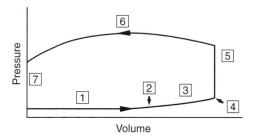

Figure 17-1. The micturition cycle presented as a pressure–volume plot with seven critical points. *1*, The normal bladder accommodates increasing urine volume without a significant increase in pressure. *2*, At around 200 ml the first sensation of bladder fullness is appreciated. *3*, This is mediated primarily by tension receptors within the bladder wall and not by increasing detrusor pressure. There then follows a period of voluntary postponement of micturition until voluntary voiding is initiated. *4*, Relaxation of the pelvic floor and urethra precedes initiation of a detrusor contraction. There is a short initial period of isometric detrusor contraction *5*, before the bladder neck opens. *6*, Normal voiding follows and is achieved by maintenance of a sustained and relatively constant detrusor contraction throughout the voiding phase. *7*, With the bladder completely empty, the voiding phase ends and the detrusor relaxes. Some patient may have a short "aftercontraction" as the detrusor continues to contract during bladder neck closure. The cycle then begins again. (From reference 4, with permission of Professor Stuart Stanton.)

socially, and only then, the normal individual can initiate a voluntary detrusor contraction to begin voiding (Figure 17-1, point 4). There is a short period of isometric detrusor contraction (longer in the male) as pressure builds up before the vesical neck and urethra are completely open (Figure 17-1, point 5), after which bladder volume decreases as a sustained detrusor contraction empties the bladder (Figure 17-1, point 6). Finally, flow ceases, the bladder neck closes, the pelvic floor regains its resting tone, and the detrusor relaxes as the cycle begins over again (Figure 17-1, point 7).

Simply put, uninhibited detrusor contractions represent an abnormal and premature shift of the bladder cycle from the filling (storage) phase to the emptying phase, with resultant involuntary loss of urine.

The two phases of the bladder cycle are evaluated clinically by using a cystometrogram. The cystometrogram is an attempt to reproduce the patient's symptoms under controlled clinical conditions while pressure measurements are made. It is nothing more than an attempt to reproduce the bladder cycle in the urodynamics laboratory.[3,36] However, the cystometrogram is not a "black box" into which a patient can be dropped in order to get a diagnosis as if by magic. A cystometrogram is not meaningful taken out of its clinical context. In many ways, a cystometrogram is merely an extension of the physical examination. Urodynamic results that do not reproduce the patient's complaint should always be regarded with suspicion.

Since the bladder is an intraabdominal organ, the pressure measured within the bladder is a summation of the abdominal forces surrounding the bladder and the intrinsic pressure generated by activity of the detrusor muscle. As a result, simple measurement of bladder pressure by itself may not always produce an accurate reflection of detrusor muscle activity.[37,38] A more precise evaluation of detrusor activity is given by calculating the "true", "subtracted", or "intrinsic" detrusor pressure, which is determined from the formula

$$P_{det} = P_{ves} - P_{abd}$$

where P_{det} is the detrusor pressure, P_{ves} is the pressure measured in the bladder, and P_{abd} is abdominal pressure, approximated clinically by using the pressure measured by a catheter placed in either the vagina or the rectum[39] (Figure 17-2). The bladder is filled while all pressures are measured simultaneously. During filling, there should be no detrusor activity. Continuous bladder filling uncovers more detrusor activity than does intermittent or incremental bladder filling.[40,41]

Cystometry can be performed using either gas or fluid as the filling medium. The use of carbon dioxide gas is popular because it is clean, economical, and easy to use, but it often produces false positive resultsults because of the high incidence of bladder irritation induced by the formation of carbonic acid.[42] Gas cystometry on rare occasions can produce a gas embolus, does not allow leakage of medium from the bladder to be detected, does not change bladder mass during filling, and prevents the performance of pressure-flow voiding studies.[3] We agree with Abrams[36] that "the CO_2 cystometer should become a relic of the urodynamic museum".

Cystometry, using a fluid such as water, is more physiological, minimizes artifactual irritation of the urothelium, allows leakage of bladder contents to be

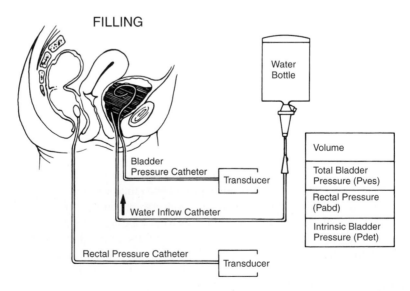

Figure 17-2.   Filling cystometry. Pressure catheters are in place in the bladder and rectum. An additional filling catheter has been placed in the bladder. Volume infused, total bladder pressure, rectal (abdominal) pressure, and subtracted detrusor pressure (intrinsic bladder pressure) are recorded. (From reference 3, with permission.)

observed, provides a better evaluation of bladder sensation (mass, temperature, etc.), and allows a clinical assessment of bladder emptying to be made. If radio-contrast material is used and the study is performed with fluoroscopy, the anatomy of the bladder and urethra can be visualized at the time of the study.[37] Cystometry can also be carried out using natural or provoked diuresis, further eliminating unphysiologic artifacts. If rapid diuresis is induced, the prevalence of detrusor instability appears to be greater and to occur at lower detrusor pressures in women with motor urge incontinence.[43]

The diagnosis of detrusor instability is made when symptomatic unstable phasic contractions are demonstrated during the filling (storage) phase of the cysto-metrogram, irrespective of their amplitude[4] (Figure 17-3). An earlier suggestion by the International Continence Society that these contractions reach a threshold of 15 cm of water to be significant has been abandoned[44] in light of the demonstration that "subthreshold" contractions can be significant.[45] Detrusor contractions that produce no symptoms are clinically irrelevant. A gradual increase in detrusor pressure during cystometery without phasic contractions represents low bladder

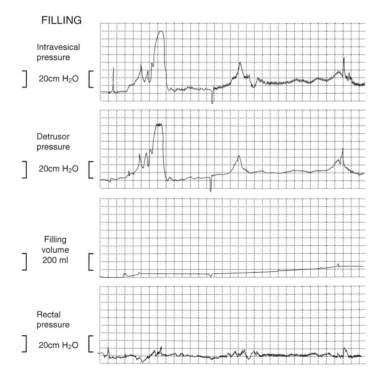

Figure 17-3. Subtracted filling cystometrogram showing uninhibited detrusor contractions. In this patient very little water has been infused into the bladder, which has nonetheless responded to filling by contracting briskly. Intravesical pressure and detrusor pressure both rise rapidly, while rectal pressure remains constant, demonstrating that the pressure rise is due to detrusor muscle contraction rather than abdominal straining.

compliance ($\Delta v/\Delta p$) rather than detrusor instability. Although these conditions are often confused with one another, they are not the same. Altered bladder compliance is often seen if the bladder is filled faster than it can accommodate, an artifact due to poor urodynamic technique that needs recognition for what it is rather than treatment for what it is not. If bladder filling is stopped in such cases, the detrusor pressure will fall progressively as bladder accommodation "catches up" with the volume of fluid that has been infused. In rare cases where the resting detrusor pressure is >40 cmH$_2$O, further investigation of the upper urinary tract is warranted, since pressures of this magnitude have been associated with deterioration of renal function in children with myelodysplasia.[46]

Because cystometry provides only a relatively a short-lived window on bladder function, it is important to realize that the investigator's comments can only be directed toward the results of a particular study. A "stable cystometrogram" where detrusor contractions are not demonstrated is not the same thing as a "stable bladder", since contractions may be present during other times and other circumstances. Just because uninhibited detrusor contractions have not been demonstrated during cystometry does not mean that they are not a problem for a particular patient. The relative lack of sensitivity of the standard cystometrogram in detecting detrusor activity has been emphasized by the research that has been done with continuous ambulatory urodynamic monitoring.

Ambulatory urodynamic studies performed by Bhatia and coworkers[47] revealed that abnormal detrusor contractions were present in many patients who had previously had stable cystometrograms. Kulseng-Hanssen and Klevmark[48] demonstrated detrusor instability in an additional 57% of patients compared to conventional stationary cystometry. Virtually all other authors have found similar results.[49–53] It appears that ambulatory urodynamic studies produce far more evidence of detrusor over activity than do conventional uro-dynamic studies. Heslington and Hilton[54,55] have found similar findings in asymptomatic volunteers, raising the question of whether or not some of these findings represent either artifact or bladder irritation from microtip transducer catheters used for several hours.

The experience of continuous ambulatory urodynamic monitoring, as well as that of studies that have evaluated cystometry in various positions or levels of physical activity, suggests that increased physical provocation during testing uncovers more detrusor instability than does static cystometry.[53,54] Petros and Ulmsten[56,57] performed a provocative handwashing test in patients with history of urge incontinence, and found it quite useful as a diagnostic test. Almost invariably urge symptoms were followed by a rise in detrusor pressure and a fall in urethral pressure, suggesting a premature activation of a micturition reflex. Geirsson and colleagues[58,59] used an "ice-water" infusion of the bladder as an adjunctive urodynamic test, and showed a significant correlation between abnormal bladder sensation on filling and inability to inhibit micturition in patients with overactive bladders. The normal, stable bladder should not contract despite ice-water provocation. Other adjunctive tests for detecting detrusor instability, such as acceleration of the flow rate and evaluation of detrusor contraction shortening times, and trigonal sensitivity testing, have not become popular.[60–62]

Creighton and coworkers[63] found distal urethral electrical conductance testing correlated well with the urodynamic diagnosis of detrusor instability. In this test an electrode placed in the urethra was able to detect minute opening of the bladder neck by detecting the ingress of urine from the bladder. Similar studies by Wyndaele,[64] who evaluated bladder fullness and its relationship to the electrical stimulation sensory threshold found that patients with detrusor instability perceived bladder fullness at lower volumes than did normal controls, but that the electrical stimulation threshold was the same in both groups and was independent of motor function.

If complex multichannel urodynamic studies are not available, simple urodynamic studies can still provide considerable useful diagnostic information. Sand and coworkers[41] concluded that standing retrograde incremental water cystometry done on two occasions is accurate in diagnosing detrusor instability in a population with a high prevalence of this condition. Fonda and coworkers[65] found that simple cystometry at the bedside had a 75% specificity and 88% sensitivity in diagnosing detrusor instability. Similarly, Wall and colleagues[66] compared the diagnostic efficacy of observing urine loss during simple bladder filling (without pressure measurement) and a cough stress test, with multichannel substracted cystometry. Urge incontinence that occurred during simple bladder filling proved to be a reliable predictor of detrusor instability with a 64% sensitivity, 86.8% specificity, 83.3% positive predictive value, and 70.2% negative predictive value. Even though the absence of detrusor instability was less reliable in excluding detrusor overactivity, simple bladder filling can replace complex urodynamic testing, particularly when the proposed treatment carries a low risk. In many cases, it is helpful in selecting patients who need more extensive evaluation.

Although some authors recommend performing urodynamic studies on all female patients with urinary incontinence,[67] we believe that a degree of clinical judgment is essential, particularly in a climate of increasingly limited resources in medicine. To a large extent, the importance of a precise diagnosis depends upon the possible consequences of the proposed therapy. We believe that a firm urodynamic diagnosis is important in patients who are contemplating surgery for their condition, but a patient who gives a coherent history of frequency, urgency, and urge incontinence—particularly if stress incontinence cannot be demonstrated clinically—can probably be given a trial of medical and behavioral therapy for her condition without the expense of a full urodynamic evaluation. Once diagnosed, the unstable detrusor will remain qualitatively unstable over a prolonged period of time (up to 8 years) if followed with serial cystometry and left untreated.[68]

ETIOLOGY

The cause of detrusor instability remains unknown. Bladder function is controlled by a complex and poorly understood neural system that includes the cerebral cortex, brainstem, spinal cord, sacral micturition center, and peripheral nerves innervating the bladder. Any defects, congenital or acquired, structural or metabolic, within this network can affect bladder functioning.[69] In the majority of cases, no neurologic cause can be discovered for the detrusor overactivity, but patients with urinary incontinence should be screened for occult neuropathology, since the consequences of these conditions can be significant.

The prevalence of urinary incontinence increases dramatically with age, and urge incontinence due to bladder overactivity is the main cause of incontinence in the elderly. Del Carro and associates[70] subjected patients with detrusor instability and age-matched controls to to extensive neurophysiological tests. All patients had normal tests without significant difference, suggesting the absence of damage to central sensory or motor pathways in detrusor instability, but alteration of suprasegmental mechanisms could not be excluded. Parys and co-workers[71] studied the sacral reflex latencies in women presenting with an onset of bladder dysfunction since undergoing a simple hysterectomy. While detrusor instability was diagnosed in 47% compared to controls, 80% showed abnormal nerve conduction.

The bladder is innervated by the sympathetic hypogastric nerve and the parasympathetic pelvic nerve. The striated urethral sphincter receives efferent innervations from the pudendal nerve. It is plausible to postulate that detrusor overactivity is due, at least in part, to some disorder of neuroregulation, possibly involving neurotransmitters or neuromodulators. Sympathetic control of the bladder is exercised theough α-adrenergic receptors, which are found pre-dominately in the urethra and the bladder base, and by β-adrenergic receptors in the bladder body that mediate detrusor relaxation. Bladder biopsy studies suggest that there may be an increased density of adrenergic receptors in patients with detrusor instability. Beyond the principal neurotransmitters, nonadrenergic noncholinergic neuromodulators also appear to be involved in detrusor control through the actions of peptide-containing nerves. For example, vasoactive intestinal polypeptide (VIP), a powerful smooth muscle relaxant, has been found in the normal bladders in abundance but appears to be markedly decreased in overactive bladders. VIP may act to reduce the basal detrusor tension and spon-taneous activity in the bladder filling phase, suggesting a deficiency predisposes patients with this condition to develop detrusor overactivity.[72] Supporting evidence for the activity of other neuromodulators such arginine vasopression has not been forthcoming,[73] however endogenous opiods do appear to play a role in lower urinary tract control. Administration of naloxone, an opioid antagonist, causes a rise in detrusor pressure along with decreases in bladder capacity and urethral closure pressure.[74] Intravenous administration of apomorphine appears to induce a hyperactive bladder response in anesthetized rats by stimulating brainstem and spinal cord micturition centers.[75] The neurochemistry of detrusor control remains an area in which much additional research is required.

Prostaglandins may also be involved in involuntary detrusor muscle activity. Bergman and colleagues[76] studied prostaglandin production in detrusor muscle biopsies from women with idiopathic detrusor instability. Prostaglandin F_2-α and the stable metabolites of prostacyclin (6-keto-prostaglandin F_1-α) and thromboxane-A_2 (thromboxane-B_2) were measured after *in vitro* incubations. A significant reduction of 6-keto-prostaglandin F_1-α without differences in the production of prostaglandin F_2-α and thromboxane-B_2 suggest that deficient prostacyclin production may be involved in detrusor instability.

The relationship of inflammatory bladder responses such as those that are seen in patients with interstitial cystitis to detrusor overactivity has rarely been investigated. Histamine provokes detrusor contractions in *in vitro* preparations, leading Moore and coworkers[77] to assess mast cell counts in patients with refractory instability. Elevated mast cell counts were found in 29% of these patients. The significance of these findings remains unclear, but it may suggest that some overactive bladders are more sensitive to irritating substances in the urine. Creighton and Stanton[78] investigated the effects of 200 mg of caffeine citrate on the cystometrograms of women with proven detrusor instability and asymptomatic controls. The group with detrusor instability showed a statistically significant increase in detrusor pressure on filling after caffeine administration, but no difference in volume at first sensation, height of contraction or capacity. Caffeine produced no abnormalities in the cystometrograms of asymptomatic normal women. Kieswetter[79] found that women with urgency syndromes had lower electrical sensitivity thresholds that did normal controls, and Creighton and colleagues[80] found that women with sensory urgency or detrusor instability had similarly abnormal perceptions of bladder fullness and maximal bladder capacity than controls.

Jeffcoate and Francis[9] pointed out the importance of the social environment in the development of normal bladder control. They suggested that "functional bladder disturbances commonly affect more than one member of a family and are *acquired by example*". Others have taken the other side of the "nature" vs "culture" debate. Birch and Miller[81] studied the familial incidence of primary nocturnal enuresis and found a significant genetic component among twins. They described a family of adults with detrusor overactivity that spanned three generations, and suggested that, in some cases, the overactive detrusor followed an autosomal dominant inheritance pattern. In other cases, detrusor instability may simply be due to a failure of final maturation of cortical control over the micturition reflex.[82]

On a more simple scale, it should not be forgotten that acute urinary tract infections can mimic the symptoms of detrusor instability or indeed cause unstable detrusor contractions themselves.[83] Chronic infection is unlikely to cause detrusor instability; it is more likely that patients with detrusor instability are carelessly diagnosed as having "chronic cystitis".[10] Local irritation or stimuli increases the sensitivity of the bladder sensory nerve endings causing abnormal stimulation responses like urgency and frequency.[9]

Outflow obstruction is commonly suspected as a cause of detrusor instability in men. Strips of detrusor muscle from patients with obstruction and detrusor overactivity showed an increased sensitivity to acetylcholine *in vitro* when compared to detrusor muscle strips from patients with obstruction but without documented destrusor instability. Harrison and colleagues[84] postulated that outflow obstruction might cause subsequent nerve damage and detrusor instability. Unless they have undergone previous bladder neck suspension surgery, outflow obstruction is rare in women and this is unlikely to be a cause of detrusor instability in most females with this condition.

On the other hand, several studies have noted the presence of urethral relaxation or electrical silence of the pelvic floor just prior to the start of an uninhibited detrusor contraction.[56,58] It is unclear if this is a "trigger" mechanism, the first coordinated response of a prematurely activated bladder micturition reflex, or an entirely unrelated event. McGuire[85] showed that this could occur in incontinent patients with acontractile bladders after overdistention. Koonings and Bergman[86] observed two groups of women with detrusor instability who had a drop in urethral pressure before or after a detrusor contraction. They concluded that women who had urethral relaxation before the detrusor contraction had a different pathophysiology from "classic detrusor instability", since 88% of these women did not improve with anticholinergic therapy. They proposed treating them with α-agonists as well, with some success. Similarly, Wise and co-workers[87] found that 42% of patients with detrusor instability had a spontaneous fall in maximum urethral pressure of at least one-third over a 2-minute period. They suggested that these patients had primary urethral dysfunction as a cause of their symptoms, and proposed treating them with an α-adrenergic agonist in addition to, or instead of anticholinergic therapy, to enhance urethral closure.

In some patients coital activity provokes urgency and sometimes urge incontinence, particularly with orgasm. Hilton[88] noted an increased prevalence of detrusor instability in women who complained of urinary incontinence with orgasm. Such patients may have aberrant innervation or abnormalities of neuromodulators that activate a reflex micturition pathway through parasympathetic activity at the time of sexual climax. Not surprisingly, this phenomenon has been difficult to study, but the phenomenon has been reproduced in the urodyanamics laboratory.[89]

An open or incompetent bladder neck has often been suggested as a precipitating cause of uninhibited detrusor activity. The distal urethral electrical conductance studies mentioned above suggest that subtle bladder neck opening correlates well with urinary urgency, but Sutherst and Brown[90] were unable to provoke a detrusor contraction by rapidly infusing saline into the posterior urethra.

The role of generalized pelvic muscular weakness in the genesis of detrusor instability was studied by Penders and coworkers[91] in a group of patients who had unstable detrusors, pelvic floor hypotonia, and stress urinary incontinence with normal urethral closure. These patients improved through pelvic muscle rehabilitation therapy. Patients with mixed incontinence often seem to improve symptoms of both stress and urge incontinence with therapy of this kind, suggesting some kind of neuromuscular synergism in mixed conditions.[92]

In short, though there are many theories about detrusor overactivity, and while there is some experimental evidence in support of each theory, the vast majority of clinical cases do not have a clear etiology. Although known relevant neurologic causes can be found for some cases of detrusor overactivity, the etiology of most cases remains unknown and subject only to speculation. We suspect that further research will reveal that there are many different factors contributing to this frustrating clinical condition.

EPIDEMIOLOGY

As with other forms of urinary incontinence, patient embarassment about the condition and the general inattentiveness of physicians in addressing the problem have led to serious under reporting of the scope and magnitude of the problem of detrusor overactivity. Turner-Warwick[2] estimated that some form of detrusor instability affected up to 10% of the population between the ages of 10 and 50. The prevalence of detrusor instability ranges from 9% to 55% according to the population studied. In patients who have undergone previous unsuccessful surgery for stress incontinence, the prevalence of detrusor instability is also variable, but tends to be high. In all studies of female urinary incontinence detrusor overactivity is a major contributing cause. At least 25% of patients with neurological impairment will have detrusor overactivity, and for conditions such as multiple sclerosis or Parkinson's disease, the prevalance of detrusor hyperreflexia is between 70% and 95%.[93,94] Among patients with a history of childhood nocturnal enuresis, there is a link with later detrusor instability, but this appears to be higher for males than for females.[95]

The prevalence of detrusor instability increases with age, increasing after the menopause to become a major cause of suffering and disability among the elderly. Incontinence is a major precipitating event for nursing home admissions, and is very common in long-term care facilities.[96] In a clinical and cystometric study of non instutionalized elderly women, Diokno and colleagues[97] reported a prevalence of detrusor instability of 4.9% among continent and a prevalence of 12.2% among incontinent elderly women. This is probably the best estimate of the overall prevalence of detrusor overactivity in community-dwelling elderly women to date.

Many workers have suspected that there is a link between detrusor instability and mental instability in women, since many of these patients seem to have high degrees of neuroticism. In generally, carefully done studies have not given much support to this hypothesis. Macaulay and coworkers[98] found that women with detrusor instability were anxious and lacked self-esteem, as did women with sensory urgency. The patients with detrusor instability appeared to be as depressed as a control group of psychiatric inpatients. Moore and Sutherst[99] found that patients with detrusor instability responded better to medical therapy if they had lower psychoneurotic scores, but Walters and colleagues[100] did not find any difference in personality between women with detrusor instability and genuine stress incontinence on the Minnesota Multiphasic Personality Inventory, but compared to continent controls, women with detrusor instability had higher scores for hypochondriasis, depression, and hysteria. These authors concluded that psychosexual abnormalities were associated more with incontinence in general than with detrusor instability in particular.

Women with detrusor instability represent a diverse population with a wide variety of symptoms and urodynamic findings. Women with mixed incontinence, for example, may represent a distinct subpopulation with characteristics different from those women who have incontinence on the basis of pure detrusor instability.[101] Further research that attempts to describe other discrete subpopulations of patients with detrusor instability may improve our understanding of this troublesome clinical problem.

TREATMENT

Treatment approaches for patients with detrusor overactivity fall into four major categories: behavioral intervention, drug therapy, electrical stimulation, and surgery. Use of any one of these management strategies is not exclusive; indeed, it is our experience that these patients often need multiple forms of therapy in order to obtain the best results. In practical terms, behavioral modification and drug therapy are the treatments that are most likely to be practical for the average clinician in practice. Electrical stimulation and specialized denervation surgery at present are most appropriately employed in a tertiary level university research setting.

Behavorial Management

The rationale for behavioral therapy is that most cases of idiopathic detrusor instability are due to loss of previously established cortical control of voiding. The purpose of bladder behavior modification is to reestablish cortical control and to reestablish a normal voiding pattern. In essence, bladder behavioral modification programs are refresher courses in "potty training" for adults. These programs may be combined with pharmacologic therapy and patient counseling if other stressful life situations are part of the overall clinical picture.

"Bladder drill" is the most common way in which bladder retraining is accomplished. It involves placing patients on a rigid timed voiding schedule in which the intervals between voids are gradually increased until a normal voiding pattern has been achieved (every 2 to 3 hours). The process is simply, straightforward, and effective. It works for patients with motor urge incontinence or sensory urgency. In a motivated and cooperative patient, the symptoms of urgency, frequency, and urge incontinence can be controlled effectively and fairly quickly, and for long periods of time.

It works like this. The patient is instructed to empty her bladder upon awakening, and then to void at set intervals throughout the day. Initially, the interval between voids is about 1 hour; in some patients it may be necessary to start with voids as often as every 30 minutes. Patients must only void at the scheduled times, whether or not they feel the urge to urinate. Once they have managed the initial schedule for 1 week, the interval between voids is increased by 15 minutes, and increased by a similar interval of time each week until they have reached an interval between voids of about 2.5 hours. A frequency/volume bladder diary provides documentation of voiding patterns and can be used to reinforce the patient's motivation for bringing her errant bladder back under voluntary control. Verbal instruction should be accompanied by a written protocol and frequent encouragement for the physician and supportive nursing personnel.

Frewen[102] was the first to report on the results of a bladder drill training regimen in women with urge incontinence. Initially he hospitalized patients for a 10-day course of intensive behavioral training and concurrent drug therapy, but subsequently moved to an outpatient program of bladder drill that produced a symptomatic cure in 87% of his patients. These success rates have been maintained for up to 6 years in motivated patients—but motivation is the key. The validity and usefulness of behavioral modification regimens of this kind have been repeated and published in many reports.[103] Concurrent drug therapy does not reduce the number of incontinent episodes but might be superior in reducing frequency due to detrusor instability in the very elderly people.[104] Whether or not concurrent drug therapy is used, enthusiastic reassurance and long-term support enhance the effectiveness of therapy and contribute to patient compliance with the regimen. When used on an outpatient basis, the cost of therapy is minimal. Fantl and coworkers[92] have recommended that bladder training should be part of the initial treatment of all women with urinary incontinence, a sentiment with which we do not disagree.

A number of other behavioral interventions have been recommended for women with detrusor instability, including psychotherapy, hypnosis, acupuncture, and biofeedback.[103] Of these, the only therapy that appears to be clinically useful is biofeedback, in which the patient learns to suppress detrusor contractions by manipulating an auditory or visual signal. Biofeedback regimens are labor-intensive and require the use of specialized equipment, but appear to be effective. Audiotaped pelvic-floor muscle exercises are also effective in women with urge, stress or mixed incontinence.[105]

Drug Therapy

Patients who are unable or who are unwilling to participate in a behavioral modification program can be treated pharmacologically. For example, patients with neuropathic detrusor overactivity may be improved by a timed-voiding regimen, but rarely respond completely to behavioral therapy alone. These patients, as well as patients who are not motivated enough to pursue bladder drill resolutely, often benefit from drug therapy.

Numerous pharmacologic agents have been used to treat detrusor overactivity. All of these agents interfere in some manner to alter the control of bladder contractility. This may be done by altering control in the central nervous system; by blocking the action of acetylcholine (the main neurotransmitter involved in detrusor contractility); by a direct relaxant effect on smooth muscle; or by regulating other substances that are believed to modulate bladder control. The major pharmacologic categories of these drugs are anticholinergics, spasmolytics, tricyclic antidepressants, calcium antagonists, prostaglandin synthetase inhibitors, and a variety of drugs used in small series of clinical trials that constitute little more than anectodal information about their utility or lack thereof. Table 17-1 shows the drugs used most commonly in the treatment of detrusor instability.

Table 17.1.   Drugs most useful in the treatment of detrusor overactivity

Drug	Dosage
Oxybutynin chloride	2.5–10 mg by mouth 3–4 times per day
Propantheline bromide	15–30 mg by mouth 3–4 times per day
Dicyclomine	20 mg by mouth 3–4 times per day
Hyoscyamine sulfate	0.125–0.25 mg by mouth 3–5 times per day
Imipramine hydrochloride	10–25 mg by mouth 2–3 times per day

Anticholinergic Drugs

Acetylcholine is the main neurotransmitter involved in bladder contraction and in the functioning of many other organ systems. The prototypical anticholinergic drug is atropine, a belladonna alkaloid with competitive antimuscarinic activity. For a variety of pharmaologic reasons, it has not been possible to develop an anticholinergic drug that acts exclusively on the bladder. Therefore, all anticholinergic drugs used to treat detrusor overactivity (including most of the drugs listed as "spasmolytics", "tricyclic antidepressants", or "calcium antagonists") have generalized anticholinergic properties that produce common—indeed, expected—side-effects, including development of a "dry-mouth" due to suppression of salivary and oropharyngeal secretions; "constipation" due to decreased gastrointestinal motility; an increase in heart rate due to vagal blockade; and transient "blurred vision" due to inhibition of the sphincter of the iris and the ciliary muscles of the lens of the eye. Drugs with anticholinergic properties should not be prescribed for patients with narrow-angle glaucoma, and must be used cautiously in patients with significant cardiac arrhythmias.

Belladona was first proposed to control urinary urgency and frequency in 1936. Problems with the potency of atropine led to develop synthetic quaternary ammonium analogs, which interfere with nicotinic ganglion transmission as well as with muscarinic receptors, but have fewer side effects. Methantheline bromide, initially used in the treatment of peptic ulcer disease, was discovered to lead to urinary retention in some patients, and explorations of its effectiveness as a urinary drug followed. Propantheline bromide (Pro-Banthine; Searle) was then developed as a more potent agent with fewer side effects. Two other quaternary ammonium compounds have been used widely in Europe: emepronium bromide, and emepronium carrageenate. Both drugs have gradually been withdrawn from the European market and probably will not become available in the United States. Scopolamine has been used in the treatment of detrusor instability, but has been found to be not tolerated well, even when used transdermally.[106] Hyoscyamine derivatives, which have long been available as anticholinergic-drugs, are currently marketed with some enthusiasm for the treatment of detrusor instability. Since these drugs were already available there has been little interest by drug companies or clinicians in evaluating them in clinical trials to assess their objective effectivenss in treating urge incontinence.

Spasmolytics

Spasmolytics are drugs that have a direct relaxant effect on smooth muscle. In spite of their being classified in this manner, all of them posess significant anticholinergic properties. The most common drugs are flavoxate hydrochloride (Urispas; Smith, Kline, and French), oxybutynin chloride (Ditropan; Marion) and dicyclomine hydrochloride (Bentyl; Lakeside).

Flavoxate hydrochloride is a smooth muscle relaxant with analgesic and local anesthetic effects. It inhibits phosphodiesterase activity and increases intracellular adenosine monophosphate, a mediator of smooth muscle relaxation. In general, this drug has been disappointing and rarely appears to be useful clinically.[108]

Oxybutynin chloride is a tertiary amine compound with a strong musculo-tropic antispasmodic and local anesthetic effects. In addition, it possesses moderate anticholinergic and antihistaminic properties. It is rapidly absorbed, and almost completely metabolized when given orally, with a wide margin of safety. Of all of the drugs currently available for suppressing detrusor con-tractility, it appears to be the most powerful and has been found to be as effective as, or superior to, propantheline both in objective cystometric studies as well as in subjective patient response to treatment.[107] Unfortunately, oxybutynin brings with it a high incidence of side effects that many patients find intolerable for more than short periods of time.

Dicyclomine hydrochloride acts as a competitive antagonist of acetylcholine at muscarinic receptor sites. It has been used in the treatment of a variety of gastrointestinal disorders including irritable bowl syndrome. Although dicyclomine has been found to be effective in relieving symptoms of frequency, urgency, and urge incontinence in women with detrusor instability,[109] it has never become popular in the treatment of urge incontinence.

Tricyclic Antidepressants

Tricyclic antidepressants are a heterologous group of compounds that share a three-ring molecular core and have similar therapeutic effects in the treatment of depression.[103] Imipramine (Tofranil; Ciba-Geigy), a dibenzazepine derivative, is the oldest, best-studied prototype of this class, which now includes desipramine, amitryptiline, nortryptiline, and doxepin. It remains unclear precisely how these drugs works on the central nervous system, but they appear to potentiate the action of biogenic amines by blocking their reuptake at nerve terminals. These compounds have anticholinergic, spasmolytic, and local anesthetic actions on the bladder.

Imipramine has long been used in the treatment of nocturnal enuresis in children. It is the most common tricyclic antidepressant used in the treatment of detrusor instability. It is especially useful to add if nightime symptoms are part of the patient's complaints. It also seems to have an additive effect when used in conjunction with other drugs, and its effectiveness may be enhanced by behavioral therapy.[110] The usual oral dose is in the range of 10 to 25 mg t.i.d., 25 to 50 mg b.i.d., or up to 100 mg as a single dose at night. These doses are much lower than those used in treating clinical depression. The amount needed should be titrated to the patient's symptoms. The initial dose should be low, and should be increased gradually.

The tricyclic antidepressants have similar anticholinergic side effects. They may cause sedation, drowsiness, and confusion. The tricyclics can produce significant cardiovascular side effects including orthostatic hypotension and conduction disturbances with bundle branch block. They should be used cautiously in patients who have preexisting cardiovascular disease.

Calcium Channel Blockers

The entry of calcium ions from the extracellular space is an important step in the excitation and contraction of any muscle, and this holds true as well for the activation of urinary bladder smooth muscle. Drugs that inhibit the influx of calcium ions may therefore play a role in the treatment of detrusor instability. For example, the antihypertensive and antianginal drug nifedipine (Procardia; Pfizer) has been shown to improve symptoms, to increase bladder capacity, and to reduce the frequency and amplitude of uninhibited detrusor contractions in women with detrusor instability.[111] Similar results have been obtained using other calcium antagonists such as verapamil and flunzarizine.[112,113]

More promising results were obtained using terodiline hydrochloride (Mictrol; Kabi-Vitrum), a calcium-channel blocker with antimuscarinic anticholinergic activity, originally developed in Scandinavia as an antianginal agent. This drug had some popularity in the late 1980s in the treatment of detrusor instability due to its long half-life (60 hours), combined anticholinergic and calcium antagonist effects, low serum clearance and almost complete absorption. It could be given in doses of 12.5–25 mg b.i.d. and even only once per day in many cases, giving it a great advantage over the shorter-acting and poorly absorbed anticholinergic preparations, even though it took up to 10 days to achieve steady-state serum levels. Several studies showed[114–123] that terodiline decreased frequency of urination and incontinent episodes in a wide range of patients, and the drug promised to be of great potential benefit to incontinent patients.

The side effects of terodiline were related primarily to its anticholinergic and calcium antagonist properties, but these were generally less severe than with the other agents used for detrusor overactivity. Unfortunately, the drug was withdrawn from the European market prior to its introduction into the United States after several patients with preexisting cardiac disease develop serious cardiac arrhythmias.[124] A reformulated version of the drug may eventually become available.

Prostaglandin Synthetase Inhibitors

Prostaglandins are biochemical intermediaries in many physiological processes and human tissues, including the bladder. *In vitro* studies have shown that prostaglandins can make isolated strips of bladder muscle contract[125] suggesting that they could play a role in patients with detrusor instability. A small number of clinical studies have shown that these drugs may have some usefulness, but the overall results have been disappointing and the incidence of side effects has been high.[103] One group of patients who may benefit from prostaglandin synthetase inhibitors are women with irritable bladder symptoms around the time of menstruation. Wall and Warrell[126] reported an otherwise asymptomatic patient who suffered from cyclic urge incontinence that began with the onset of menstruation. She was cured of her symptoms by taking mefenamic acid (Ponstel; Parke-Davis) 500 mg orally b.i.d. for 7 days, starting 3 days before menstruation. The authors suggested that this patient had a low-compliance bladder that was precipitated into detrusor instability by perimenstrual prostaglandin synthesis and release. Since many women seem to have irritative bladder symptoms around the time of menstruation, this condition may prove to be more prevalent than is currently suspected.

Estrogens

Cytological studies of urine sediment have shown correlations between the estrogen status of vaginal epithelial cells and cells present in the bladder and urethra.[127] Estrogen receptors have been identified in the female lower urinary tract,[128] prominent in the urethra but rare in the trigone and bladder body. Detrusor instability is more prevalent in the elderly and irritable bladder symptoms are common in the postmenopausal women. The possibility of a link between estrogen deprivation and detrusor instability suggests that estrogen replacement therapy may be useful in postmenopausal women with lower urinary tract symptoms.[129,130] For example, estorgen therapy appears to enhance the response of the female urethra to α-adrenergic stimulation, a fact which has a potential role in the conservative management of stress incontinence.[131–133] While there is no data that really shows any appreciable effect of estrogen on detrusor funcgtion, estrogen therapy does appear to be beneficial for women with atrophic urethritis and sensory urgency.[134] It may therefore play an indirect role in managing patients with unstable bladders by decreasing sensory "triggers" in some patients and by enhancing the quality of life by decreasing local irritation.

Miscellaneous Drugs

A variety of other drugs have been tried with variable success rates in the treatment of detrusor instability. Among the drugs that have been tried clinically are baclofen, bromocriptine, β-agonists, dimethylsulfoxide, prazosin, mazindol, lignocaine, propiverine, pinacidil, and cromakalin.[135–146] None of these drugs has been used in enough patients or with enough efficacy to suggest that they have a place in the current clinical management of patients with detrusor overactivity.

Electrical Stimulation

The fact that muscle contracts when stimulated by an electrical current led to the idea that continuous or intermittent low-voltage electrical stimulation of the pelvic floor might have a role in treating patients with urinary incontinence. Experimental evidence suggests that intravaginal electrical stimulation activates inhibitory nerve fibers in the sympathetic hypogastric nerve while inhibiting parasympathetic excitatory neurones in the pelvic nerve.[147] This creates a reflex inhibition of detrusor function, and provided the impetus for examining the role of electrical stimulation in the treatment of detrusor instability.

The electrical stimulus is delivered through "plug" electrodes, usually through the vagina, sometimes through the rectum.[103] The precise mechanism of action is unclear, but it seems probable that prolonged electrical stimulation leads to "reeducation" by a neuronal reorganization at a central or peripheral level that results in the restoration of normal reflex patterns.[148]

The main difficulty with electrical stimulation therapy is poor patient acceptance of the devices needed to supply the electrical current to the pelvic floor and bladder. The devices must be worn intravaginally or intrarectally for several hours each day, if not continuously. Many patients reject them for psychological or aesthetic reasons. Attempts have been made to overcome this problem by experimenting with intermittent stimulation regimens, with mixed results.[103,149] At the present time electrical stimulation appears to be most useful as adjunctive therapy in the armamentarium of specialized centers that deal with large numbers of complicated patients and who are capable of evaluating such patients on clinical research protocols.

Surgical Treatment

In rare cases, detrusor overactivity can be treated surgically. Surgical treatment is not appropriate as a first-line therapy, but may be indicated in carefully selected patients who have failed more conservative attempts at managing their incontinence. The surgical procedures used in the treatment of this condition are designed to improve continence by inhibiting the bladder's contractile capabilities, either by denervating the bladder or by augmenting its capacity.[150,151] Many patients who might be candidates for these procedures have significant neurologic disorders that require specialist care. The surgical treatment of detrusor overactivity should only be undertaken in specialist centers that are used to dealing with complex cases and that are prepared to deal with the complications of these operations, which can be significant.

The least invasive form of surgical treatment for detrusor instability is bladder distension under anesthesia. This form of therapy was first used in 1972 by Helmstein, who tried to treat bladder carcinoma by hydrodistension.[103] The idea was that overdistension of the bladder would cause tissue anoxia by reducing the blood flow to the tumor cells, which were thought to be more susceptible than the healthy bladder tissues. It was also felt that this technique could cause partial denervation of the bladder. Under conduction anesthesia, the bladder was distended for several hours to a pressure that approximated the patient's systolic blood pressure. While early reports showed encouraging results but most other series have not suggested comparable levels of improvement. The technique does not appear to benefit patients with neuropathic detrusor hyperreflexia, and some patients have been made worse. There is about an 8% chance of bladder rupture with this technique,[152] and at least one reported death due to a myocardial infarction after the procedure.[153] Despite attempts to modify the technique, it has not proven particularly helpful in managing most cases of detrusor instability.[103,154]

Another therapy that enjoyed transient popularity was bladder denervation using subtrigonal injections of 6% aqueous phenol under cystoscopic guidance. Although short-term follow-up in the initial series was encouraging, the long-term results have been disappointing, and several fistulae have resulted as complications. This technique has largely been abandoned as a result.[103,155,156]

Other surgical attempts at bladder denervation have included selective blockade of the sacral nerves, selective sacral neurectomy, and transvaginal denervation by resection of the inferior hypogastric nerve plexus along the inferior vesical artery at the bladder base.[157–159] None of these techniques has been used extensively.

Direct operations on the bladder have been used to treat detrusor overactivity as well. Turner-Warwick and Ashken[160] pioneered a bladder transection operation described as "cystocystoplasty" in which the entire bladder was transected above the level of the trigone and ureteric orifices in order to sever its nerve supply but leave the sensation of the trigone intact.[161] Modifications using posterolateral transections or endoscopic resections have been tried,[162,163] but the effectiveness of these procedures remains uncertain.

The most successful surgical procedures for intractable detrusor contractility involve augmentation cystoplasty. In these cases the bladder is opened and its capacity is increased by sewing a segment of cecum, ileum, or stomach into the bladder, increasing its capacity while at the same time introducing a non-contracile segment that acts as a "damper" on involuntary bladder contractions when they do occur. This resolves the problem in many cases; however, many of these patients continue to have difficulty with bladder emptying, electrolyte imbalance, mucus production in the bladder from the gastrointestinal segment that has been interposed into the bladder, and persistent contractile activity of the bowel segment.[164,165] In rare cases, complete urinary diversion using any one of number of sophisticated reconstructive procdures might be considered.[166]

MANAGEMENT OF MIXED INCONTINENCE

Detrusor instability often coexists with genuine stress incontinence. Precise preoperative cystometric diagnosis should confirm the diagnosis to avoid "failures" from selecting patients improperly for surgery. In general, the presence of concurrent detrusor instability is a poor prognostic factor in the success of operations for stress incontinence. Detrusor instability can resolve postoperatively, but it may also worsen. Sometimes it arises *de novo* in a previously asymptomatic patient. In patients with mixed symptomatology, it is often unclear how much of their problem is due to which component of their bladder dysfunction. As a clinical rule of thumb, it is important to try to determine which component bothers the patient more before therapy is undertaken, and to treat the worst symptom first, usually with conservative therapy.

Generally speaking, the outcome of surgery for stress incontinence in patients with mixed incontinence is poorer than the outcome of surgery in patients whose only problem is genuine stress incontinence. Therefore, it seems prudent to offer most patients with mixed incontinence a trial of conservative therapy for detrusor instability and reassess their situation in a month or two.[167] Some patients will improve; in these cases nothing further will often need to be done. Patients who do not have an optimal response can then be offered an attempt at surgical correction of the anatomical defect responsible for their stress incontinence, such as urethral hypermobility or intrinsic sphincteric deficiency. McGuire[168] suggested that large numbers of patients who had mixed incontinence and were cured of their stress incontinence by surgery also reported that their urge incontinence went away postoperatively as well. However, it is important to appreciate that there are few reliable urodynamic predictors of success of failure in these cases, and that some patients' symptoms of urgency, frequency, and urge incontinence get considerably worse after an operation.[169]

CONCLUSIONS AND RECOMMENDATIONS

The initial evaluation of any woman suspected of having detrusor overactivity does not differ from the initial evaluation of any woman with incontinence in general. She should have a thorough and detailed medical history taken from her, with special attention paid to the nature, duration, and ranking of her symptoms. She should have a complete physical examination, including a neurological screening examination. An attempt should be made to demonstrate incontinence in women with this complaint, particularly the presence of stress incontinence. The urine should be examined and, where appropriate, sent for culture and/or cytology. After voiding, the amount of residual urine should be measured. If the residual urine volume is elevated, this should be treated by placing the patient on a regimen of clean intermittent self-catheterization, after which her symptoms should be reevaluated. As a general rule, all incontinent patients should be encouraged to keep a frequency-volume bladder chart for at least 24 hours. Patients with documented frequency, urgency, urge incontinence and a small functional bladder capacity can be presumed to have an overactive bladder. Once this basic body of information has been obtained, we believe that a number of clinical decisions can be made without the need to undertake full urodynamic studies.

Women with complaints of urinary frequency and urgency *but without incontinence* rarely benefit from urodynamic studies. These women should probably undergo cystourethroscopy to rule out a bladder or urethral lesion, but in the absence of a positive finding, most of these women can be treated using some form of bladder retraining.

Women who say that their primary complaint is urge incontinence can be treated with a combination of bladder drill and anticholinergic drugs, particularly if stress incontinence is not a complaint or if stress incontinence cannot be demonstrated on physical examination. The vast majority of these patients will improve within 4–6 weeks on the conservative regimen mentioned above. If not, they may be candidates for further evaluation using urodynamic studies. The mainstay of treatment in these patients should be bladder retraining, supplemented with the minimum amount of pharmacologic agent needed to treat their symptoms. Patients should be encouraged to titrate the dose of drug needed freely and on their own. The medications used for detrusor overactivity are safe and the maximum tolerated dose is limited by side effects more often than any serious drug toxicity. The physician should encourage this for the simple reason that patients will do this anyway; virtually no one takes anticholinergic drugs at high doses for long periods of time because the side effects are so unpleasant. Doctors should learn to take advantage of this inevitable fact to bring their patients into partnership with them in treating this condition.

Patients with neuropathic detrusor hyperreflexia are less suited for behavioral treatment and usually require long-term anticholinergic therapy combined with timed-voiding regimens. In these patients the purpose of the timed-voiding program is to keep the bladder volume below the threshold that triggers a detrusor contraction, rather than to reestablish cortical control of volitional voiding. Many of these patients will also require a program of intermittent catheterization to eliminate the elevated residual urine volumes that are common in patients with neurologic disease.

Because the need for precise diagnostic knowledge is largely dependent upon the risks of the proposed treatment, we tend to reserve urodynamic studies for patients who are potential surgical candidates, such as patients who have a major complaint of stress incontinence, those in whom stress incontinence is demonstrable, or those patients whose clinical presentation is confusing. Where mixed incontinence is documented, we usually prefer to treat the urge component first to see what response is obtained, before undertaking surgery. Since cystometry is not 100% accurate in picking up patients with detrusor instability, caution should still be used in treating patients with stress incontinence who give a strong history of urgency and urge incontinence as well.

Patients with refractory urge incontinece who cannot be managed successfully using behavioral therapy or one or two pharmacologic agents may benefit from referral to a tertiary care center where other treatment modalities are available. Only a small percentage of patients are appropriate candidates for surgical bladder denervation or augmentation cystoplasty.

REFERENCES

1. Hodgkinson CP, Ayers MA, Drukker BH. Dyssynergic detrusor dysfunction in the apparently normal female. *Am J Obstet Gynecol* 1963; **87**: 717.
2. Turner-Warwick RT. Observations on the function and dysfunction of the sphincter and detrusor mechanism. *Urol Clin North Am* 1979; **6**: 13.
3. Wall LL, Addison WA. Basic cystometry in gynecologic practice. *Postgrad Obstet Gynecol* 1988; **8(Suppl 26)**: 1.
4. Abrams P, Blaivas JG, Stanton SL, Standardization of terminology of lower urinary tract function. *Neurourol Urodynam* 1988; **7**: 403.
5. Turner-Warwick RT, Milroy EJ. A reappraisal of the value of routine urological procedures in the assessment of urodynamic function. Symposium on clinical urodynamics. *Urol Clin North Am* 1979; **6**: 63.
6. George NJR, Barnard RJ, Blacklock NJ. Frequency/volume charts revealing physiological abnormalities. *Proceedings of the Eleventh Annual Meeting of the International Continence Society*, 1981: 67–68.
7. Cooper CE. Giggle micturition. *Clin Dev Med*. Heineman, London 1973; **48/49**: 61–65.
8. Glahn BE. Giggle incontinence (enuresis risoria): A study and an aetiological hypothesis. *Br J Urol* 1979; **51**: 363.
9. Jeffcoate TNA, Francis WJA. Urgency incontinence in the female. *Am J Obstet Gynecol* 1966; **94**: 604.
10. Rees DLP, Whitfield HN, Islam AKM, et al. Urodynamic findings in adult females with frequency and dysuria. *Br J Urol* 1975; **47**: 853.
11. Rees DLP, Whickham JEA, Whitfield HN. Bladder instability in women with recurrent cystitis. *Br J Urol* 1978; **50**: 524.
12. Qvist N, Kristensen ES, Nielsen KK, et al. Detrusor instability in children with recurrent urinary tract infection and/or enuresis. *Urol Int* 1986; **41**: 196.
13. Diokno AC, Wells TJ, Brink CA. Urinary incontinence in elderly women: Urodynamic evaluation. *Am J Geriatr Soc* 1987; **35**: 940.
14. Cantor TJ, Bates CP. A comparative study of symptoms and objective urodynamic findings in 214 incontinent women. *Br J Obstet Gynaecol* 1980; **87**: 889.
15. Farrar DJ, Whiteside CG, Osborne JL, et al. A urodynamic analysis of micturition symptoms in the female. *Surg Gynecol Obstet* 1975; **141**: 875.
16. Koefoot RB, Webster GD. Urodynamic evaluation in women with frequency, urgency symptoms. *Urology* 1983; **6**: 648.
17. Whiteside CG, Arnold EP. Persistent primary enuresis: A urodynamic assessment. *Br Med J* 1975; **1**: 364.
18. Hindmarsh JR, Byrne PO. Adult enuresis. A symptomatic and urodynamic assessment. *Br J Urol* 1980; **52**: 88.
19. McGuire EJ, Savastano JA. Urodynamic studies in enuresis and the non-neurogenic neurogenic bladder. *J Urol* 1984; **132**: 299.
20. Norgaad JP. Urodynamics in enuretics. I:reservior function. *Neurourol Urodynam* 1989; **8**: 199.

21. Rogers MD, Gittes RF, Dawson DM, et al. Giggle incontinence. *JAMA* 1982; **247**: 1446.
22. Webster GD, Sihelnik SA, Stone AR. Female urinary incontinence: The incidence, identification and characteristics of detrusor instability. *Neurourol Urodynam* 1984; **3**: 235.
23. Korda A, Kriger M, Hunter P, et al. The value of clinical symptoms in the diagnosis of urinary incontinence in the female. *Aust NZ J Obstet Gynaecol* 1987; **27**: 149.
24. Sand PK, Hill RC, Ostergard DR. Incontinence history as a predictor of detrusor instability. *Obstet Gynecol* 1988; **71**: 257.
25. Jarvis GJ, Hall S, Stamp S, et al. An assessment of urodynamic examination in incontinence women. *Br J Obstet Gynaecol* 1980; **87**: 893.
26. Fantl JA, Hurt WG, Dunn LJ. Dysfunctional detrusor control. *Am J Obstet Gynecol* 1977; **129**: 299.
27. Arnold EP, Webster JR, Loose H, et al. Urodynamics of female incontinence: Factors influence the results of surgery. *Am J Obstet Gynecol* 1973; **117**: 805.
28. Cardozo LD, Stanton SL. Genuine stress incontinence and detrusor instability: A review of 200 cases. *Br J Obstet Gynaecol* 1980; **87**: 184.
29. Hilton P, Stanton SL, Algorithmic method for assessing in urinary incontinence in elderly women. *BMJ* 1981; **282**: 940.
30. Ouslander J, Staskin D, Raz S, et al. Clinical versus urodynamic diagnosis in an incontinent geriatric female population. *J Urol* 1987; **137**: 68.
31. Eastwood HDH, Warrell R. Urinary incontinence in the elderly female: Prediction in diagnosis and outcome of management. *Age Ageing* 1984; **13**: 230.
32. Bergman A, Bader K. Reliability of the patient's history in the diagnosis of urinary incontinence. *Int J Gynaecol Obstet* 1990; **32**: 255.
33. Haeusler G, Hanzal E, Joura E, et al. Differential diagnosis of detrusor instability and stress incontinence by patient History: the Gaudenz-Incontinence Questionnaire revisited. *Acta Obstet Gynaecol Scand* 1995; **74**: 635.
34. Turner-Warwick RT. Some clinical aspects of detrusor dysfunction. *J Urol* 1975; **113**: 539.
35. Moolgaoker AS, Ardran GM, Smith JC, et al. The diagnosis and management of incontinence in the female. *J Obstet Gynaecol Br Comm* 1972; **79**: 481.
36. Abrams P. Detrusor instability and bladder outlet obstruction. *Neurourol Urodyn* 1985; **4**: 317.
37. Bates CP, Whiteside CG, Turner-Warwick RT. Synchronous cine/pressure/flow cystourethrography with special reference to stress and urge incontinence. *Br J Urol* 1970; **42**: 714.
38. Sutherst JR, Brown MC. Comparison of single and multichannel cystometry in diagnosing bladder instability. *BMJ* 1984; **288**: 1720.
39. Wall LL, Hewitt JK, Helms MJ. Are vaginal and rectal pressures equivalent approximations of one another for the purpose of performing subtracted cystometry? *Obstet Gynecol* 1995; **85**: 488.
40. Low JA, Mauger GM, Drajovic J. Diagnosis of the unstable detrusor: Comparison of an incremental and continuous infusion technique. *Obstet Gynecol* 1985; **65**: 99.
41. Sand PK, Brubaker LT, Novak T. Simple standing incremental cystometry as a screening method for detrusor instability. *Obstet Gynecol* 1991; **77**: 453.
42. Lewis SD. Carbon dioxide versus electronic urethrocystometry for the detection of detrusor dyssynergia. *Am J Obstet Gynecol* 1979; **133**: 371.
43. van-Venrooij GE, Boon TA. Extensive urodynamic investigation: interaction among diuresis, detrusor instability, urethra relaxation, incontinence and complaints in women with a history of urge incontinence. *J Urol* 1994; **152**: 1535.
44. Bates P, Bradley WE, Glen E, et al. First report on the standardization of terminology of lower urinary tract function. *Br J Urol* 1976; **48**: 39.
45. Coolsaet BLRA, Elhilali MM. Detrusor overreactivity. *Neurourol Urodyn* 1985; **4**: 309.

46. McGuire EJ, Woodside Jr, Borden TA. Upper urine tract deterioration in patients with myelodysplasia and detrusor hypertonia: A follow-up study. *J Urol* 1983; **129**: 823.
47. Bhatia NN, Bradley WE, Haldeman S. Urodynamics: Continuous monitoring. *J Urol* 1982; **128**: 963.
48. Kulseng-Hanssen S, Klevmark B. Ambulatory urethro-cysto-rectometry: A new technique. *Neurourol Urodyn* 1988; **7**: 119.
49. McInerney PD, Vanner TF, Harris SA, Stephenson TP. Ambulatory urodynamics. *Br J Urol* 1991; **67**: 272.
50. Webb RJ, Ramsden PD, Neal DE. Ambulatory monitoring and electronic measurement of urinary leakage in the diagnosis of detrusor instability and incontinence. *Br J Urol* 1991; **68**: 148.
51. Porru D, Usai E. Standard and extramural ambulatory urodynamic investigation for the diagnosis of detrusor instability-correlated incontinence and micturition disorders. *Neurourol Urodyn* 1994; **13**: 237.
52. Robertson AS, Griffiths C, Neal DE. Conventional urodynamics and ambulatory monitoring in the definition and management of bladder outflow obstruction. *J Urol* 1996; **155**: 506.
53. Hebert DB, Ostergard DR. Vesical instability: Urodynamic parameters by microtip transducer catheters. *Obstet Gynecol* 1982; **60**: 331.
54. Heslington K, Hilton PA. Ambulatory urodynamic monitoring. *Br J Obstet Gynaecol* 1996; **103**: 393.
55. Heslington K, Hilton PA. Ambulatory monitoring and conventional cystometry in asymptomatic female volunteers. *Br J Obstet Gynaecol* 1996; **103**: 434.
56. Petros PE, Ulmsten U. Bladder instability in women: A premature activation of the micturition reflex. *Neurourol Urodyn* 1993; **12**: 359.
57. Petros PE, Ulmsten U. Tests for detrusor instability in women. *Acta Obstet Gynecol Scan* 1993; **72**: 661.
58. Geirsson G, Fall M, Lindstrom S. The ice-water test: A simple and valuable supplement to routine cystometry. *Br J Urol* 1993; **71**: 681.
59. Geirsson G, Lindstrom S, Fall M. The bladder cooling reflex in man: Characteristics and sensitivity to temperature. *Br J Urol* 1993; **71**: 675.
60. Cucchi A. Acceleration of flow rate as a screening test for detrusor instability in women with stress incontinence. *Br J Urol* 1990; **65**: 17.
61. Cucchi A. Bladder contractility and idiopathic detrusor instability in males. *Neurourol Urodyn* 1994; **13**: 627.
62. Frazer MI, Haylen BT. Trigonal sensitivity testing in women. *J Urol* 1989; **141**: 356.
63. Creighton SM, Plevnik S, Stanton SL. Distal urethral electrical conductance (DUEC): A preliminary assessment of its role as a quick screening test for incontinent women. *Br J Obstet Gynaecol* 1991; **98**: 69.
64. Wyndaele JJ. [Is the lower urinary tract sensation different in patients with bladder instability?]. *Prog Urol* 1992; **2**: 220.
65. Fonda D, Brimage PJ, D'Astoli M. Simple screening for urinary incontinence in the elderly: Comparison of simple and multichannel cystometry. *Urology* 1993; **42**: 536.
66. Wall LL, Wiskind AK, Taylor PA. Simple bladder filling with a cough stress test compared with subtracted cystometry for the diagnosis of urinary incontinence. *Am J Obstet Gynecol* 1994; **171**: 1472.
67. Demuylder X, Claes H, Neven P, et al. Usefulness of urodynamic investigations in female incontinence. *Eur J Obstet Gynaecol Reprod Biol* 1992; **44**: 205.
68. Ziv E, Krieger MS, Howick VA, et al. The natural history of idiopathic detrusor instability: A 12-year follow-up. *Neurourol Urodyn* 1988; **7**: 187.
69. Hald T, Bradley WE: *The Urinary Bladder Neurology and Dynamics.* Baltimore: Williams & Wilkins, 1982.
70. DelCarro U, Riva D, Comi GC, et al. Neurophysiological evaluation in detrusor instability. *Neurourol Urodyn* 1993; **12**: 455.

71. Parys BT, Woolfenden KA, Parsons KF. Bladder dysfunction after simple hysterectomy: Urodynamic and neurological evaluation. *Eur Urol* 1990; **17**: 129.
72. Kinder RB, Mundy AR. Inhibition of spontaneous contractile activity in isolated human detrusor muscle strips by vasoactive intestinal polypeptide. *Br J Urol* 1985; **57**: 20.
73. Berggren T, Andersson KE, Lundin S, et al. Effect and content of arginine vasopressin in normal and obstructed rat urinary bladder: An in-vivo and in-vitro investigation. *J Urol* 1993; **150**: 1540.
74. Murray KHA, Feneley RCL. Endorphins-a role in lower urinary tract function? The effect of opioid blockage on the detrusor and urethral sphincter mechanism. *Br J Urol* 1982; **54**: 638.
75. Kontani H, Inoue T, Sakai T. Effects of apomorphine on urinary bladder motility in anesthetized rats. *Jpn J Pharmacol* 1990; **52**: 59.
76. Bergman A, Stanczyk FZ, Lobo RA. The role of prostaglandins in detrusor instability. *Am J Obstet Gynecol* 1991; **165**: 1833.
77. Moore KH, Nickson P, Richmond DH. Detrusor mast cells in refractory idiopathic instability. *Br J Urol* 1992; **70**: 17.
78. Creighton SM, Stanton SL. Caffeine: Does it affect your bladder? *Br J Urol* 1990; **66**: 613.
79. Kieswetter H. Mucosal sensory threshold of urinary bladder and urethra measured electrically. *Urol Int* 1977; **32**: 437.
80. Creighton SM, Pearce JM, Robson I, et al. Sensory urgency: How full is your bladder? *Br J Obstet Gynaecol* 1991; **98**: 1287.
81. Birch BR, Miller RA. Primary nocturnal enuresis: A urodynamic study spanning three generations. *Scand J Urol Nephrol* 1995; **29**: 2854.
82. Meullner SR. Development of urinary control in children. *JAMA* 1960; **171**: 1256.
83. Bhatia NN, Bergman A. Cystometry: Unstable bladder and urinary tract infection. *Br J Urol* 1986; **58**: 134.
84. Harrison SCW, Hunnam GR, Furman P, et al. Bladder instability and denervation in patients with bladder outflow obstruction. *Br J Urol* 1987; **60**: 519.
85. McGuire EJ. Reflex urethral instability. *Br J Urol* 1978; **50**: 200.
86. Koonings PP, Bergman A. Urethral pressure changes in women with detrusor instability: Bladder or urethral pathologic process? *Urology* 1991; **37**: 540.
87. Wise BG, Cardozo LD, Cutner A, et al. Prevalence and significance of urethral instability in women with detrusor instability. *Br J Urol* 1993; **72**: 26.
88. Hilton P. Urinary incontinence during sexual intercourse: A common, but rarely volunteered symptom. *Br J Obstet Gynaecol* 1988; **95**: 377.
89. Khan Z, Bhola A, Starer P. Urinary incontinence during orgasm. *Urology* 1988; **21**: 279.
90. Sutherst JR, Brown M. The effect on the bladder pressure on sudden entry of fluid into the posterior urethra. *Br J Urol* 1978; **50**: 406.
91. Penders L, Vanstalle-Nelissen G. [Bladder instability and kinesitherapy: The concept of deficient bladder instability]. *Acta Urol Belg* 1990; **58**: 103.
92. Fantl JA, Wyman JF, McClish DK, et al. Efficacy of bladder training in older women with urinary incontinence. *JAMA* 1991; **265**: 609.
93. Hebjorn S, Anderson JT, Walter S, et al. Detrusor hyperreflexia: A survey of its etiology and treatment. *Scand J Urol Nephrol* 1976; **10**: 103.
94. Khan Z, Starer P, Bhola A. Urinary incontinence in female Parkinson's disease patients: Pitfalls of diagnosis. *Urology* 1989; **33**: 486.
95. Moore KH, Richmond DH, Parys BT. Sex distribution of adult idiopathic detrusor instability in relation to childhood bedwetting. *Br J Urol* 1991; **68**: 479.
96. Yu LC, Rohner TJ, Kaltreider DL, et al. Profile of urinary incontinent elderly in long term care institutions. *J Am Geriatr Soc* 1990; **38**: 433.
97. Diokno AC, Brown MB, Brock BM, et al. Clinical and cystometric characteristics of continent and incontinent non-institutionalized elderly. *J Urol* 1988; **140**: 567.

98. Macaulay AJ, Stern RS, Stanton SL. Psychosocial aspects of 211 female patients attending a urodynamic unit. *J Psychosom Res* 1991; **35**: 1.
99. Moore KH, Sutherst JR. Response to treatment of detrusor instability in relation to psychoneurotic status. *Br J Urol* 1990; **66**: 486.
100. Walters MD, Taylor S, Schoenfeld LS. Psychosexual study of women with detreusor instability. *Obstet Gynecol* 1990; **75**: 22.
101. Wiskind AK, Miller KF, Wall LL. One hundred unstable bladders. *Obstet Gynecol* 1994; **83**: 108.
102. Frewen WK. A reassessment of bladder training in detrusor dysfunction in the female. *Br J Urol* 1982; **54**: 372.
103. Wall LL. Diagnosis and management of urinary incontinence due to detrusor instability. *Obstet Gynecol Surv* 1990; **45**: 1S.
104. Szonyi G, Collas DM, Ding YY, et al. Oxybutynin with bladder retraining for detrusor instability in elderly people: A randomized controlled trial. *Age Ageing* 1995; **24**: 287.
105. Nygaard IE, Kreder KJ, Lepic MM, et al. Efficacy of pelvic floor muscle exercises in women with stress, urge and mixed urinary incontinence. *Am J Obstet Gynecol* 1996; **174**: 120.
106. Cornella JL, Bent AE, Ostergard DR, et al. Prospective study utilizing transdermal scopolamine in detrusor instability. *Urology* 1990; **35**: 96.
107. Meyhoff HH, Gerstenberg TC, Nordling J. Placebo: The drug of choice in female motor urge incontinence? *Br J Urol* 1983; **55**: 34.
108. Holmes DM, Montz FJ, Stanton SL. Oxybutynin versus propantheline in the management of detrusor instability: A patient-regulated variable dose trial. *Br J Obstet Gynaecol* 1989; **96**: 607.
109. Awad SA, Bryniak S, Dowie JW, et al. The treatment of the uninhibited bladder with dicyclomine. *J Urol* 1977; **117**: 161.
110. Castleden CM, Duffin HM, Gulati RS. Double-blind study of imipramine and placebo for incontinence due to bladder instability. *Age Ageing* 1986; **15**: 299.
111. Rud T, Andersson KE, Ulmsten U. Effects of nifedipine in women with unstable bladders. *Urol Int* 1979; **34**: 421.
112. Mattiasson A, Ekstrom B, Andersson KE. Effects of intravesial instillation of verapamil in patients with detrusor hyperactivity. *Neurourol Urodyn* 1987; **6**: 253.
113. Palmer JH, Worth PHL, Exton-Smith AN. Flunarizine: A once-daily therapy for urinary incontinence. *Lancet* 1981; **2**: 279.
114. Tapp A, Fall M, Norgaard J, et al. Terolidine: A dose-titrated, multicenter study for the treatment of idiopathic detrusor instability in women. *J Urol* 1989; **142**: 1027.
115. Norton P, Karram M, *Wall L*, Rosenschweig B, Benson T, Fantl A. idiopathic detrusor instability. *Obstet Gynecol* 1994; **84**: 386.
116. Tulloch AGS. The drug treatment of the unstable bladder. *Br J Urol* 1979; **51**: 359.
117. Wiseman PA, Malone-Lee J, Rai GS. Terodiline with bladder retraining for treating detrusor instability in elderly people. *BMJ* 1991; **302**: 994.
118. Elmer M, Norgaard JP, Djurhuus JC, et al. Terodiline in the treatment of diurnal enuresis in children. *Scand J Prim Health Care* 1988; **6**: 119.
119. Hennessy A, Robinson LQ, Weston P, et al. A comparison between oxybutynin and terodiline in patients with multiple sclerosis. *Neurourol Urodyn* 1988; **7**: 195.
120. Kinn AC, Brekkan E, Jansson A, et al. Terodiline for patients with urinary incontinence in neurogenic bladder disorders: Efficacy and tolerance. *Neurourol Urodyn* 1988; **7**: 196.
121. Andersen JR, Lose G, Norgaard M, et al. Terodiline, emperonium bromide or placebo for treatment of female detrusor overactivity? A randomized double-blind, crossover study. *Br J Urol* 1988; **61**: 310.
122. Beisland HO, Fossberg E. The effects of terodiline on severe motor urge incontinence in geriatric patients. *J Am Geriatr Soc* 1985; **33**: 29.

123. Langtry HD, Mctavish D. Terodiline: A review of its pharmacological properties, and therapeutic use in the treatment of urinary incontinence. *Drugs* 1990; **40**: 748.
124. Thomas SH, Higham PD, Hartigan-Go K, et al. Concentration dependent cardiotoxicity of terodiline in patients treated for urinary incontinence. *Br Heart J* 1995; **74**: 53.
125. Abrams P, Feneley RCL. The actions of prostaglandins on the smooth muscle of the human urinary tract in-vitro. *Br J Urol* 1976; **47**: 909.
126. Wall LL, Warrell DW. Detrusor instability associated with menstruation: Case report. *Br J Obstet Gynaecol* 1989; **96**: 737.
127. Del Castillo EB, Argonz J, Mainini CG. Cytological cycle of the urinary sediment and its parallelism with the vaginal cycle. *J Clin Endocrinol* 1948; **8**: 76.
128. Iosif CS, Batra S, Ek E, et al. Estrogen receptors in the human female lower urinary tract. *Am J Obstet Gynecol* 1981; **141**: 817.
129. Salmon UJ, Walter RI, Gerst SH. The use of estrogens in the treatment of dysuria and incontinence in post-menopausal women. *Am J Obstet Gynecol* 1941; **42**: 845.
130. Siegel I, Zelinger BB, Kanter AE. Estrogen therapy for urogenital conditions in the aged. *Am J Obstet Gynecol* 1962; **84**: 505.
131. Schreiter F, Fuchs D, Stockamp K. Estrogenic sensitivity of alpha-receptors in the urethral musculature. *Urol Int* 1976; **31**: 13.
132. Hilton P, Stanton SL. The use of intravaginal oestrogen cream in genuine stress incontinence. *Br J Obstet Gynaecol* 1983; **9**: 940.
133. Wilson PD, Faragher B, Butler B, et al. Treatment with oral piperazine oestrone sulphate for genuine stress incontinence in postmenopausal women. *Br J Obstet Gynaecol* 1987; **94**: 568.
134. Fantl JA, Wyman JF, Anderson RL, et al. Postmenopausal urinary incontinence: Comparison between non-estrogen-supplemented and estrogen-supplemented women. *Obstet Gynecol* 1988; **71**: 823.
135. Taylor MC, Bates CP. A double-blind crossover trial of braclofen: A new treatment for the unstable bladder. *Br J Urol* 1979; **51**: 504.
136. Abrams PH, Dunn M. A double-blind trial of bromocriptine in the treatment of idiopathic bladder instability. *Br J Urol* 1979; **51**: 24.
137. Lindholm P, Lose G. Terbutaline (Bricanyl) in the treatment of female urge incontinence. *Urol Int* 1986; **41**: 158.
138. Anderson JT, Walter, Vejlsgaard R. A clinical and bacteriological trial with dimethylsulfoxide (DMSO) in the treatment of severe detrusor hyperreflexia. *Scand J Urol Nephrol* (Suppl) 1981; **60**: 63.
139. Jensen D. Uninhibited neurogenic bladder treated with prazosin. *Scand J Urol Nephrol* 1981; **15**: 229.
140. Wall LL, Addison WA. Prazosin-induced stress incontinence. *Obstet Gynecol* 1990; **75**: 558.
141. Higson RH, Smith JC, Hills W. Intravesical lignocaine and detrusor instability. *Br J Urol* 1979; **51**: 500.
142. Blau U, Retzke U. Treatment of symptomatology of urge and urge incontinence with propiverine. *Zentralbl Gynakol* 1984; **106**: 981.
143. Malmgrem A, Andersson KE, Sjogren C et al. Effects of pinacidil and cromakalim (BRL 34915) on bladder function in rats with detrusor instability. *J Urol* 1989; **142**: 1134.
144. Seki N, Karim OM, Mostwin JL. Effect of pinacidil on the membrane electrical activity of guinea pig detrusor muscle. *J Pharmacol Exp Ther* 1992; **263**: 816.
145. Hedlund H, Mattiasson A, Andersson KE. Effects of pinacidil on detrusor instability in men with bladder outlet obstruction. *J Urol* 1991; **146**: 1345.
146. Nurse RE, Restorick JM, Mundy AR. The effect of cromakalim on the normal and hyperreflexic human detrusor muscle. *Br J Urol* 1991; **68**: 27.
147. Lindstrom S, Fall M, Carlsson CA, et al. The neurophysiological basis of bladder inhibition in response to intravaginal electrical stimulation. *J Urol* 1983; **129**: 405.

148. Fall M. Does electrostimulation cure urinary incontinence? *J Urol* 1984; **131**: 664.
149. Lamhut P, Jackson TW, Wall LL. The treatment of urinary incontinence with electrical stimulation in nursing home patients: A pilot study. *J Am Geriatr Soc* 1992; **40**: 48.
150. Torrens MJ. The role of denervation in the treatment of detrusor instability. *Neurourol Urodyn* 1985; **4**: 353.
151. Mundy AR. The surgical treatment of detrusor instability. *Neurourol Urodyn* 1985; **4**: 352.
152. Higson RH, Smith JC, Whelan P. Bladder rupture: An acceptable complication of distension therapy? *Br J Urol* 1978; **50**: 529.
153. Lloyd SN, Lloyd SM, Rogers K, et al. Is there still a place for prolonged bladder distention? *Br J Urol* 1992; **70**: 382.
154. McCahy PJ, Styles RA. Prolonged bladder distension: Experience in the treatment of detrusor overactivity and interstitial cystitis. *Eur Urol* 1995; **28**: 325.
155. Wall LL, Stanton SL. Transvesical phenol injection of the pelvic nerve plexuses in females with refractory urge incontinence. *Br J Urol* 1989; **63**: 465.
156. Bennani S. [Evaluation of sub-trigonal injections in the treatment of the hyperactive bladder]. *Ann Urol Paris* 1994; **28**: 13.
157. Awad SA, Flood HD, Acker KL, et al. Selective sacral cryoneurolysis in the treatment of patients with detrusor instability/hyperreflexia and hypersensitive bladder. *Neurourol Urodyn* 1987; **6**: 307.
158. Opsomer RJ, Klarskov P, Holm-Bentzen M, et al. Long term results of superselective sacral nerve resection for motor urge incontinence. *Scand J Urol Nephrol* 1984; **18**: 101.
159. Ingelman-Sundberg A. Partial denervation of the bladder. *Acta Obstet Gynecol Scand* 1959; **38**: 487.
160. Turner-Warwick RT, Ashken MH. The functional results of partial, sub-total and total cystoplasty with special reference to ureterocaecocystoplasty, selective sphincter-otomy and cystocystoplasty. *Br J Urol* 1967; **39**: 3.
161. Staskin DR, Parsons KF, Levin RM, et al. Bladder transection: A functional, neuro-physiological, neuropharmacological and neuroanatomical study. *Br J Urol* 1981; **53**: 552.
162. Mundy AR. Long-term results of bladder transection for urge incontinence. *Br J Urol* 1983; **55**: 642.
163. Lucas MG, Thomas DG. Endoscopic bladder transection for detrusor instability. *Br J Urol* 1987; **59**: 526.
164. Mundy AR. The surgical approach to the treatment of incontinence due to drug resistant detrusor instability with particular reference to "clam" ileocystoplasty. *World J Urol* 1986; **4**: 45.
165. Hasan ST, Marshall C. Robson, WD, et al. Clinical outcome and quality of life following enterocystoplasty for idiopathic detrusor instability and neurogenic bladder dysfunction. *Br J Urol* 1995; **76**: 551.
166. King LR, Stone AR, Webster GD. *Bladder Reconstruction and Continent Urinary Diversion*, 2nd ed. St. Louis: Mosby, 1991.
167. Karram MM, Bhatia NN. Management of coexistent stress and urge urinary incontinence. *Obstet Gynecol* 1989; **73**: 4.
168. McGuire EJ. Bladder instability and stress incontinence. *Neurourol Urodyn* 1988; **7**: 563.
169. Chin YK, Stanton SL. A follow-up of silastic sling for genuine stress incontinence. *Br J Obstet Gynaecol* 1995; **102**: 143.

PART VI

OTHER LOWER URINARY TRACT AND PELVIC FLOOR DISORDERS

CHAPTER 18

Urethral diverticulum

MARY T. McLENNAN

INCIDENCE

The first documented treatment of a suburethral diverticulum was in 1786 and described by William Hey in 1805.[1] At Johns Hopkins Hospital from 1894 to 1956 there were approximately 109 reported cases.[2] From 1955 to 1979, Ginsburg and Genadry[3] noted 110 cases. The apparent increase in the incidence of the disease since 1956 at both Johns Hopkins and worldwide most likely reflects the increased awareness of the entity and the increase in pickup through newer diagnostic techniques, most notably the use of the double-balloon catheter. Davis and Cian[4] first described positive pressure urethrography using a double-balloon catheter in 1956.

The true incidence is largely unknown, as most reports have included patients with lower urinary tract symptoms. Using positive pressure urethrography, Andersen[5] noted a 3% incidence among 300 asymptomatic females presenting for evaluation of carcinoma of the cervix. Using a similar technique, Adams[6] noted a 4.7% incidence among 129 asymptomatic females. Stewart and colleagues[7] noted a 40% incidence among 40 patients being evaluated for lower urinary tract complaints, and Davis and Robinson[8] reported a 1.9% incidence for patients being admitted to a general urology service.

Most patients present after the age of 20, and the most common age group is 30–40 years.[3,9,10] Most studies have noted a high incidence among black females (3.6–6.1);[3,10,11] however, Leach and Bavendam[9] noted equivocal rates. It is a disease of both multiparous and primiparous patients.[8–10]

ETIOLOGY

Most authors now agree that the origin is acquired not congenital. The evidence to support this lies in the fact that diverticula have rarely been described in children.[2,8] Congenital diverticula tend to be anterior in location, which is in contrast to the usual location described. Ginsburg and Genadry[3] in their review of 70 patients noted the youngest was 17 years and Peters and Vaughan[10] noted one of 30 patients under the age of 20 years. Davis and TeLinde[2] noted no patient under the age of 20 in their series of 121 patients.

Diverticula are thought to arise from the paraurethral glands. Obstruction of the glands leads to abscess formation. The abscess ruptures into the urethra, and a communication is established back to the urethral lumen. Continued infection, inflammation, and presence of urine with voiding in the cavity leads to epithelialization and formation of a true sac. Huffman[12] in 1948 constructed wax models of infected urethras. Microscopic studies of several sections confirmed the presence of a complex network of paraurethral glands. Most were located in the distal one-third of the urethra and opened postlaterally.

Birth trauma as an etiologic factor has been largely abandoned. The incidence among nulliparous patients has been reported at 18–39%.[8,10,13] Peters and Vaughan[10] noted no relationship with increasing parity.

ASSOCIATED FACTORS

Microbiology

It is difficult to determine whether infection is a cause or effect or both. Peters and Vaughan[10] noted a 61% incidence of documented gonococcal infection in patients with complete records. Unfortunately, only 11 of their original 32 patients had complete data, which may account for this apparent high incidence.

The most common organisms isolated in the urine are the typical uropathogens—*Escherichia coli, Streptococcus faecalis, Staphylococcus aureus, Klebsiella, Proteus*, and *Pseudomonas*.[2,8,14] Rarely have microbial studies been performed on the diverticula contents themselves.

Location

Most diverticula occur in the midurethra (47–89%).[5,8,15,16] Leach and Bavendam[9] noted 18.9% in the proximal urethra, 70.3% in the midurethra, and 10.8% distally. Ginsburg and Genadry[3] noted 18.7% proximally, 48.9% midurethra, and 34.4% distally when the urethra was analyzed in thirds.[8]

Multiple diverticula have been noted in 9–54%.[8,15,16] Each diverticulum may have multiple openings (4–33%).[8,9,16] Size may vary from 0.5 to 6 cm.[3]

Before the current imaging techniques were available, most diverticula were thought to arise posteriorly and have the ostium posteriorly. MacKinnon and coworkers,[17] in a series of 204, noted only 9 with the ostium opening anteriorly or antrolaterally. These figures may change with the advent of magnetic resonance imaging (MRI). While not particularly good at visualizing the ostium, it is superior to other techniques in detecting and characterizing the diverticulum. Kim and colleagues[15] noted an anterolateral location in one-third of the 13 cases none of which was seen with conventional imaging.

Contents

Cancer arising from a diverticulum is rare with 34 cases reported in the literature.[18] Adenocarcinoma is the most common (21 cases), with the remainder transitional cell (4 cases) and squamous (9 cases).[18,19]

It is important to attempt to make this diagnosis preoperatively, as diverticulectomy alone has the highest recurrence rates (67%).[18] A single case of endometriosis of a diverticular sac has been reported.[20] Calculi can be identified in 3–13% of diverticula.[9,21]

SYMPTOMS

The typical patient does not present to the office with complaints of a painful vaginal mass that, when compressed, expels pus or urine. With the exception of one series by Hoffman and Adams,[22] fewer than 20% of patients present with a mass.[22] Most often they present with symptoms common to many of the lower urinary tract disorders.

The most frequent presenting complaints are of irritative voiding symptoms in approximately 60% (range: 11–100%).[8,9,13,22–24] A history of recurrent urinary tract infection is often noted (33–80%).[8,9,17,22] The classic symptom of postvoid dribbling is present in approximately one-third of patients (15–90%).[8,9,13,18,22–24] Incontinence both stress and urge may be the only presenting symptom.[8,9,11,13,22–24] Leach and Bavendam[9] did note that on urodynamic evaluation of their 37 patients, 32% had documented genuine stress incontinence, 8% detrusor instability, and 16% both. These issues need to be addressed separately.[9] Only a small number in each series were asymptomatic. A cross-section of symptoms is presented in Table 18-1.

Hematuria is the most common presenting symptom of carcinoma in a diverticulum; however, 7–35% of patients with diverticula have hematuria.[8,13,23,24] Also, all the general irritative symptoms have been described in cases of carcinoma.[18,19] In most cases, a palpable mass is present; however, McLoughlin[25] reported a case of carcinoma *in situ* indicating the need for a tissue diagnosis in all cases.

DIAGNOSIS

The ability to diagnose this disorder was well summarized by Davis and Cian in 1956. "There is convincing evidence that this lesion is one of those conditions which is found in the direct proportion to the activity with which it is sought."[4]

The diagnosis should be considered in any patient presenting with recurrent urinary tract infection especially refractory cystitis, and in patients with irritative voiding symptoms. Assessment includes a full history, directed neurologic examination and pelvic examination. The anterior vaginal wall should be

Table 18-1. Presenting symptoms (percent)

	No. of patients	Dysuria	Frequency urgency	Recurrent UTI	Mass	Postvoid dribbling/ pain	Urethral pain	Incontinence stress	Incontinence urge	Pus from urethra	Dyspareunia	Hematuria	Asymptomatic
Leach & Bavendam[9]	37	10.8	—	40.5	16	13.5	—	51	35	—	19	—	—
Ginsburg & Genadry[3]	70	90	90	51	—	5.7	—	—	—	20	—	—	—
Rozsahegyi et al.[23]	50	80	100	80	—	—	45	25	—	—	70	35	—
Peters & Vaughan[10]	32	69	34	—	6	—	3	6	3	—	9	13	20
Davis & Robinson[8]	120	32	58	33	—	32	30	9	—	—	32	17	1.6
Pathak & House[13]	45	47	42	—	18	22	26	22	4	31	13	7	—
Kittredge et al.[24]	27	52	44	—	—	15	—	30	—	—	15	—	11
Hoffman & Adams[22]	60	58	—	—	45	90	—	70	—	—	20	18	—
Mackinnon et al.[17]	204	73	66	46	12	—	29	17	25	—	14	17	—
Davis & TeLinde[2]	121	63	83	—	—	13	—	25	—	1.6	24	26	7.4

examined with the patient straining with a Sims speculum or half a Graves speculum retracting posteriorly. This may help the diverticulum to come more easily into view. With a speculum in place, the urethra and paraurethral tissue should be palpated and compressed while the external urethral meatus viewed to determine if any pus or urine can be expelled. Examination of the urethra should be repeated with the speculum removed as a small high- or mid diverticulum may be easier to palpate without the instrument. Clinically, if a diverticulum is noted, further investigations should be performed to determine the number, location, size of the diverticulum, information not readily available on examination only. As stated previously, multiple diverticula can occur in up to 51% of cases.[8,15,16] If no mass is palpable but clinical suspicion high, investigations should also be performed for confirmation.

Urethroscopy, voiding cystourethrogram (VCUG), and positive pressure urethrography (DBC study) are most commonly performed. There are also a number of recent reports on the role of MRI[15,26] and a renewed interest in ultrasonography.[27,28] The adjunctive use of urethral pressure profilometry has been studied by some.[16,29–31] Ideally, urethroscopy should be performed with a 24F "female urethroscope". The larger caliber allows better visualization and the shortened beakless sheath makes the procedure much more comfortable for the patient. The urethroscope should be placed initially in the bladder and with one finger in the vagina, the urethra occluded, and the urethroscope slowly withdraw. Occlusion with the vaginal finger permits much better distension of the urethra and also allows for the compression and expression of any purulent material or urine from the diverticulum (Figure 18-1). This may aid in locating the ostium. Most reports note a diagnostic rate of 56–78%.[3,8,9,15] The ostium may be missed if the diverticulum is infected, edematous, or obstructed.

Voiding cystourethrography (VCUG) is highly reliable in making the diagnosis. In 32 patients, Peters and Vaughan[10] noted a 100% detection rate. Leach

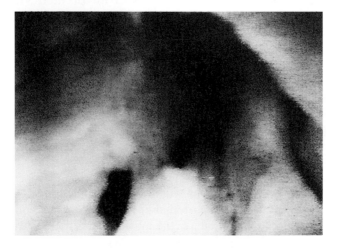

Figure 18-1. Urethroscopy: proximal diverticulum with 2 openings (*right*).

and Bavendam[9] noted only one case in 37 (3%) and Ginsburg and Genadry[3] two in 60 cases (3%) where further testing was essential for the diagnosis. Lee and Keller[32] noted a lower sensitivity of 65%. A standing oblique VCUG under fluoroscopic control allows for better definition of the size, location, and number of diverticula (Figure 18-2). A postvoid film may be helpful as the diverticulum may fill with voided contrast material.

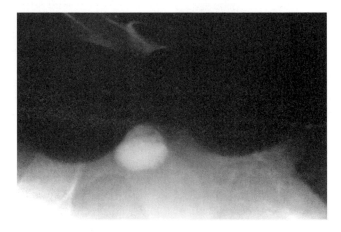

Figure 18-2.   Voiding cystourethrogram.

Positive pressure urethrography (DBC study) is considered by most as the gold standard. Initially described in 1956 by Davis and Cian[4] it involves the placement of a sliding balloon catheter into the urethra. The proximal balloon is inserted into the bladder and filled with 20 ml of fluid via a connector identical to a Foley catheter. The distal balloon is movable over the main catheter shaft. It is filled with 30 ml of fluid via an intracath needle and clamped. It is pulled snugly up against the external urethral meatus in an effort to prevent spillage. Under fluoroscopic guidance, undiluted contrast material (5–10 ml) is injected into the main catheter sleeve. Fluoroscopy enables positioning of the patient so that the three-dimensional relationship of the diverticulum to the urethra can be assessed (Figures 18-3, and 18-4). Unfortunately, the proximal balloon may obscure the base and may make it difficult to determine the relationship of the diverticulum to the bladder base. Kølhorn and Glickman[33] reported on a technique where the balloons were inflated with diluted contrast material (proximal 25% concentration and external 50% concentration). An undiluted contrast medium was then injected into the main catheter. They reported the variation in the contrast medium allowed more precise delineation of the position of the diverticulum to the bladder base and external urethral meatus.[33] Accuracy of the DBC has been reported at 80–100%.[32–34] A number of physicians recommend this test only

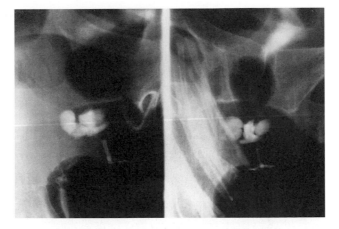

Figure 18-3. Double balloon catheter study: multiple diverticula.

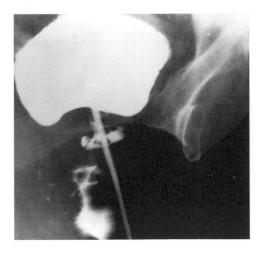

Figure 18-4. Double balloon catheter study: single diverticulum.

when all others fail to make the diagnosis as it is uncomfortable for the patient, technically more difficult, and the catheter is not readily available in all departments.

Vaginal ultrasound has improved the diagnostic accuracy of ultrasound as a tool for the diagnosis of diverticula.[27,32,34–36] It has the advantage of being non-invasive, well tolerated, and allows assessment of the size, shape, and contents of the diverticulum. Baert[27] noted that even if the diverticulum doesn't fill during VCUG, a slitlike or cystlike fluid filled cavity can clearly be differentiated from the surrounding urethra (Figure 18-5). Its other advantage is in the evaluation of the diverticula contents. However, the largest series to date

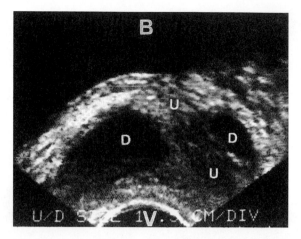

Figure 18-5. Endovaginal ultrasound: large diverticulum. *B*, bladder; *U*, urethra; *D*, diverticulum; *v*, transducer in the vagina. (From reference 27, with permission.)

consisted of only six patients. Further investigation of this as a diagnostic tool needs to be made.

The most recent reports have been on MRI. MRI can readily identify the urethra from the surrounding vagina and periurethral tissues.[15,26,37] The imaging should include thin section axial T1- and T2-weighted images and sagittal T2-weighted images (Figure 18-6).[12,26,30] Kim and coworkers.[15] in a study of 13 patients showed it superior to all other techniques in detecting and characterizing the diverticulum. It can detect the unfilled sac thereby showing the complete contents with the lesion. It also allows excellent visualization of the contents. It is, however, poor at detecting ostea or differentiating multiple sacs from septate ones. Contrast enhanced MR images help in differentiating tumor from stone. Unfortunately, the cost is three times that of a VCUG and thus should be reserved for patients where clinical suspicion is high and investigations negative or in patients where the contents of the sac are suspicious.

Urethral pressure profilometry has been looked at as a preoperative tool to determine the relationship of the diverticulum to the urethral sphincter. This potentially may help predict those patients at risk of postoperative incontinence. It has been noted that patients with diverticula have a biphasic urethral closure pressure profile. (Figure 18-7). The depression was thought to represent the ostea.[29–31] Many authors now consider this may represent other structural changes in the urethral wall secondary to surrounding inflammation, fibrosis or damage due to the diverticulum itself. Leach and Bavendam[9] noted a biphasic curve in 72% of their 37 patients. Summit and Stovall[16] noted depressions in 100% of their patients, but also noted this finding in two-thirds of their patients without diverticulum. They also noted that the depression involved from 41% to 64% of the functional length and felt it poorly represented the ostium.[16]

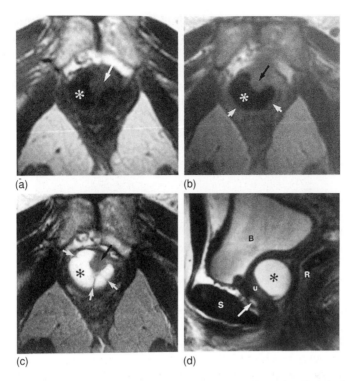

Figure 18-6. (a) Axial. T1-weighted MRI shows a low-signal intensity diverticulum (*) within enlarged urethra. (b) Contrast-enhanced, axial. T_1-weighted MRI shows enhancement of displaced urethra (➡) and diverticular wall (⇨). (c) Axial, T_2-weighted MRI shows high density fluid in urethral diverticulum (*) with several septa (⇨). Black arrow = displaced urethra. (d) Sagittal. T_2-weighted MRI show a large diverticulum (*) in the posterior aspect of the urethra (U) and a small diverticulum (⇨) in anterior aspect. (From reference 15, with permission.)

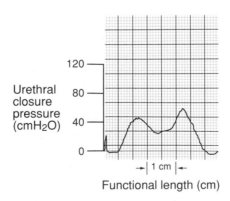

Urethral closure pressure (cmH₂O)

Figure 18-7. Urethral closure pressure profile.

Currently urethral pressure profilometry is helpful in detecting those with pre-operative genuine stress incontinence (6–70%) and may alter surgical management but has not proven useful as a tool for detecting those asymptomatic patients likely to develop genuine stress incontinence after surgery.

In a small number of cases a small diverticulum may be suspected or palpated but not identified by any of the above imaging techniques. The suspicious area can be cleaned and a fine-gauge needle introduced into the area and after aspiration of pus or urine, contrast material directly injected. Anteroposterior and lateral x-rays can be taken to outline the diverticula.[33]

TREATMENT

Asymptomatic diverticula without palpable stones or tumors may be managed expectantly. The patient should be counseled that should a urinary tract infection develop with associated peridiverticulitis she may experience extreme discomfort and the surrounding inflammation may make dissection at a later date more difficult.

Many techniques have been described, but most involve a vaginal approach with either complete or partial excision of the diverticular wall.[3,9–11,38] The basic surgical technique is the same as that of a fistula repair-dissection; closure with as many layers as possible, and closure without tension.

A weighted speculum is placed in the vagina and a Foley catheter in the urethra. The patient is covered preoperatively with broad-spectrum antibiotics. The anterior vaginal mucosa is infiltrated with a dilute vasoconstrictor solution (e.g., 20 units Pitressin/100 ml of normal saline). An inverted U incision with the apex above the diverticulum is made. This flap is then dissected inferiorly with the use of fine instruments, for example plastic surgery instruments. It is important to make this layer thick enough to be viable but thin enough that a number of layers can be created. The endopelvic fascia covering the diverticulum is then visualized and incised vertically or transversely depending on the number of layers the operator feels can be dissected free. If the patient has had previous infection, this may be densely adherent to the diverticular wall. With the use of fine Metzenbaum scissors and often aided with the use of a No. 15 scalpel, this endopelvic fascia layer can be separated. If the diverticulum is inadvertently entered, a pediatric Foley catheter (6–8F) can be inserted into the opening and inflated. This greatly enhances the ease of dissection and most times we will electively do this. Once the endopelvic fascia is deflected, traction on the pediatric Foley may make another layer over the diverticulum evident. Incision of this layer in the transverse plane is made and the flaps dissected. The key to success with minimal complications is layers, layers, layers. The diverticulum is then fully dissected and opened until the communication with the urethra is visualized. It is important to isolate the opening into the urethra. This is then closed longitudinally with either continuous or interrupted 4/0 polyglycolic suture. It is our preference to use an interrupted technique as the suture line is more secure should an infection develop (Figure 18-8). If breakdown of suture occurs with a continuous suture then the whole area is at risk. A second implicated layer can be placed. Excess diverticula sac is excised. Many authors believe it is important to dissect and excise as much of this sac as possible to decrease the risk of recurrence.[39] The deeper fascial layers are closed in a horizontal manner with interrupted 4/0 sutures. The superficial fascial layer is then closed vertically in a similar manner. This provides a double fascial layer over the diverticulum for support with all suture lines running at right angles to the previous ones. This provides minimal tension on the suture lines. The inverted U is then advanced without tension and closed with 2/0 adsorbable sutures. If a number of layers of fascia cannot be dissected, then the end of the U vaginal flap can be denuded of its vaginal mucosa and used as a patch that can be sutured in place. The shorter U is then further freed and advanced without tension.

A variation of this technique was reported by Tancer and colleagues[40] and Hajj and Evans.[41] They sutured a portion of the diverticular wall in a double/breasted fashion to support the urethral closure and obliterate the diverticular cavity. No fistula occurred after this technique. Rozsahegyi and associates[23] closed the ostium with a purse string suture and then enclosed the vaginal wall. Most people advocate the use of multiple layers to decrease the risk of fistula.[9,10,42] Downs[43] described a technique for large diverticulum where extensive dissection is avoided and a portion of the sac is left and marsupialized to the vaginal mucosa.

For diverticula of the distal two-thirds of the urethra, Edwards and Beebe[44] and Parks[45] incised the urethra from the external meatus to the diverticulum, excised the diverticulum, debrided the edges and closed the urethra in layers. Spence and Duckett[45] described marsupialization of distal diverticula. Scissors are placed in the urethra and the urethra opened from the external urethral meatus to the diverticula ostium. The edges of the diverticulum are sutured to the edges of the vaginal mucosa in a running fashion. It effectively creates a large meatotomy. This procedure can be done as an outpatient and has minimal morbidity. Incision and drainage can be used for acute infection.[47] Excision may need to be performed at a later date. Dissection may be more difficult due to scarring at the incision site.

A number of techniques can make dissection easier. We prefer the use of a pediatric Foley catheter.[33,48] No imaging technique has proved useful intraoperatively. Recently Chancellor and coworkers[49] reported on the use of intraoperative endoluminal ultrasound. They felt it helped to determine the surgery by not only defining the size, shape, and location of the diverticulum, but by defining the extent of periurethral inflammation, wall thickness, and the distance from the diverticular wall to the urethral lumen (Figure 18-9).

If the patient has associated genuine stress incontinence, concomitant surgery for this can be performed without adding to the complication rate. Leach and Bavendam[9] noted no complications in their 22 patients who had simultaneous bladder neck suspensions compared to the eight patients treated with

(a)

(b)

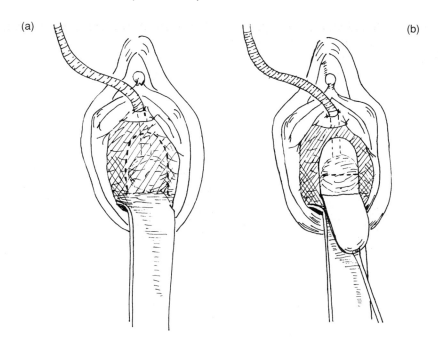

(c)

(d)

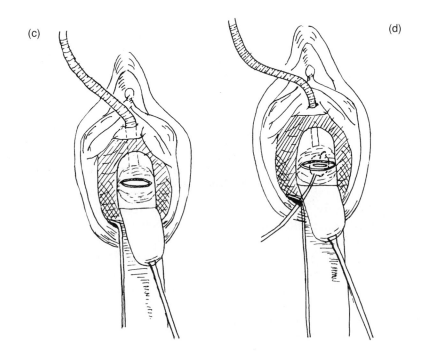

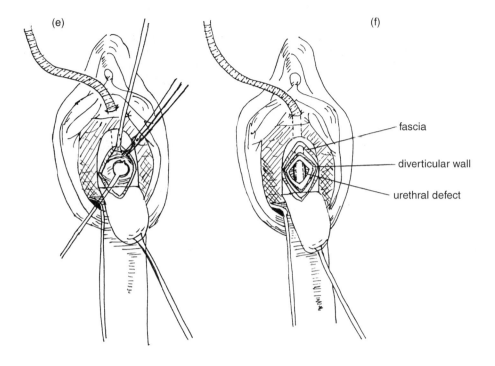

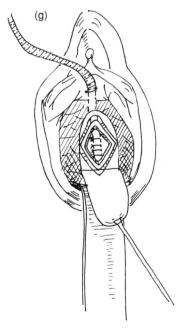

Figure 18-8. Excision of urethral diverticulum. (a) Inverted U-shaped incision with apex distal to diverticulum. (b) Transverse incision in fascia over diverticulum. (c) Fascia over diverticulum dissected around the diverticulum. (d) Stab incision into the wall and pediatric Foley catheter placed and balloon inflated to outline the sac. (e) Traction on the Foley catheter aids in dissection around the diverticulum. (f) Opening into the urethra exposed and indwelling Foley catheter visualized (note layer of fascia and diverticular wall dissected free). (g) Closure of the urethral defect with interrupted absorbable sutures.

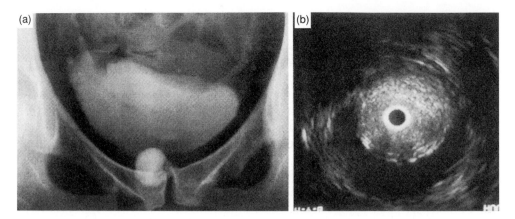

Figure 18-9.   Endoluminal ultrasonography. (a) Large urethral diverticulum. (b) Ultrasound image of large horseshoe-shaped diverticulum. (From reference 49, with permission.)

diverticulectomy alone. If the patient has a large diverticulum involving the urethral sphincter area or a diverticulum necessitating a lot of pelvic dissection, an associated sling procedure using organic material can be considered. Synthetic material should not be used because of the high risk of erosion and fistula formation. If the tissue is poor, especially in the presence of surrounding inflammation, or closure without tension impossible, then a Martius graft can be placed between the fascia and the vaginal wall.

Patients are typically discharged home 1 to 2 days postoperatively with a Foley catheter. Many authors place both a transurethral Foley and a suprapubic catheter. A voiding cystourethrogram can be done postoperatively at 7–10 days. If extravasation is identified suprapubic drainage can be continued and a repeat study performed in 1 week. Young and colleagues[50] noted no extravasation on any patient after the second VCUG, but Leach and Bavendam[9] noted an average of 15 days to catheter removal with the range of 7–28 days.

RESULTS

There have been no randomized trials of one treatment versus another. The largest series have reported on excision of the diverticulum. Ginsburg and Genadry[39] amalgamated several large series together. Of the 414 combined patients, complications developed in 17%. Recurrence of the diverticulum and recurrent urinary tract infections were the most common complications. Their own series had the highest recurrence rate at 20%.[3] The majority of recurrences occurred within 3 years. They felt a number may have been due to missed or developing diverticula underscoring the need for adequate preoperative imaging.

Fistula formation is surprisingly rare (Table 18-2). A significant number of patients may develop postoperative genuine stress incontinence though this may reflect a nondiagnosed condition preoperatively. Leach and Bavendam[9] noted no cases of genuine stress incontinence postoperatively in patients where the diagnosis had been excluded preoperatively by appropriate testing. Thus appropriate preoperative evaluation is imperative in attempting to achieve post-operative continence. Peters and Vaughan[10] noted that rarely did patients have persistent unexplained urinary tract infection. Those with recurrent infections usually had a recurrence of the diverticulum or calculus or some other identifiable cause. Those patients with recurrent urinary tract infections post-operatively should be investigated for probable cause.

Only a small number of patients have been treated by marsupialization alone. In a total of 23 patients reported to date,[3,46,51] there were no cases of recurrence, recurrent urinary tract infections, fistula, or stricture. One person had mild genuine stress incontinence not requiring treatment. Patient selection limiting this procedure to distal diverticula is of paramount importance.

Table 18-2. Postoperative complications (percent)

	No. of patients	Recurrence	Fistula	Postoperative GSI	Stricture	Recurrent UTI
Leach & Bavendam[9]	29	3	0	0	0	—
Ginsburg & Genadry[3]	64	20	1.6	6	1.6	—
Davis & Robinson[8]	98	1	4	—	—	—
Pathak & House[13]	42	—	—	—	—	3
Tancer et al.[40]	34	0	0	0		
Hoffman & Adams[22]	60	—	1.7	6.7	1.7	—
Davis & TeLinde[2]	84	12	—	—	—	13

CONCLUSIONS

A high index of clinical suspicion combined with physical examination, VCUG, cystoscopy, and possibly a double balloon catheter study will diagnose the majority of urethral diverticula. MRI can be used where x-ray findings are equivocal and suspicion high. Appropriate assessment of preoperative genuine stress incontinence will minimize the risk of postoperative incontinence. Recurrence rates are significant and patients must be counseled appropriately. All other complications following repair are rare.

REFERENCES

1. Hey W. *Practical Observations in Surgery*. Philadelphia: J. Humphreys. 1805: 303.
2. Davis H. TeLinde R. Urethral diverticula: An assay of 121 cases. *J Urol* 1958; **80**: 34–39.
3. Ginsburg DS, Genadry R. Suburethral diverticulum: Classification and therapeutic considerations. *Obstet Gynecol* 1983; **61**: 685–688.
4. Davis H, Cian L. Positive pressure urethrography: A new diagnostic method. *J Urol* 1956; **75**: 753–757.
5. Andersen M. The incidence of diverticula in the female urethra. *J Urol* 1967; **98**: 96–98.
6. Adams WE. Urethrography. *Bull Tulane Med Fac* 1964; **23**: 107–109.
7. Stewart M. Bretland PM. Stidolph NE. Urethral diverticula in the female urethra. *Br J Urol* 1981; **53**: 353–359.
8. Davis BL, Robinson DG. Diverticula of the female urethra: Essay of 120 cases. *J Urol* 1970; **104**: 850–853.
9. Leach GE, Bavendam TG. Female urethral diverticula. *Urology* 1987; **30**: 407–415.
10. Peters WA, Vaughan ED. Urethral diverticulum in the female: Etiological factors and post-operative results. *Obstet Gynecol* 1976; **47**: 549–552.
11. Benjamin J, Elliott L, Cooper JF, Bjornson L. Urethral diverticulum in adult female: Clinical aspects, operative procedure, and pathology. *Urology* 1974; **3**: 1–7.
12. Huffman JW. The detailed anatomy of the paraurethral ducts in the adult human female. *Am J Obstet Gynecol* 1948; **55**: 86–101.
13. Pathak U, House M. Diverticulum of the female urethra. *Obstet Gynecol* 1970; **36**: 789–794.
14. Spraitz A, Welch J. Diverticulum of the female urethra. *Am J Obstet Gynecol* 1965; **91**: 1013–1016.
15. Kim B, Hricak H, Tanagho EA. Diagnosis of urethral diverticula in women: Value of MR Imaging. *AJR* 1993; **161**: 809–815.
16. Summitt, RL, Stovall TG. Urethral diverticula: Evaluation by urethral pressure profilometry, cystourethroscopy, and the voiding cystourethrogram. *Obstet Gynecol* 1992; **80**: 695–699.
17. MacKinnon M, Pratt J, Pool T. Diverticulum of the female urethra. *Surg Clin North Am* 1959; **39**: 953.
18. Patanaphan V, Prempree T, Scwchand W, Hafiz MA, Jaiwatana J. Adenocarcinoma arising in female urethral diverticulum. *Urology* 1983; **22**: 259–264.
19. Cea PC, Ward JN, Lavengood RW, Gray GF. Mesonephric adenocarcinomas in urethral diverticula. *Urology* 1977; **10**: 58–61.
20. Palagiri A. Urethral diverticulum with endometriosis. *Urology* 1978; **11**: 271–272.
21. Presman D, Rolnick D, Zumerchek J. Calculus formation within a diverticulum of the female urethra. *J Urol* 1964; **91**: 376–377.
22. Hoffman M, Adams W. Recognition and repair of urethral diverticula. *Am J Obstet Gynecol* 1965; **92**: 106–111.
23. Rozsahegyi J, Magasi P, Szule E. Diverticulum of the female urethra: A report of 50 cases. *Acta Chir Hung* 1984; **15**: 33–38.
24. Kittredge R, Bienstock M, Finby N. Urethral diverticula in women. *AJR Radium Ther Nucl Med* 1966; **98**: 200–207.
25. McLoughlin MG. Carcinoma in situ in urethral diverticulum: Pitfalls of marsupialzation alone. *Urology* 1975; **6**: 343.
26. Hricak H, Secaf E, Buckley DW, Brown JJ, Tanagho EA, McAninch JW. Female urethra: MR imaging. *Radiology* 1991; **178**: 527–535.
27. Baert L. Willemen P, Oyen R. Endovaginal sonography: New diagnostic approach for urethral diverticula. *J Urol* 1992; **147**: 464–466.

28. Pavlica P, Viglietta G, Losinno F, Veneziano S, Dalla Rovere S. Diverticulae of the female urethra: A radiological and ultrasound study. *Rad Med* 1988; **75**: 521–527.
29. Bhatia NN, McCarthy TA. Ostergard DR. Urethral pressure profiles of women with urethral diverticula. *Obstet Gynecol* 1981; **58**: 375–378
30. Reid RE, Gill B, Laor E, Tolia BM, Freed SZ. Role of urodynamics in management of urethral diverticula in females. *Urology* 1986; **28**: 342–346.
31. Drutz HP. Urethral diverticula. *Obstet Gynecol Clin North Am* 1989; **16**: 323–829.
32. Lee TG, Keller FS. Urethral diverticulum: Diagnosis by ultrasound. *AJR*: 1977; **128**: 690–691.
33. Kølhorn EI, Glickman MG. Technical aids in investigation and management of urethral diverticula in the female. *Urology* 1992; **40**: 322–325.
34. Greenberg M, Stone D, Cochran ST, et al. Female urethral diverticula: Double-balloon catheter study. *AJR* 1981; **136**: 259–264.
35. Wexler JS, McGovern TP. Ultrasonography of the female urethral diverticulum. *AJR* 1980; **134**: 737–740.
36. Reuter KL, Young SB, Colby J. Transperitoneal sonography in assessment of a urethral diverticulum. *J Clin Ultrasound* 1992; **20**: 221–223.
37. Klutke C, Golomb J, Barbaric Z, Raz S. The anatomy of stress incontinence: Magnetic resonance imaging of the female bladder neck and urethra. *J Urol* 1990; **143**: 563–566.
38. Leach GE, Schmidbauer H, Hadley HR, et al. Surgical treatment of female urethral diverticulum. *Semin Urol* 1986; **4**: 33–34.
39. Ginsburg DS, Genadry R. Suburethral diverticulum in the female. *Obstet Gynecol Surg* 1984; **39**: 1–7.
40. Tancer ML, Mooppan MU, Pierre-Louis C, Kim H, Ravski N. Suburethral diverticulum treatment with partial ablation. *Obstet Gynecol* 1983; **62**: 511–513.
41. Hajj SN, Evans MI, Diverticula of the female urethra. *Am J Obstet Gynecol* 1980; **136**: 335.
42. Lee RA. Diverticulum of the female urethra: Post-operative complications and results. *Obstet Gynecol* 1983; **61**: 52–58.
43. Downs RA. Urethral diverticula in females. Alternative surgical treatment. *Urology* 1987; **39**: 201–203.
44. Edwards E, Beebe R. Diverticula of the female urethra. *Obstet Gynecol* 1955; **5**: 729.
45. Parks J. Section of the urethral wall for correction of urethrovaginal fistula and urethral diverticula. *Am J Obstet Gynecol* 1965; **93**: 683.
46. Spence H, Duckett J. Diverticulum of the female urethra: Clinical aspects and presentation of simple operative technique for cure. *J Urol* 1970; **104**: 423–437.
47. Ellik M. Diverticulum of female urethra: New method of ablation. *J Urol* 1957; **77**: 243–244.
48. Moore TU. Diverticulum of female urethra: Improved technique of surgical incision. *J Urol* 1952; **68**: 611–616.
49. Chancellor MB, Liu J-B, Rivas DA, Karasick S, Bagley DH, Goldberg BB. Intraoperative endo-luminal ultrasound evaluation of urethral diverticula. *J Urol* 1995; **153**: 72–75.
50. Young GPH, Weahle GR, Raz S. Female urethral diverticulum. In: Raz S (ed). *Female Urology*. Philadelphia: W.B. Saunders, 1996: 477–489.
51. Lichtman A, Robertson J. Suburethral diverticula treated by marsupialization. *Obstet Gynecol* 1976; **47**: 203–206.

CHAPTER 19

Anal incontinence

ROBERT L. HARRIS AND STEVEN E. SPEIGHTS

Anal incontinence refers to the involuntary loss of flatus or feces. Although a benign disorder, it can be socially, psychologically, and emotionally devastating and may lead to institutionalization for some patients.[1] The disorders of anal control are poorly understood and remain underreported by patients and many times unrecognized or ignored by physicians.[2] Recently there has been increased interest in the study of these disorders, and reports suggest that problems of control are more significant and more common than previously reported.[3-5] However, even with increasing awareness, there is no current standardization for the definition of disorders of anal continence so it has been difficult to generate meaningful and reproducible data.

EPIDEMIOLOGY

Much is published but little is known about the incidence and prevalence of anal incontinence and how it affects those who suffer from it. It is clear that women, especially multiparous women, the elderly, and institutionalized persons are particularly victimized.[6,7] In the community, the prevalence of anal incontinence has been reported to be around 2%.[3,8] It is more common in males in younger age groups and females in the older age groups. Between 7% and 18% of healthy adults acknowledge incontinence of gas or feces.[9,10] In hospitalized or institutionalized elderly patients, the prevalence ranges from 17% to 66%.[10-14] Incontinence of urine and anal contents may occur concomitantly, and double incontinence has been shown to be 12 times as likely as anal incontinence alone.[8] Differing definitions of anal incontinence probably account for most of the variability among reported prevalence rates. However, an additional factor may be the patient's reluctance to admit to anal incontinence. In one study, 10% of urine-incontinent patients denied anal incontinence on initial questioning, only to admit the problem to medical personnel on follow-up questioning.[15]

SOCIOECONOMIC AND PSYCHOLOGICAL IMPACT

The management of anal incontinence presents a great burden both to those who suffer with the problem and to their care-givers. The direct cost is based on prevalence rates, number of episodes of incontinence, laundry and disposable undergarments, and increased nursing time requirements. To embark on a complete diagnostic evaluation for diarrhea is very expensive and it is not uncommon that many patients who complain of diarrhea, actually have incontinence of liquid stool but are unwilling to admit to this on initial questioning.[2,16] Treatment and subsequent preventive therapy for breakdown of excoriated skin from fecal contamination, and investigation and treatment of vaginal and urinary symptomatology secondary to bacterial exposure from frequent contamination with feces is also costly. Anal incontinence is a common reason for institutionalization of the elderly, which represents a large financial burden for society, and the number of persons placed in nursing home care is expected to increase in future years.[17] The total cost to society for anal incontinence is unknown.

The psychological impact of anal incontinence is poorly studied. Certainly, defecation is an extremely private function and inability to control bowel function is a profound personal problem. Social isolation and alienation is not uncommon and may be reinforced by physicians or other medical personnel who will not or cannot discuss the problem.[15,18] The loss of bowel control, which is a basic function learned in early childhood, often signifies a loss of independence and is associated with aging in a negative manner. This may result in lower self-esteem, a sense of inadequacy or helplessness, and even clinical depression. Nonetheless, severity of illness resulting from anal incontinence is highly subjective and to assume that anal incontinence represents an independent causal relationship with psychological dysfunction is only speculative at this point as no data are currently available to address this. In women with urinary incontinence, however, there has been shown a degree of similar negative psychological impact.[18,19] Also, women with incontinence report more sexual dysfunction, including decreased libido and dyspareunia.[20,21] Embarrassment about odor and fear of coital incontinence also may cause or worsen sexual dysfunction.

ANORECTAL CONTINENCE

Functional Anatomy

Complex coordination of the striated and smooth muscles of the pelvis along with precise sensory input from the anorectum is required for continence. Normal continence is also dependent on many other factors; stool volume, stool consistency, colonic transit, distensibility of the rectum, function of the anal canal, and adequate mental function. The relative contribution of each is not known but abnormalities in any of these may lead to incontinence.[22] For example, even with normal muscular and neurologic function, a person may not be able to maintain control if a large bolus of liquid stool is presented to the anal canal suddenly. Similarly, with radiation proctitis or inflammatory bowel disease, the rectum may become poorly distensible precluding a normal reservoir and resulting in incontinence.[23-25]

Muscles important for maintenance of continence are the puborectalis and external anal sphincter (EAS), both striated muscles, and the internal anal sphincter (IAS), which is smooth muscle. Solid stool remains above the anal canal by constant activity of the puborectalis which originates at the pubic bone and passes beside the vagina and rectum to fuse behind the anorectal junction and form a sling that maintains stool high in the pelvis (Figure 19-1). The puborectalis and EAS maintain constant muscular tone and are thus dominated by type 1 (slow-twitch) fibers. A smaller proportion of type 2 (fast-twitch) fibers also exists for quick response. Puborectalis action is responsible for the somewhat acute angle between the rectal and anal canals and thus is somewhat effective in maintaining continence of solid stool even in the event of sphincter separation. There is some evidence that receptors within the puborectalis sense passage of feces from the rectum to the anal canal and modulate the muscle's resting activity.[26] The EAS and IAS maintain continence below the level of the puborectalis and are especially important in the control of gas and liquid stool. The vectors of force in the sphincter complex that work together to maintain continence include the anteriorly directed puborectalis, posterior attachments of the EAS to coccyx, and anteriorly directed attachment of superficial EAS to the perineal body. At rest the anal canal is kept closed by the constant tonic activity of the EAS and IAS.[6] The IAS is responsible for about 80% of the resting tone with the EAS and vascular cushions in the anal canal lining accounting for the remainder.[27-28] This is further supported by the correlation of decreasing maximal basal pressures, as measured by manometry, with IAS defects; as well as decreased maximum squeeze pressure with EAS defects.[29] Although a voluntary sphincter contraction can only be maintained for a short time, this nearly doubles the pressure of the anal canal. The vascular cushions in the lining of the anal canal act as an important barrier against mucus and fecal material by

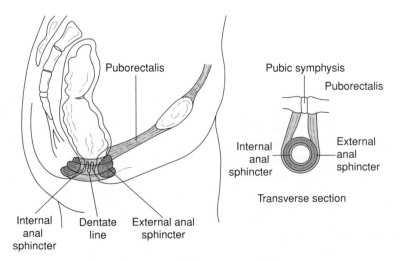

Figure 19-1.   Diagram of the rectum, anal canal, sphincteric muscles, and puborectalis muscle.

encouraging an hermetic closure of the anal canal. This may be lost in patients with hemorrhoids thus allowing fecal soiling and spotting.[30] Therefore, passive fecal incontinence, that is, the loss of feces without the patient's awareness, and incontinence at rest are related to IAS dysfunction and somewhat to the anatomy of the anal canal, whereas urge incontinence, that is, the loss of feces due to an inability to suppress defecation, and the inability to maintain continence in times of sudden distention are related to EAS dysfunction.[4,29,31] Continence of liquid stool requires adequate function of both the internal and external sphincters but normal EAS function is imperative in this situation.

The IAS is the thickened downward prolongation of the circular smooth muscle layer of the rectum. These smooth muscle fibers form dense bundles in an oblique arrangement which produces a high pressure zone in the anal canal 2.5 to 5 cm in length.[32] The EAS has been described as having deep, superficial, and subcutaneous components, but some believe it best considered as a continuous, circumferential mass as these three divisions are not always clearly demarcated at least with anal endosonography (AES) and magnetic resonance imaging (MRI).[33–35] When viewed as having three parts, the deep EAS is a continuation of the puborectalis posteriorly, the superficial component is imaged in the midcanal, and the subcutaneous component at the anal verge (Figure 19-2a).[34,36] There is debate on the size and thickness of the sphincters and on the best method of measurement. Both MRI and AES have been used for imaging of the sphincteric complex and one study directly compared the two methods[37]; their measurements reflecting those of many other reports.[38] Almost all agree that the sphincteric complex is thinner anteriorly (between 2 and 4 mm) and thicker posteriorly (between and 6 and 10 mm). This has been demonstrated by anatomic dissection[39] and confirmed by several authors using AES and MRI.[34,37,40] Variations in width measurements are also noted, but most agree that the EAS measures 2–3 cm over its entire craniocaudad length anteriorly and 3 cm posteriorly.[38]

Innervation

Striated pelvic floor muscles are innervated by motor neurons from the second and third sacral segments. The EAS is innervated by the inferior hemorrhoidal branches of the pudendal nerve, with one in three also having another branch from S4. The puborectalis may be innervated by perineal branches of the pudendal nerve or by branches of the sacral plexus.[42] The IAS is under autonomic control; sympathetic fibers being excitatory and parasympathetic fibers inhibitory. Unlike the EAS and puborectalis, the IAS cannot be controlled voluntarily as its function is mediated by reflex arcs at the spinal cord level.[27,28]

The rectum has very few intraepithelial ganglion cells. Both myelinated and nonmyelinated fibers are close to the rectal mucosa but none are in the epithelium, which explains its relative in-sensitivity to painful stimuli. The rectum is very sensitive to distention but the mechanism of this response is unknown.[42] Current belief is that these receptors are not located in the rectal

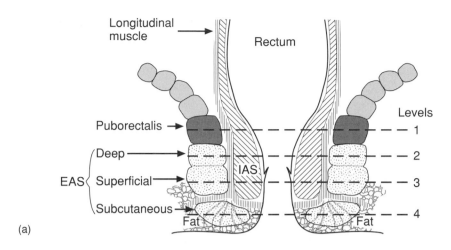

(a)

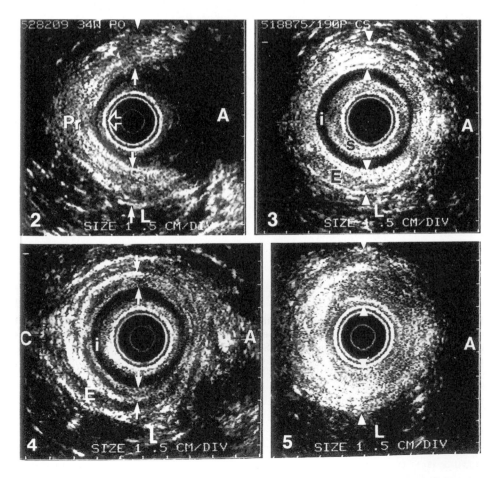

wall, but possibly in the pelvic floor. This is supported by the observation of normal continence and reflexes in patients who have undergone restorative proctocolectomy or coloanal anastamosis.[43,44]

In contrast to the rectum, the anal canal is sensory-rich. The main sensory input is below S2 and sensory impulses from the anal canal travel through the inferior hemorrhoidal branches of the pudendal nerve to S2–S4. The anal canal and perianal skin is sensitive to pain, temperature and touch similar to that of the tip of the index finger.[41]

Physiology of Defecation

Since the anal canal maintains a high pressure zone even at rest, which is primarily from IAS action, stool is usually maintained above the anal canal and is not typically present on digital examination.[30] As colonic contents pass into the rectum and it distends, the IAS relaxes. This reflex is independent of cerebral influence. As these contents pass into the upper anal canal, the lower anal canal is kept closed by contraction of the EAS, which is primarily under conscious control. Sampling of the contents to distinguish solid, liquid, or gaseous fecal material, then occurs. Once the contents have been sampled, if the person chooses not to defecate or release flatus, further contraction of the EAS and puborectalis allows the IAS to regain tone. Together these actions allow contents to be propelled out of the anal canal and back up into the rectum until the reflex again occurs.[27,28,30,31,41] The exact mechanism that allows discrimination between solid, liquid, and gas is not known.

ETIOLOGIES OF ANAL INCONTINENCE

Anal incontinence may have a variety of causes, most of which are outlined in Table 19-1.

Figure 19-2. (a) Schematic representation of the anal canal illustrating the various levels at which measurements of muscle thickness were taken. Level *1* = puborectalis muscle; level *2* = deep (proximal) external anal sphincter (EAS); level *3* = superficial (mid) EAS; level *4* = subcutaneous (distal) EAS. (Modified and published with permission). (b) Sonographic image at level *1* (a) of the puborectalis (*Pr*) muscle. *A* anterior; *L* left. The bright double ring (*open arrow*) is the reflection of the probe cone. The *closed arrows* indicate the sites of measurement of muscle thickness on each side. (c) Image at level *2* (a) of the deep external anal sphincter (*E*) with arrows indicating sites of measurement. *A* anterior; *L* left. *s* submucosa; the internal anal sphincter (*i*) appears as a hypoechoic ring. (d) Image at level *3* (a) of the superficial external sphincter (EAS) which appears elliptical compared with the circular deep EAS (c). *A* anterior; *L* left. The sites of measurement of the relatively hyperechoic longitudinal muscle are demonstrated by *arrows*. *C* anococcygeal ligament. External anal sphincter (*E*); Internal sphincter (*i*). (e) Image at level *4* (a) of the dense hyperechoic subcutaneous EAS. *Arrows* indicate lateral thickness. *A* anterior; *L* left.

Table 19-1.   Etiologies of anal incontinence

Normal pelvic floor
    Diarrheal states
        Infectious diarrhea
        Inflammatory bowel disease
        Short-gut syndrome
        Laxative abuse
        Radiation enteritis
    Overflow
        Impaction
        Encopresis
        Rectal neoplasms
    Neurologic conditions
        Congenital anomalies
        Multiple sclerosis
        Dementia
        Cerebrovascular accidents
        Diabetic neuropathy
        Neoplasms of brain, spinal cord, cauda equina
Injuries and abnormal pelvic floor
    Congenital anorectal malformation
    Trauma
        Obstetrical injury
        Accidental injury
        Anorectal surgery
    Aging
    Pelvic-floor denervation
        Vaginal delivery
        Chronic straining at stool
        Rectal prolapse
        Descending-perineum syndrome

Obstetric Injury

Of women with anal incontinence, clearly obstetric trauma is the most important cause. Damage to the continence mechanism may occur through direct muscular damage, damage to the motor or sensory innervation of the pelvic floor and anal canal, or in combination. It is postulated that delivery of the fetal head through the pelvis may damage the pudendal nerve by compression as it exits Alcock's canal or that injury may occur secondary to stretching of the nerve as the head bulges the perineum during the second stage of labor.[45,46] Direct muscular damage usually occurs as an anterior disruption of the sphincter. In a study of 62 women with fecal incontinence related to obstetrical procedures, anal endosonography (AES) revealed an external anal sphincter (EAS) defect in 90% and an internal anal sphincter (IAS) defect in 65%.[47] Deen and colleaques[36] reported that of 42 women with fecal incontinence, obstetric trauma was identified as the only predisposing factor in 35 of these patients; 30 of whom exhibited a morphologic defect in the sphincter complex on AES. In 22 of these patients with a history of a perineal tear and/or an episiotomy, 21 (95%) had a sphincter defect.

Using AES, manometry, perineometry, nerve latencies, and bowel symptoms (urgency, anal incontinence), Sultan and colleagues[48] evaluated 202 consecutive women who had been pregnant more than 34 weeks. All were studied during the 6 weeks preceding delivery, 150 patients who returned 6 weeks after delivery, and 32 with abnormal findings 6 months after delivery. Of 127 women who delivered vaginally, 79 were primiparous (none with fecal urgency or sphincter defects before delivery) and 48 were multiparous (19 had a defect before delivery); 13 (10%) developed one or both bowel symptoms. With the exception of one primiparous patient, sphincter defects were demonstrated on all women who experienced either fecal urgency or anal incontinence after delivery. The maximal resting anal pressures and maximal squeeze pressures fell significantly in both primiparous and multiparous women; even though there was considerable overlap of values between women with and without symptoms. Perineal descent increased significantly in both groups also and the 36 women with abnormal descent on straining after delivery had significantly longer pudendal nerve terminal motor latencies (PNTML) postpartum than the 35 with normal descent. However, there was no association between bowel symptoms and increased perineal descent or prolonged PNTML. Internal anal sphincter defects developed in 3 women, although their perinea were intact. External anal sphincter defects were detected only in those who underwent episiotomy or who sustained a spontaneous perineal tear. Only 3% of primiparous women and no multiparous women had clinically recognized third-degree or fourth-degree tears at time of delivery. However, 28 (35%) of the primiparous women had postdelivery sphincter defects by AES as did 21 (44%) of the multiparous women, most of whom had only one previous delivery, suggesting that the risk of sphincter damage is greatest during the first vaginal delivery (19 of 41 had defects before this delivery). Anal endosonogrpahic examination also suggested that the structural damage to the sphincters was permanent, since the defects were present at 6 months and, again, the incidence of defects among primiparous women after delivery was similar to that among multiparous women before delivery. None of the 23 women who underwent cesarean section had any bowel symptoms or any change in anal pressure. This is documented again by Sultan and colleagues[49] in another prospective evaluation of 20 women who underwent elective cesarean section at term. The authors found no change in anal pressures or sphincter morphology in any of these women. There also appears to be some correlation with forceps delivery and pudendal nerve and anal sphincter damage.[48,50,51] However, no data are currently available to determine whether this is primarily due to direct damage from the instrument itself or from damage secondary to the indication for its use.

Perineal Descent

Abnormal perineal descent (PD) occurs when the weakened pelvic floor lies at a lower level than normal. Excessive descent has been defined as downward movement of >2.5 cm and as descent of the plane of the perineum beyond the plane of the ischial tuberosities.[55,56] Amount of PD may be measured by use of a perineometer or by cinedefecography. Increased PD occurs in many patients with idiopathic fecal incontinence and is a common finding in patients with constipation and rectal pain.[57] Besides obstetric injury associated with a prolonged second stage of labor, significant PD thought to be the result of chronic, repeated straining, as with chronic constipation, which forces the anterior rectal wall to protrude into the anal canal thus creating a sensation of incomplete defecation. This then results in more straining and worsening of the problem.[58] Present evidence implicates that pudendal nerve injury is the main cause of anal sphincter weakness with associated anal incontinence in these patients. This appears to be the result of damage to motor as well as sensory innervation.[59,60]

Age

The effect of age on anorectal function has been studied. Findings with increasing age include increased perineal descent at rest and with straining, slowed pudendal nerve conduction, and decreased anal resting and maximal squeeze pressures.[61,62] Estrogen receptors have been identified in the EAS,[63] however the interrelations of aging and menopausal effects on anorectal incontinence, even though obviously important, are difficult to define from currently available data.

Diabetes

Peripheral and autonomic neuropathies may develop in up to 20% of patients with diabetes. From a standpoint of anal control, this can result in an increased conscious threshold of rectal sensation and difficulty with reflex EAS contraction in response to distention of the rectum. Autonomic neuropathy may result in chronic diarrhea producing further difficulty maintaining fecal continence.[64]

Traumatic Causes

Direct trauma to the sphincteric mechanism may cause incontinence. The most common direct injury to the sphincteric mechanism occurs as a result of iatrogenic damage.[65,66] For example, the incidence of continence disorders ranges from 30% to 50% after partial internal sphincterotomy and fistulotomy. Soiling and impaired control for gas may occur in up to 45% of these patients.[67,68] These same disorders also occur in anorectal procedures where the sphincters are not divided. These include anal stretch procedures, for example, anal dilatation and surgical retraction, with 15–25% of patients experiencing continence problems.[69] Hemorrhoidectomy is another example, after which as many as 20% of patients report similar problems.[70] With a history of rectal prolapse, a loss of feeling of urge is common and specific symptoms in these patients incontinent due to pelvic floor denervation is as high as 70%. From neurophysiologic studies, it is known that only about 3% of patients with obstetric sphincter ruptures and incontinence have significant denervation injury, whereas denervation injury frequently occurs in iatrogenic incontinence (20–30%).[65] Therefore, it very likely that incontinence after anorectal surgery, even after sphincter-cutting procedures, is caused by denervation rather than local muscular sphincter damage or disruption. Incontinence due to causes other than iatrogenic or obstetric injury is very rare (<10%). These causes include accidents complicated by pelvic fractures, perineal lacerations and sexual trauma. Most are complicated, that is, multiple lacerations of the sphincters and/or pelvic nerve injury, thus most require a more radical surgical intervention such as gracilis or gluteus transposition.[71]

Radiation Injury

Another uncommon cause of anal incontinence is radiation injury. The rectum is the most common site of injury after pelvic irradiation and more than 70% of patients with severe chronic injury suffer from rectosigmoid involvement. Doses of 3000–4000 cGy over 3–4 weeks causes early damage (edema and hyperemia) of the mucosa in 50–70% of patients.[23] Common symptoms include incomplete evacuation, diarrhea, tenesmus, and incontinence. Later changes, that is, ulceration, fibrosis, stricture, fistula, occur between 12 and 48 months. Symptoms include the above plus, rectal bleeding, pain, and constipation. Proctosigmoiditis due to radiation damage may cause incontinence. This is diagnosed by sigmoidoscopy which shows erythema, telangiectasia, ulceration, and necrosis. A double-contrast barium enema usually demonstrates loss of distensibility of the rectum and colon. Up to 75% of patients will be responsive to conservative medical therapy including rectal steroids, low-residue diets, and antidiarrheals. Other causes of incontinence due to radiation injury include fistulas, of which rectovaginal is the most common, followed by colovesical; small bowel enteritis resulting in malabsorption, diarrhea, and incontinence; and strictures which narrow the lumen and decrease capacity with resultant frequent evacuation, tenesmus, and incontinence.[24] Direct damage to the rectum from radiation results in decreased motility and a reduction in rectal volumes and compliance. This decreases its proprioceptive ability producing frequency, urgency, and urge incontinence. The internal anal sphincter is often damaged resulting in a significant reduction in anal canal resting pressure and physiologic length and the rectosphicteric reflex is reduced.[25] Both of these actions are probably a function of decreased compliance and damage to the myenteric plexus and/or direct damage to pelvic floor receptors. The external anal sphincter is relatively unaffected.

Congenital Abnormalities

Rarely, the obstetrician may encounter a newborn with a congenital malformation; most commonly imperforate anus. Imperforate anus occurs in one of every 4000–5000 newborns and is slightly higher in males. The anal canal is absent in most types anorectal malformations therefore "normal" bowel function does not occur. There is a spectrum of defects with "low" or infralevator defects, that is, malformations only with effects distally, having a better prognosis than "high" or supralevator defects, such as a bladder-neck fistula.[72] Most have different degrees of development of muscle structures and thus different degrees of rectal proprioception. Many are unable to discriminate gas, liquid, and solid because there is no anal canal. If the rectum is located within the sphincteric mechanism, patients are able to detect distension as measured by balloon inflation, so their main enemy is liquid stool that may leak without distending rectum. Voluntary sphincters are present in most and the quality depends on the severity of the defect. For example, with rectal atresia, the sphincter quality is almost normal, whereas with cloacae the sphincter quality is very poor. Complex malformations most often have an abnormally dilated distal rectum and severe constipation. This is a primary hypomotility disorder of the rectosigmoid resulting in incapacity to empty completely. There is a correlation between the degree of original dilation and severity; the more severe dilation occurring in lower defects and in cases without a fistula. The sacrum is the most frequently deformed bony structure. More than two missing sacral segments is poor prognostic sign for continence and hemisacrum is a bad prognostic sign. The most frequent malformation seen in females is imperforate anus with rectovestibular fistula.[73]

Most defects can be diagnosed by perineal inspection. Initial clues include a prominent midline skin tag just below which an instrument can be passed into an orifice. Other findings include a midline raphe; subepithelial meconium fistula, which looks like a black ribbon placed in the middle of the perineum; the presence of meconium coming out through small orifice anterior to anal dimple; a very narrow anus (anal stenosis); or an anal membrane, which is a thin epithelial membrane through which meconium can be seen. All of these represent low defects, which may be treated with perineal anoplasty without a protective colostomy.[74] A colostomy is required for a flat bottom which is usually a reflection of poor muscle structures and usually associated with very high defects. Meconium in the urine represents some form of communication between the urinary tract and rectum and also requires colostomy. Decisions concerning opening of colostomy should never be made prior to 24 hours of life because when a baby is born, the abdomen is not distended initially. It takes 16–24 hours before abdominal distension and an increase in intraluminal colonic pressure occurs. This pressure forces meconium into the urinary tract or a tiny perineal fistula or allows intestinal gas to reach the very end of blind rectal pouch, which affects management decisions.[75,76] From 20% to 54% of patients have associated urogenital defects.[72,73] The higher the malformation (supralevator), the more frequently urologic abnormalities are associated. Low defects (infralevator) have less than a 10% chance of associated urologic abnormalities. Patients with persistent cloacae or rectovesical fistulas have up to 90% chance of associated urologic abnormalities.

All anorectal malformations can be surgically corrected by the posterior sagittal approach.[77] The common denominator of infralevator defects is that the rectum opens in an abnormal orifice located anterior to the center of the sphincter. All perineal fistula have universally good results with the most common sequela being constipation. Vestibular fistulas reach fecal control in >95%. Supralevator defects have a poor prognosis. With rectobladder-neck fistulas, most have abnormal sacrums and if the sacrum is good, only 20–30% have voluntary bowel movements by age 3. The remainder are incontinent for life. With cloacae, if there is a good sacrum then there is good chance for some voluntary control, although all still suffer degrees of malfunction resulting in different degrees of soiling between bowel movements. If the common channel is ≥3 cm and/or the sacrum is abnormal, these patients are usually incontinent for life. Urinary control is variable but not usually normal, again dependent on the status of the sacrum and any damage secondary to surgical dissection.[78]

EVALUATION

History and Physical Examination

A meticulous history and complete physical examination are essential in determining the cause of anal incontinence in a particular patient.[5] After the existence of incontinence has been established, the onset, duration, frequency, severity, and other circumstances surrounding the incontinent episodes should be addressed. Whether the incontinence involves flatus, liquid, or solid stool or any combination is important information and can give clues as to where the deficit lies. A history of fecal urgency or urge incontinence or inability to control only liquid stool and flatus may indicate a deficit in EAS function. A history of inability to control solid stools may implicate abnormalities in the puborectalis or, if the patient complains of no warning of impending defecation, then a sensory deficit may exist. Patients with sensory deficits may have fecal soiling as may patients with IAS defects, anal fissures, hemorrhoids, and anal polyps. A history of chronic and/or bloody diarrhea, or rectal pain should prompt a consideration of inflammatory bowel disease and these patients should undergo an adequate evaluation including endoscopy of the lower bowel. With new onset of any unusual bowel or bladder symptomatology, a neurologic abnormality should always be considered and ruled out.

The obstetrician-gynecologist proficient at pelvic examination can glean much information from inspection and palpation of the vagina and perineum and the rectum and anus. Initially, the underpants should be examined for soiling and staining. Then, any erythema, dermatitis, evidence of poor hygiene or other abnormality of the skin of the perineum or perianal area should be noted.

Scars from previous episiotomies or tears may be present. A patulous, gaping anus may indicate severe loss of function. A rectovaginal fistula should immediately be ruled out. Rectal prolapse may not be apparent on resting examination in the supine position so the patient should be asked to perform the Valsalva maneuver and possibly be examined while standing if the history is worrisome for rectal prolapse. Significant perineal descent can also be noted with this technique. Neurologic examination should assess the integrity of S2–S4. To test the motor function of the EAS, the anal reflex can be evoked by lightly stroking the perianal skin and observing the concentric contraction of the EAS or, by tapping the clitoris, the bulbocavernosus reflex as well as the anal reflex can be elicited. If these are unsuccessful or indeterminate, the cough reflex can be used, which should result in a reflex contraction of the EAS and levator ani immediately before the cough. Sensory function, that is, the ability to discern rectal distention or contraction, is very difficult to determine on physical examination, and if history indicates that function may be compromised, further tests will be needed to determine if a sensory deficit exists. In any event, symmetric sensation over the vulva and perineum as tested by light touch and pinprick should be present.

Integrity of the EAS and puborectalis should be evaluated with observation and palpation both at rest and with voluntary contraction. A concentric contraction of the EAS and an upward and inward movement of the perineum and EAS, secondary to contraction of the puborectalis muscle, should occur when the patient is asked to voluntarily contract her sphincter. This can be assessed on digital examination (Figure 19-3). An intact EAS that has a weak resting tone

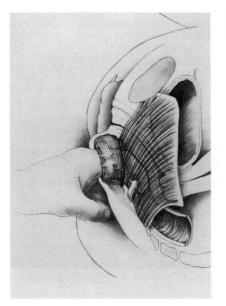

Figure 19-3. Digital assessment of the external anal sphincter and puborectalis muscles.

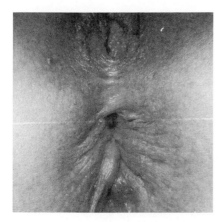

Figure 19-4. The "dovetail" sign.

and a weak voluntary contraction may be suggestive of significant pudendal neuropathy. When the sphincter is separated such as in chronic third-degree and fourth-degree lacerations, this separation is almost always anterior and may result in complete loss of the perineal body or in separation of the EAS with an otherwise relatively normal appearing perineal body.[79,80] With voluntary contraction, the separated ends of the EAS may create a dimpling in the perianal skin. A "dovetail" appearance of the anal skin resulting from loss of the anterior radial creases between the separated ends of the EAS has been described[6] (Figure 19-4). In addition to neuropathy associated with a weak contraction of an intact EAS, if there is no dimpling with voluntary contraction, neuropathy should also be considered. Simple digital examination can also be useful in the diagnosis of fecal impaction, which is a common cause of soiling and staining, especially in the elderly. If a rectovaginal fistula is identified, it is important to document integrity of the continence mechanism fully as coexistent sphincteric injury has been reported in 8.3% and 32% of patients who presented with complaints of fecal incontinence.[81,82]

Anal Manometry

Anal manometry is still one of the most common investigations used in assessing anorectal function. Although anal sphincter function can be estimated on digital examination, the accuracy of this measurement is limited.[83] Important manometric parameters of sphincteric function include measurement of the resting anal canal pressure and the maximum anal canal pressure with voluntary squeeze.[84,85] Length of the anal canal and presence or absence of the rectoanal inhibitory reflex can also be ascertained with use of anal manometry.[86] A pull-through technique is most commonly used, measuring resting and squeeze pressures with one of several different catheters; air or water filled micro-balloons, sleeve catheters or water perfused catheters, or microtransducers.

Multilumen perfused catheters assess anal canal pressures on a cross-sectional or directional basis and give a representative pressure for each quadrant of the anal canal. Computerized cross-sectional analysis then permits accurate localization of segmental pressure defects that correspond to anatomic disruption of the sphincter.[87]

Electrophysiologic Testing

The tonic activity of the pelvic floor and EAS results in continuous electrical activity that can be recorded with electrodes. Electromyography (EMG) of the anal sphincter and puborectalis muscle demonstrates integrity of their innervation. With the use of single-fiber or concentric needle EMG techniques, identification of neuropathic or myopathic changes can be determined.[46] Concentric needle EMG is useful in mapping the ends of the EAS when a separation exists.[88,89] PNTML is also used to determine evoked potential; increased delay implying damage to the pudendal nerve.[90]

Ultrasonography

Anal endosongraphy (AES) is performed using a 7 or 7.5 MHz rectal probe which has a hard sonolucent plastic cone filled with degassed water. It is about 4 cm in length with an external diameter of 1.7 cm. AES has been critically evaluated in terms of its ability to correctly identify normal and abnormal anatomy and to influence management (Figure 19.2b).[34,91,92] Also, results of AES have been shown to be reproducible both among and between examiners.[93] Dissection studies have shown a close correlation between endosonographic images and anatomical structures. Anal endosonogrpahy has also lessened the need for other investigations, such as electromyography, to identify external anal sphincter defects. The ultrasound image of a defect correlates well with absent electromyographic activity, and the former is more accurate at picking up lesions. Law and coworkers[88] compared concentric needle EMG and AES in mapping EAS defects in 15 patients with fecal incontinence. Both examinations showed defects in 12 patients and no defects in 3. All defects in the 12 patients were localized to the same quadrant using both techniques. Burnett and associates[89] related sonographic findings directly to EMG in an investigation of 13 patients where AES was used to localize the defect prior to needle insertion thus lessening the number of needle insertions required. These authors also voiced concerns regarding the depth of needle insertion. The anal canal radio-logically averages 4 cm in length and as previously mentioned, many defects occur only in the mid to deep EAS. Allowing for skin thickness, it is to be expected that the deep aspects of the EAS may be beyond the needle insertion depth unless inserted to at least 3 cm. Sultan compared clinical examination, manometry, EMG, and AES in 12 patients with fecal incontinence undergoing sphincter repair.[91] During operation tissue biopsy or removal of the defect was performed to allow histologic confirmation by pathology. Combined operative and histological examination identified an EAS defect in 9 of the 12 patients. Anal endosonography correctly identified all 9 defects and the 3 normal sphincters. The accuracy of clinical examination was 50% and that of both EMG and anal manometry was 75%. In addition, AES identified a defect of the IAS in 8 patients.

Until the recent advent of AES, evaluation of a patient with anorectal incontinence included a complete clinical examination, anal manometry, and evaluation of the innervation of the pelvic floor musculature by EMG. After this evaluation, the patient was classified as having idiopathic (neurogenic) incontinence or traumatic incontinence. Sometimes, however there is no clear correlation between these data and the clinical findings in patients in whom the surgeon suspects an existing sphincter defect. This lack of correlation is important because direct sphincter repair in general has better results than postanal repair.[94]

With the addition of AES it appears that a significant number of patients with suspected idiopathic incontinence do have sphincter defects. Using AES, Setti Carraro and colleagues[95] found clinically undetected defects in 19 of 30 patients examined after postanal repair. Anal endosonography affords several advantages in the evaluation of patients with anorectal incontinence, most notably a radial image to portray the extent of any defect. The accuracy of EMG in defining a defect in the muscle is well accepted but its usefulness may be limited by the number of needle insertions. Anal endosongraphy is quick, relatively easy to perform, its results reproducible, and it causes minimal patient discomfort.

There has been some concern regarding distortion of soft tissue and compression of sphincter musculature with use of the endoanal probe. This has led to attempts at visualization with endovaginal sonography[96,97] and transperineal scanning. Initial reports are promising but much more data are needed to determine its reliability and clinical usefulness.

Magnetic Resonance Imaging

Magnetic resonance imaging has been used in dynamic assessment of the pelvic floor and provides excellent visualization of anatomy (Figure 19.5).[98–100] Imaging of the sphincteric complex using an endorectal coil provides precise visualization[35,38,101] However, its clinical usefulness in defining defects has yet to be determined and when compared to AES, it is elaborate and costly and, based on limited data, does not seem to provide additional information.[37] Further data are needed to establish its application from a clinical and research standpoint.

Evacuation Proctography

Evacuation proctography, or defecography, radiographically evaluates defecation by video fluoroscopic imaging during simulated defecation. It is useful in diagnosing and quantifying rectoceles, enteroceles, and perineal descent and may demonstrate rectal prolapse and intussuseption. However, outside of providing information about anismus or spastic pelvic floor, it adds little to the evaluation of anal incontinence when compared to other previously mentioned modalities.[102,103]

THERAPY

The treatment of fecal incontinence includes medical therapy, behavioral therapy and biofeedback, and surgery. If any underlying gastrointestinal condition exists, it is probably prudent to treat the condition prior to embarking on an intense evaluation for other causes of incontinence, for example, steroids for inflammatory bowel disease, anticholinergics for irritable bowel syndrome and manual removal with subsequent prompted regular evacuation for fecal impaction. If the incontinence persists after adequate therapy for the presumed primary problem, then other options should be explored.

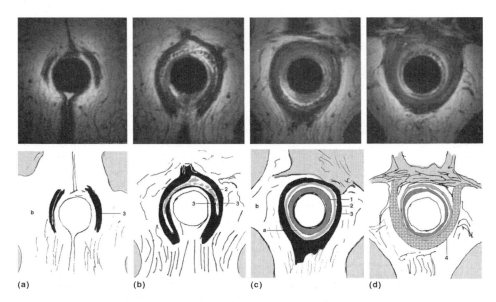

Figure 19-5. Axial T2-weighted contrast-enhanced fast field-echo MR images (30/13) and corresponding drawings. (a) Section through the lowest part of the external sphincter shows two halves of the external sphincter *3* embedded in the ischioanal space *b*; note the multiple septa within this space. (b) Section obtained slightly cranial to (a). Between the two folds of the external sphincter *3*, small bundles of the fan-shaped longitudinal muscle layer *2* are visible. Anteriorly, the two halves of the external sphincter are connected to each other. (c) Section obtained slightly cranial to (b). Compare the signal intensity of the internal sphincter *1* with that of the other structures. The external sphincter *3* is circular anteriorly while it has a thickened extension posteriorly. Anterolaterally and to the left, outer fibers of the external sphincter are in contact with fibers of the superficial perineal muscle of the urogenital diaphragm. The intersphincteric space *a* and the longitudinal layer *2* are well displayed. (d) Section obtained slightly cranial to (c). Fibers of the puborectal muscle *4*, which acts as a sling, also are in contact with the urogenital diaphragm anteriorly.

Nonsurgical Management

Mild incontinence often responds to relatively simple interventions. Dietary changes include attempts at reducing stool bulk by implementing a low residue diet, keeping a diary of foods that tend to make their symptoms worse and avoiding these foods. Decreasing carbonated beverage intake and avoiding sipping and slurping of hot foods or drinks may decrease flatulence as 75% of flatus comes from swallowed air.[6] A priority should be to treat any diarrhea as solid stools are much easier to control than liquid stools. In patients with borderline sphincter function, to convert to solid stool from liquid stool may render that patient continent. For chronic diarrhea and incontinence, loperamide and diphenoxylate are effective in producing solid stools and reducing frequency and amount of stools.[104,105] However, loperamide does this more effectively and has an additional benefit of increasing the resting pressure of the IAS.[106] Even patients with severe or chronic anal incontinence are candidates for a trial of nonsurgical therapy and may benefit a great deal from the intervention. Empiric nonsurgical therapy is especially important in patients with pudendal neuropathy as this is predictive of poor outcome after sphincter repair and postanal repair has shown mixed results.[54,94,95,107]

If incontinence persists despite pharmacologic and dietary manipulation, then biofeedback therapy may be an option if the patient is motivated, has some sensitivity to rectal distention, and is able to at least weakly contract the EAS. Biofeedback uses patient's immediate visualization of the results of her efforts in hopes of producing future more effective and efficient efforts.[108] Biofeedback is most successful when used for motor response, although sensory and reservoir function can also be treated with this modality.[108,109] As many as 70% to 80% of patients gain significant benefit from biofeedback therapy.[110] However, initial good results may deteriorate over time.[111] Functional electrical stimulation has been attempted for patients with urinary incontinence and may prove useful for certain patients with anal incontinence, although no data are currently available.[112]

Surgical Management

Since the pathogenesis of anal incontinence is multifactorial and incompletely understood, it is no surprise that surgical intervention remains a significant challenge for the obstetrician/gynecologist and many times results in less than excellent success. Those patients with a severe dysfunction resulting in loss of formed stool are most likely to benefit from surgical intervention. Repair of congenital malformations has previously been discussed. In patients with rectal prolapse, surgical correction may improve symptoms of incontinence and soiling. The Parks postanal repair has been used in patients with pelvic floor and anal sphincter neuropathy.[54,94,95,107] However, its usefulness and success is limited and this procedure probably should be reserved only for the patient with significant neuropathy and an intact external anal sphincter who has failed nonsurgical therapy.

Other more complex procedures that have been used with varying success for severe incontinence, include gluteus and gracilis muscle transpositions, artificial sphincters, and silastic anal slings. Detailed descriptions of these are beyond the scope of this chapter.

The most common problem that most obstetrician/gynecologists are likely to encounter is the obstetric sphincter disruption. Again, obstetric injury most often results in anterior disruption of the sphincter. Of immediate concern is whether the defects are adequately repaired initially. Sultan and colleagues[51] reported that of 34 women with third-degree tears after delivery (defined as sphincter tear or into rectal mucosa) who underwent primary repair, 16 (47%) had defecatory symptoms and 14 (41%) had anal incontinence. AES showed sphincter defects in 29 (85%) of these women. Most of the defects were along either the midanal or deep components of the sphincter or along its full thickness. The findings of Sultan's group are similar to those of other authors.[36,52] This has important surgical implications. Whereas the subcutaneous component of the EAS is easily recognized at operation, deeper defects may be masked by this seemingly intact subcutaneous portion of the sphincter. This holds true for primary and secondary repairs and surgery should have the primary aim of identifying the disrupted external and internal sphincters and restoring their continuity. Whether the ends of the sphincter are brought together with an overlapping or end to end technique,[79,80] the goal of the repair is to anatomically and functionally restore the anal canal. It is likely to be important that the anal sphincters are exposed along the entire length of the anal canal so that deeper defects are revealed and with appropriate reconstruction performed along at least a 3 cm craniocaudad distance.[35] This more physiologic repair should result in decreased incontinence. If the rectovaginal septum and perineal body are significantly attenuated, these should also be repaired. However, care must be taken not to add extreme bulk to this area to prevent subsequent dyspareunia or other dysfunction of the posterior vagina. A excellent, detailed description of technique is found elsewhere.[113] There is a relative paucity of information on management of subsequent deliveries after previous sphincter disruption. Bek and Laurberg[53] reported on 56 women who had experienced a subsequent vaginal delivery after complete obstetric tear with repair of the anal sphincter immediately following the first delivery; 23 (41%) had transient anorectal incontinence directly after the complete tear, and 4 had permanent anorectal incontinence; anorectal incontinence developed in 9 (39%) after the next delivery, and this was permanent in four (17.4%). In the 29 women without anorectal incontinence after complete tear, two had transient incontinence of flatus but for <14 days after the next delivery. Of the four with permanent incontinence after initial complete tear, one had worsening incontinence after subsequent delivery and the other three remained unchanged. Transient anal incontinence after a complete tear was significantly associated with development of anal incontinence after the next delivery. The major long-term problem for these patients was incontinence of flatus. Laurberg and coworkers,[54] in a report of delayed repairs noted that in five of the patients with only slight anorectal incontinence after the delivery in which the sphincter tear occurred, the problem was greatly aggravated after subsequent vaginal delivery. These authors and others[52] agree that future vaginal delivery after sphincter disruption with subsequent anorectal incontinence should prompt one to counsel the patient regarding possible avoidance of future vaginal delivery.

CONCLUSION

Loss of control of bowel function is an intense problem for those who suffer with it. However, anal incontinence remains an underreported and unrecognized problem for many women. Although surgery is still the mainstay of therapy for most conditions that result in anal incontinence, other nonsurgical options are evolving and may offer good results for some. With renewed interest in the area of anal incontinence, we can anticipate improvement in understanding of pathophysiology and offer better patient care through continued research.

REFERENCES

1. Hymans DE. Gastrointestinal problems in the old. *BMJ* 1974; **1**: 107–110.
2. Leigh RJ, Turnberg LA. Faecal incontinence: The unvoiced symptom. *Lancet* 1982; **1**: 1349–1350.
3. Nelson R, Norton N, Cautley E, Furner S. Community-based prevalence of anal incontinence. *JAMA* 1995; **274**: 559–561.
4. Kamm M. Obstetric damage and faecal incontinence. *Lancet* 1994; **344**: 730–733.
5. Madoff RD, Williams JG, Caushaj PF. Fecal incontinence. *N Engl J Med* 1992; **326**: 1002–1007.
6. Toglia MR, DeLancey JOL. Anal incontinence and the obstetrician-gynecologist. *Obstet Gynecol* 1994; **84**: 731–740.
7. Kok AL, Voorhorst FJ, Burger CW, van Houten P, Kenemans P, Janssens J. Urinary and faecal incontinence in community-residing elderly women. *Age Ageing* 1992; **21**: 211–215.
8. Thomas TM, Ruff C, Karran O, Mellows S, Meade TW. Study of the prevalence and management of patients with faecal incontinence in old people's homes. *Community Med* 1987; **9**: 232–237.
9. Talley NJ, O'Keefe EA, Zinsmeister AR, Melton JL. Prevalence of gastrointestinal symptoms in the elderly: A population based study. *Gastroenterology* 1992; **102**: 895–901.
10. Johanson JF, Lafferty JL. Epidemiology of fecal incontinence: The silent affliction. *Am J Gastroenterol* 1996; **91**: 33–36.
11. Wald A. Constipation in elderly patients: Pathogenesis and management. *Drugs Aging* 1993; **3**: 220–231.
12. Tobin GW, Brocklehurst JC. Faecal incontinence in residential homes for the elderly: Prevalence, aetiology and management. *Age Ageing* 1986; **15**: 41–46.
13. Smith RG. Fecal incontinence. *J Am Geriatr Soc* 1983; **31**: 694–697.
14. Peet SM, Castleden CM, McGrother CW. Prevalence of urinary and faecal incontinence in hospitals and residential and nursing homes for older people. *BMJ* 1995; **311**: 1063–1064.
15. Herzog AR, Fultz NH. Prevalence and incidence of urinary incontinence in community-dwelling populations. *J Am Geriatr Soc* 1990; **38**: 273–281.

16. Read NW, Hartford WV, Schmulen AC, Read MG, Santa Ana C, Fordtran JS. A clinical study of patients with fecal incontinence and diarrhea. *Gastroenterology* 1979; **76**: 747–756.
17. Clarke M, Hughes AO, Dodd KJ. The elderly in residential care: Patterns of disability. *Health Trends* 1979; **11**: 17–23.
18. Wyman JF, Choi SC, Harkins SW, Taylor JR, Fantl JA. Psychosocial impact of urinary incontinence in women. *Obstet Gynecol* 1987; **70**: 378–381.
19. Norton PA. Prevalence and social impact of urinary incontinence in women. *Clin Obstet Gynecol* 1990; **33**: 295–297.
20. Hilton P. Urinary incontinence during sexual intercourse: A common, but rarely volunteered symptom. *Br J Obstet Gynaecol* 1988; **86**: 377–381.
21. Walters MD, Taylor S, Schoenfeld LS. Psychosexual study of women with detrusor instability. *Obstet Gynecol* 1989; **75**: 22–26.
22. Gaston EA. Physiologic basis for preservation of fecal continence after resection of rectum. *JAMA* 1951; **146**: 1486–1489.
23. Varma JS, Smith AN, Busuttil A. Function of the anal sphincters after chronic radiation injury. *Gut* 1987; **27**: 528–533.
24. Varma JS, Smith AN. Anorectal function following coloanal sleeve anastomosis for chronic radiation injury to the rectum. *Br J Surg* 1986; **73**: 285–289.
25. Varma JS, Smith AN, Busuttil A. Correlation of clinical and manometric abnormalities of rectal function following chronic radiation injury. *Br J Surg* 1985; **72**: 875–878.
26. Taverner D, Smiddy FG. An electromyographic study of the normal function of the external anal sphincter and pelvic diaphragm. *Dis Colon Rectum* 1959; **2**: 153–160.
27. Sweiger M. Method for determining individual contributions of voluntary and involuntary anal sphincters to resting tone. *Dis Colon Rectum* 1979; **22**: 415–416.
28. Frencker B, Euler CV. Influence of pudendal block on the function of the anal sphincters. *Gut* 1975; **16**: 482–489.
29. Felt-Bersma R, Cuesta M, Koorevaar M, Strijers RL, Meurrissen SG, Dercksen EJ, Wesdorp RI. Anal endosonography: Relationship with anal manometry and neurophysiologic tests. *Dis Colon Rectum* 1992; **35**: 944–949.
30. Lestar B, Penninckx F, Kerremans R. The composition of anal basal pressure: An in vivo and in vitro study in man. *Int J Colorect Dis* 1989; **4**: 118–122.
31. Read N, Bartolo D, Read MG. Differences in anal function in patients with incontinence to solids and in patients with incontinence to liquids. *Br J Surg* 1984; **71**: 39–42.
32. Goligher JC, Leacock AG, Brossy JJ. The surgical anatomy of the anal canal. *Br J Surg* 1955; **43**: 51–54.
33. Dalley AF. The riddle of the sphincters. The morphophysiology of the anorectal mechanism reviewed. *Am J Surg* 1987; **53**: 298–306.
34. Sultan A, Kamm M, Hudson CN, Nicholls JR, Bartram CI. Endosonography of the anal sphincters: Normal anatomy and comparison with manometry. *Clin Radiol* 1994; **49**: 368–374.
35. Aronson M, Lee R, Berquist TH. Anatomy of anal sphincters and related structures in continent women studied with magnetic resonance imaging. *Obstet Gynecol* 1990; **76**: 846–851.
36. Deen K, Kumar D, Williams JG, Olliff J, Keighley MR. The prevalence of anal sphincter defects in faecal incontinence: A prospective endosonic study. *Gut* 1993; **34**: 685–688.
37. Schafer A, Enck P, Furst G, Kahn T, Frieling T, Lubke HJ. Anatomy of the anal sphincters: Comparison of anal endosonography to magnetic resonance imaging. *Dis Colon Rectum* 1994; **37**: 777–781.
38. Hussain SM, Stoker J, Lame'ris JS. Anal sphincter complex: Endoanal MR imaging of normal anatomy. *Radiology* 1995; **197**: 671–677.
39. Oh C, Kark A. Anatomy of the external anal sphincter. *Br J Surg* 1972; **59**: 717–723.

40. Cuesta M, Meijer S, Derckson EJ, Boutkam H, Meuwissen SG. Anal sphincter imaging in fecal incontinence using endosonography. *Dis Colon Rectum* 1992; **35**: 59–63.
41. Sagar PM, Pemberton JH. Dysfunction of the posterior pelvic floor and disorders of defecation. *J Pelv Surg* 1995; **1**: 92–105.
42. Aldridge RT, Campbell PE. Ganglion cell distribution in the normal rectum and anal canal: A basis for the diagnosis of Hirshprung's disease by anorectal biopsy. *J Pediatr Surg* 1968; **3**: 475–490.
43. Beart RW, Dozois RR, Wollf BG, Pemberton JH. Mechanisms of rectal continence: Lessons from the ileoanal procedure. *Am J Surg* 1985; **149**: 31–34.
44. Sagar PM, Holdsworth PJ, Johnston D. Correlation between laboratory findings and clinical outcome after restorative proctocolectomy: Serial studies in 20 patients after end-to-end pouch-anal anastomosis. *Br J Surg* 1991; **78**: 67–70.
45. Smith ARB, Hosker GL, Warrell DW. The role of partial denervation of the pelvic floor in the aetiology of genitourinary prolapse and stress incontinence of urine. *Br J Obstet Gynaecol* 1989; **96**: 24–28.
46. Snooks SJ, Henry MM, Swash M. Faecal incontinence due to external anal sphincter division in childbirth is associated with damage to the innervation of the pelvic floor musculature: A double pathology. *Br J Obstet Gynaecol* 1985; **92**: 824–828.
47. Burnett S, Spence-Jones C, Speakman CT, Kamm MA, Hudson CN, Bartram CI. Unsuspected sphincter damage following childbirth revealed by endosonography. *Br J Radiol* 1991; **64**: 225–227.
48. Sultan A, Kamm M, Hudson CN, Thomas JM, Bartram CI. Anal sphincter disruption during vaginal delivery. *N Engl J Med* 1993; **329**: 1905–1911.
49. Sultan A, Kamm M, Hudson CN, Bartram CI. Effect of pregnancy on anal sphincter morphology and function. *Int J Colorect Dis* 1993; **8**: 206–209.
50. Sultan A, Kamm M, Bartram CI, Hudson CN. Anal sphincter trauma during instrumental delivery. *Int J Gynaecol Obstet* 1993; **43**: 263–270.
51. Sultan A, Kamm M, Hudson CN, Bartram CI. Third degree obstetric anal sphincter tears: Risk factors and outcome of primary repair. *BMJ* 1994; **308**: 887–891.
52. Nieisen M, Hauge C, Rasmussen OO, Pedersen JF, Christainsen J. Anal endosonographic findings in the follow-up of primarily sutured sphincteric ruptures. *Br J Surg* 1992; **79**: 104–106.
53. Bek K, Laurberg S. Risks of anal incontinence from subsequent vaginal delivery after a complete obstetric anal sphincter tear. *Br J Obstet Gynaecol* 1992; **99**: 724–726.
54. Laurberg S, Swash M, Henry MM. Delayed external sphincter repair for obstetric tear. *Br J Surg* 1988; **75**: 786–788.
55. Parks AG, Porter NH, Hardcastle J. The syndrome of the descending perineum. *Proc R Soc Med* 1966; **59**: 477–482.
56. Mackle EJ, Parks TG. Clinical features in patients with excessive perineal descent. *JR Coll Surg Edinburgh* 1989; **34**: 88–90.
57. Ho Y, Goh HS. The neurophysiological significance of perineal descent. *Int J Colorectal Dis* 1995; **10**: 107–111.
58. Berkelmans I, Heresbach D, Leroi A, Touchais J, Martin P, Weber J, Denis P. Perineal descent at defecography in women with straining at stool: A lack of specificity or predictive value for future anal incontinence? *Eur J Gastroenterol Hepatol* 1995; **7**: 75–79.
59. Henry MM, Parks AG, Swash M. The pelvic floor musculature in the descending perineum syndrome. *Br J Surg* 1982; **69**: 470–472.
60. Gee AS, Mills A, Durdey P. What is the relationship between perineal descent and anal mucosal electrosensitivity? *Dis Colon Rectum* 1995; **38**: 419–423.
61. Jameson J, Chia Y, Kamm MA, Speakman CT, Chye YH, Henry MM. Effect of age, sex, and parity on anorectal function. *Br J Surg* 1994; **81**: 1689–1692.
62. Laurberg S, Swash M. Effects of aging on the anorectal sphincters and their

innervation. *Dis Colon Rectum* 1989; **32**: 737–742.

63. Haadem K, Ling L, Ferno M, Graffner H. Estrogen receptors in the external anal sphincter. *Am J Obstet Gynecol* 1991; **164**: 609–610.
64. Feldman M, Schiller LR. Disorders of gastrointestinal motility associated with diabetes mellitus. *Ann Intern Med* 1983; **98**: 378–384.
65. Christiansen J, Pedersen IK. Traumatic anal incontinence: Results of surgical repair. *Dis Colon Rectum* 1987; **30**: 189–191.
66. Kuijpers HC, Schever M. Disorders of impaired fecal control: A clinical and manometric study. *Dis Colon Rectum* 1990; **33**: 207–211.
67. Khubchandani IT, Reed JF. Sequelae of internal sphincterotomy for chronic fissure in ano. *Br J Surg* 1989; **76**: 431–434.
68. Walker WA, Rothenberger DA, Goldberg SM. Morbidity of internal sphincterotomy for anal fissure and stenosis. *Dis Colon Rectum* 1985; **28**: 832–835.
69. Tuckson W, Lavery I, Fazio V, Oakley J, Church J, Milson J. Manometric and functional comparison of ileal pouch anal anastomosis with and without anal manipulation. *Am J Surg* 1991; **161**: 90–96.
70. Snooks S, Henry MM, Swash M. Faecal incontinence after anal dilatation. *Br J Surg* 1984; **71**: 617–618.
71. Baeten C, Geerdes BP, Adang EM, Heineman E, Konsten J, Engel GL, Kester AD, Spaans F. Anal dynamic graciloplasty in the treatment of intractable fecal incontinence. *N Engl J Med* 1995; **332**: 1600–1605.
72. Munn R, Schillinger. Urologic abnormalities found with imperforate anus. *Urology* 1983; **21**: 260–264.
73. Rich M. Spectrum of genitourinary malformations in patients with imperforate anus. *Pediatr Surg Int* 1988; **3**: 110–113.
74. Wilkins S. The role of colostomy in the management of anorectal malformations. *Pediatr Surg Int* 1988; **3**: 105–108.
75. Pena A. Surgical management of anorectal malformations: A unified concept. *Pediatr Surg Int* 1988; **3**: 82–85.
76. Hendren WH. Repair of cloacal anomalies: Current techniques. *J Pediatr Surg* 1986; **21**: 1159–1176.
77. Pena A, Devries PA. Posterior sagittal anorectoplasty: Important technical considerations and new application. *J Pediatr Surg* 1082; **17**: 796–811.
78. Weber J, Beuret-Blanquart F, Ducrotte P, Touchais JY, Denis P. External anal sphincter function in spinal patients: Electromyographic and manometric study. *Dis Colon Rectum* 1991; **34**: 409–415.
79. Arnaud A, Sarles JC, Sielezneff I, Orsoni P, Joly A. Sphincter repair without overlapping for fecal incontinence. *Dis Colon Rectum* 1991; **34**: 744–747.
80. Fleshman JW, Peters WR, Shemesh EI, Fry RD, Kodner IJ. Anal sphincter reconstruction: Anterior overlapping muscle repair. *Dis Colon Rectum* 1991; **34**: 739–743.
81. Hibbard LT. Surgical management of rectovaginal fistulas and complete perineal tears. *Am J Obstet Gynecol* 1978; **130**: 139–141.
82. Corman ML. Anal incontinence following obstetrical injury. *Dis Colon Rectum* 1985; **28**: 86–89.
83. Hallan RI, Marzouk DE, Waldron DJ, Womack NR, Williams NS. Comparison of digital and manometric assessment of anal sphincter function. *Br J Surg* 1989; **76**: 973–975.
84. Parks TG. The usefulness of tests in anorectal function. *World J Surg* 1992; **16**: 804–810.
85. Williams N, Barlow J, Hobson A, Scott N, Irving M. Manometric asymmetry in the anal canal in controls and patients with fecal incontinence. *Dis Colon Rectum* 1995; **38**: 1275–1280.
86. Barkel DC, Pemberton JH, Pezim ME, Phillips SF, Kelly KA, Brown ML. Scintigraphic assessment of the anorectal angle in health and following ileal pouch-anal anastomosis. *Ann Surg* 1988; **208**: 42–49.

87. Perry RE, Blatchford GJ, Christensen MA, Thorson AG, Attwood SE. Manometric diagnosis of anal sphincter injuries. *Am J Surg* 1990; **159**: 112–117.
88. Law P, Kamm M, Bartram CI. A comparison between electromyography and anal endosonography in mapping external sphincter defects. *Dis Colon Rectum* 1990; **33**: 370–373.
89. Burnett S, Speakman C, Kamm MA, Bartram CI. Confirmation of endosonographic detection of external anal sphincter defects by simultaneous electromyographic mapping. *Br J Surg* 1991; **78**: 448–450.
90. Kiff ES, Swash M. Slowed conduction in the pudendal nerves in idiopathic (neurogenic) fecal incontinence. *Br J Surg* 1984; **74**: 615–616.
91. Sultan A, Kamm M, Talbot IC, Nocholls RJ, Bartram CI. Anal endosonography for identifying external sphincter defects confirmed histologically. *Br J Surg* 1994; **81**: 463–465.
92. Sultan A, Nicholls R, Kamm MA, Hudson CN, Beynon J, Bartram CI. Anal endosonography and correlation with in vitro and in vivo anatomy. *Br J Surg* 1993; **80**: 508–511.
93. Neilsen M, Hauge C, Rasmussen OO, Sorensen M, Pedersen JF, Christainsen J. Anal sphincter size measured by endosonography in healthy volunteers: effect of age, sex, and parity. *Acta Radiol* 1992; **33**: 453–456.
94. Browning G, Motson R. Anal sphincter injury: Management and results of Parks sphincter repair. *Ann Surg* 1988; **199**: 324–328.
95. Setti Carraro P, Kamm M, Nicholls RJ. Long-term results of postanal repair for neurogenic faecal incontinence. *Br J Surg* 1994; **81**: 140–144.
96. Sandridge DA, Thorpe JM. Vaginal endosonography in the assessment of the anorectum. *Obstet Gynecol* 1995; **86**: 1007–1009.
97. Sultan AH, Loder PB, Bartram CI, Kamm MA, Hudson CN. Vaginal endosonography new approach to image the undisturbed anal sphincter. *Dis Colon Rectum* 1994; **37**: 1296–1299.
98. Goodrich MA, Webb MJ, King BF, Bampton AEH, Campeau NG, Riederer SJ. Magnetic resonance imaging of pelvic floor relaxation: Dynamic analysis and evaluation of patients before and after surgical repair. *Obstet Gynecol* 1993; **82**: 883–891.
99. Yang A, Mostwin JL, Rosenshein NB, Zerhouni EA. Pelvic floor descent in women: Dynamic evaluation with fast MR imaging and cinematic display. *Radiology* 1991; **179**: 25–33.
100. Christensen LL, Djurhuus JC, Constantinou CE. Imaging of pelvic floor contractions using MRI. *Neurourol Urodyn* 1995; **14**: 209–216.
101. deSouza NM, Puni R, Kmiot WA, Bartram CI, Hall AS, Bydder GM. MRI of the anal sphincter. *J Comput Assist Tomogr* 1995; **19**: 745–751.
102. Kelvin FM, Maglinte DDT, Benson JT. Evacuation proctography (defecography): An aid to the investigation of pelvic floor disorders. *Obstet Gynecol* 1994; **83**: 307–314.
103. Goei R. Anorectal function in patients with defecation disorders and asymptomatic subjects: Evaluation with defecography. *Radiology* 1990; **174**: 121–123.
104. Harford WV, Krejs GJ, Santa CA, Fortran JS. Acute effect of diphenoxylate with atropine (Lomotil) in patients with chronic diarrhea and fecal incontinence. *Gastroenterology* 1980; **78**: 440–443.
105. Palmer KR, Corbett CL, Holdsworth CD. Double-blind cross-over study comparing loperamide codeine and diphenoxylate in the treatment of chronic diarrhea. *Gastroenterology* 1980; **79**: 1272–1275.
106. Read M, Read NW, Barber DC, Duthie HL. Effects of loperamide on anal sphincter function in patients complaining of chronic diarrhea with fecal incontinence and urgency. *Dig Dis Sci* 1982; **27**: 807–814.
107. Cheong DMO, Vaccaro CA, Salanga VD, Waxner SD, Phillips RG, Hanson MR. Electrodiagnostic evaluation of fecal incontinence. *Muscle Nerve* 1995; **18**: 612–619.

108. Macleod JH. Biofeedback in the management of partial anal incontinence. *Dis Colon Rectum* 1983; **26**: 244–246.
109. Whitehead WE, Burgio KL, Engel BT. Biofeedback in the treatment of fecal incontinence in geriatric patients. *J Am Geriatr Soc* 1985; **33**: 320–324.
110. Guillemot F, Bouche B, Gower-Rousseau C, Chartier M, Wolschies E, Lamblin M, Harbonnier E, Cortot A. Biofeedback for the treatment of fecal incontinence. *Dis Colon Rectum* 1995; **38**: 393–397.
111. Keck JO, Staniunas RJ, Coller JA, Barrett RC, Oster ME, Schoetz DJ, Roberts PL, Murray JJ, Veidenheimer MC. Biofeedback training is useful in fecal incontinence but disappointing in constipation. *Dis Colon Rectum* 1994; **37**: 1271–1276.
112. Matzel KE, Stadelmaier U, Hohenfellner M, Gall FP. Electrical stimulation of sacral spinal nerves for treatment of faecal incontinence. *Lancet* 1995; **346**: 1124–1127.
113. Toglia MR, Elkins TE: Management of rectovaginal fistulas and the disrupted anal sphincter. In: Mann WJ, Stovall TG (eds). *Gynecologic Surgery*. New York: Churchill Livingstone, 1996.

Index

Note: Page numbers in *italic* refer to tables and/or figures